# practicing MEDICINE

## in the 21ˢᵗ century

Edited by: David B. Nash, MD, MBA
Alexandria Skoufalos, EdD
Megan Hartman, MS
Howard Horwitz, MPH

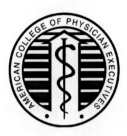

**American College of Physician Executives**
4890 West Kennedy Boulevard, Suite 200
Tampa, Florida 33609-2575
813-287-2000

ISBN: 0-924674-99-7

Library of Congress Card Number: 2006936850

Printed in the United States of America by Lightning Source, Inc., St. Louis, Missouri.

# Contents

Foreword ...........................................................................................................vii

Preface ..............................................................................................................ix

Contributors .....................................................................................................xi

# Introduction .....................................................................................xiii

David B. Nash, MD, MBA, FACP and Karisa Walker

# SECTION 1: Clinical Management

**Chapter 1**     Quality of Care: Terms, Tools, and Techniques............................1
Neil I. Goldfarb

**Chapter 2**     Ensuring the Safety of Our Patients.............................................15
Alan P. Marco, MD, MMM, CPE, FACPE and Brian M. Aboff, MD, FACP

**Chapter 3**     Preparing for Pay for Performance .............................................31
David A. MacKoul, MD, MS, FAAP, DFACMQ

**Chapter 4**     Achieving Positive Patient-Physician Relationships:
              The Importance of Patient-Centeredness....................................47
Sara L. Thier, MPH and Christopher N. Sciamanna, MD, MPH

**Chapter 5**     Succeeding as a Member of the Health Care Team....................63
Christine B. Turley, MD and Jose L. Gonzalez, MD, JD, MSEd

# SECTION 2: Information Management

**Chapter 6**     Ambulatory Information Technology .............................................77
Albert G. Crawford, PhD, MBA, MSIS

**Chapter 7**     Communication: The Key to Good Medicine .............................93
Nancy B. Finn

# SECTION 3: The Practice Environment

**Chapter 8**      Risk Management in Medical Practice Today............................113
*Rosemary Gafner, EdD*

**Chapter 9**      Health Care and the Law...........................................................129
*Sarah Freymann Fontenot, JD*

**Chapter 10**     Practicing Medicine in a Managed Care Environment.............155
*Ralph O. Bischof, MD, MBA, FAAFP*

**Chapter 11**     What Every Doctor Needs to Know
About Medicare and Medicaid ...................................................171
*Joshua J. Gagne, PharmD and Vittorio Maio, PharmD, MS, MSPH*

**Chapter 12**     Medical Malpractice Protection.................................................187
*David G. Halpern, JD and Jose L. Gonzalez, MD, JD, MSEd*

**Chapter 13**     Dealing or Succeeding with Disease Management ...................203
*Harry L. Leider, MD, MBA, FACPE, Raymond L. Wedgeworth, MA, and
Laurie Russell, MS, RN, CCM*

# SECTION 4: Practice Administration

**Chapter 14**     The Practice Setting: Office, Hospitals, and Others.................225
*Theodore D. Fraker, Jr., MD, FACC and
Alan P. Marco, MD, MMM, CPE, FACPE*

**Chapter 15**     Open Access Scheduling............................................................243
*George P. Valko, MD*

**Chapter 16**     Understanding the Referral Process..........................................257
*Stephen E. Whitney, MD, MBA, BCM and
Jerald L. Zarin, MD, MBA, FAAP*

**Chapter 17**     Practice Innovation ..................................................................277
*Michael S. Barr, MD, MBA, FACP*

# SECTION 5: Financial Management

**Chapter 18**   Joining or Starting a Medical Practice........................................301
Geoffrey T. Anders, JD, CPA, CHBC and Anne E. Jorgensen, JD

**Chapter 19**   Fundamentals of Health Care Accounting and Finance..........323
Barbara J. Grant, CPA, MST

**Chapter 20**   Documenting, Coding and Billing:
Getting it Right the First Time....................................................353
Brian M. Aboff, MD, FACP and Rosemary Bell, RN, CPC

**Chapter 21**   Physician Compensation Trends, Models, and Approaches.....377
David Edward Marcinko, DPM, MBA, CFP, CMP and
Hope Rachel Hetico, RN, MHA, CMP, CPHQ


# Future Trends..................................................................................399

Sara L. Thier, MPH


# Index................................................................................................407

# Foreword

That the actual, real-world practice of medicine in the United States continues to evolve would be considered by most to be an understatement. The advances in medical knowledge dwarf most of the expectations we set before ourselves as a profession in the 1970s. The revolution in technical and procedural abilities promised by advances in metallurgy, computing power, fiber optics, and imaging technology have resulted in parallel advances in physician skill, leading to what would have been considered wizardry a generation ago. Finally, advances in drug identification, chemical design, the mapping of the human genome, and the promise of both these advances gives rise to both the dawn of pre-emptive gene-specific pharmacologic intervention, as well as gene-specific therapeutic manipulation. And, the next 15-20 years will bring a pace of change not yet seen! These factors will coalesce with greater understanding of the central nervous system and its afflictions, as well as yet to be exploited concepts in xenotransplantation, and the continued march forward of computing power and its impact on the new tools of our profession.

That said, the actual delivery of patient care will continue to be a highly personalized process, one provided by physicians and other caregivers in an increasingly complicated, information rich environment. Physicians will need a series of new competencies in order to position themselves to successfully deliver care to their patients. This new set of competencies is largely specialty independent, and part of the General Competencies of the Physician promulgated by the Accreditation Council for Graduate Medical Education (ACGME) and espoused by most of organized medicine, including the American Board of Medical Specialties (ABMS). The adoption of these competencies provides us with the lexicon to discuss this domain of physician practice that is common to all physicians, regardless of specialty choice, geographic setting, or nature of practice.

While each physician will not require competency in all the areas explored in this text, David B. Nash and colleagues provide a broad view of the competencies that each physician may need in his or her practice over the next 15-20 years. Under the broad rubric of ACGME General Competencies, this text explores key dimensions of the exploded competencies of Practice-based Learning and Improvement (PBL&I) and Systems-based Practice (SBP). Its important contribution is that it explores these competencies from the perspective of a community-based provider, not a resident working largely in an inpatient care delivery system in a large academic medical center setting.

Exploration of broad topics such as Clinical Management are approached from the perspective of the skill set needed, regardless of specialty, to operationalize SBP and

PBL&I in any setting. Concepts of team and team management are included, recognizing that the practice of medicine, even in small group practices, will evolve to interprofessional groups, with physicians and other providers functioning together in the care of patients. Information management and knowledge flow will be essential components of each physician's practice, as they learn to incorporate information technology to provide timely access to patient information, and expert digested knowledge in their evidence-based clinical practices.

The final three sections address topics that are clearly SBP issues, but are not yet effectively dealt with in our current educational paradigm. Understanding and mastering the practice environment, rather than being controlled or paralyzed by factors in that environment, is essential to the successful practice of medicine. A solid foundation in management and fiscal issues is essential in order to survive in practice, and create an economically stable platform for the formation of a microsystem of care for a population of patients, centering on the clinical practice, and utilizing the local hospital and ambulatory care environment in which the physician practices.

This text should become required reading for senior residents in all disciplines, especially those entering clinical practice in the solo practice and small physician group setting. It will also be of value to those entering large group and academic group practice, as a firm foundation in the underpinnings of these settings is required to be successful in these environments, as well. Congratulations to Dr. Nash and his co-authors on a valuable contribution to the evolving knowledge base in these essential competencies!

**Thomas J. Nasca, MD, MACP**
*Professor of Medicine and Physiology*
*Dean, Jefferson Medical College*
*Senior Vice President and Provost,*
Thomas Jefferson University

# Preface

My co-editors and I are very pleased to be able to bring you, the reader, our multi-authored edited text entitled *Practicing Medicine in the 21ˢᵗ Century*. Thomas Jefferson University and Jefferson Medical College have been my professional home since 1990 and this is my 17ᵗʰ multi-authored edited book. In some respects, this book closes an important academic circle for me. One of my earlier efforts, *Future Practice Alternatives in Medicine*, was published 20 years ago as the first book directed at soon to-be-graduated medical students. I hope its descendant meets with the same outstanding level of success.

This book has had many parents, in a literary sense, including our key contributors from across the country. Each one was selected for his or her expertise in the field and desire to help trainees to navigate the future practice of their chosen field. While multi-authored texts can sometimes have a few rough edges, we believe that we have woven together the individual contributions from each of the authors while still allowing their unique literary "voice" to shine through. We hope you agree.

Others who have participated in the creation of this volume include my co-editors. Alexis Skoufalos and Megan Hartman, members of our education and training team within the Department of Health Policy at Jefferson Medical College, were tireless workers organizing every aspect of this nearly year-long project. Howard Horwitz has been a valued colleague at the American College of Physician Executives for many years; we wish him Godspeed at his new role at the American College of Healthcare Executives in Chicago, Illinois.

Of course, the real key contributors to this volume are the literally hundreds of medical students with whom I have had the privilege of being associated over the past seventeen years. I hope that this book reflects much of what we have learned from our junior colleagues and from their experience in the undergraduate and graduate medical education aspects of their training.

Finally, I'd like to thank the two best bosses any department chair could every hope to have. Thomas J. Nasca, MD, Dean of Jefferson Medical College, has been a stalwart supporter of our young department from its earliest stages. Thomas J. Lewis, the Chief Executive Officer of our University Hospital, has stood by our team through its entire evolutionary growth at Jefferson. Our new University President, Robert Barchi, MD, sets a high bar for faculty performance and we hope this text easily clears that hurdle.

Who should read this book? Like any multi-authored edited text covering a broad area, we believe the book deserves a wide readership. Necessarily, it is focused on the needs of young trainees, those about to enter practice and those contemplating a change in their current practice venue. The book is tightly organized into five sections, including one on clinical management, information management, the practice environment, practice administration, and financial management. It is buttressed by a thorough introduction and a concluding chapter focused on key future trends. Busy readers could, of course focus, on their specific needs, but I would recommend a cover-to-cover review. The future practice of medicine will be quite challenging and every chapter, I'm sure, will have some important take-home message for physicians at every level of training and experience.

As editor-in-chief, I take ultimate responsibility for any errors of omission or commission throughout the text. More importantly, I am very personally interested in feedback from you, our reader, as you tackle these futuristic issues. I'm grateful for my daily interaction with young persons in medicine, as they continue to energize me and stimulate our thinking as a department regarding critical issues about the organization and delivery of medical care. Our trainees are the manifestation of our connectedness in medicine from Hippocrates and Maimonides to our current leaders and, most importantly, to the leaders yet to be determined. My hope is that this book will contribute to every reader's successful career in the best of all professions. All the best to each and every one of you on your own career journey.

**David B. Nash, MD, MBA**
*Raymond C. and Doris N. Grandon Professor of Health Policy*
Chairman, Department of Health Policy
Fall 2006

# Contributors

**Brian M. Aboff, MD, FACP**
Internal Medicine Residency Program
Director
Christiana Care Health System
Newark, DE

**Geoffrey T. Anders, JD, CPA, CHBC**
President
The Health Care Group, Inc.
Plymouth Meeting, PA

**Michael S. Barr, MD, MBA, FACP**
Vice President, Practice Advocacy and
Improvement
American College of Physicians
Washington, DC

**Rosemary Bell, RN, CPC**
Senior Medical Auditor
Christiana Care Health System
New Castle, DE

**Ralph O. Bischof, MD, MBA, FAAFP**
Senior Medical Director
Department of Medical Policy
Administration
Aetna
Blue Bell, PA

**Albert G. Crawford, PhD, MBA, MSIS**
Assistant Professor
Department of Health Policy
Jefferson Medical College
Philadelphia, PA

**Nancy B. Finn**
President
Communication Resources
Needham, MA

**Sarah Freymann Fontenot, JD**
Adjunct Professor
Trinity University
Fredericksburg, TX

**Theodore D. Fraker, Jr., MD**
Associate Division Director for Clinical
Affairs and Operations
Division of Cardiovascular Diseases
The Ohio State University Medical Center
Columbus, OH

**Rosemary Gafner, EdD**
President
Medical Risk Management, Inc.
Houston, TX

**Joshua J. Gagne, PharmD**
Postdoctoral Outcomes Research Fellow
Jefferson Medical College & Ortho-McNeil
Janssen Scientific Affairs, LLC.
Philadelphia, PA

**Neil I. Goldfarb**
Director of Research
Department of Health Policy
Jefferson Medical College
Philadelphia, PA

**Jose L. Gonzalez, MD, JD, MSEd**
Vice Chair for Medical Education
University of Texas Medical Branch
Galveston, TX

**Barbara J. Grant, CPA, MST**
Principal
Gates, Moore and Company
Atlanta, GA

**David G. Halpern, JD**
Assistant Attorney General
Office of the Attorney General of Texas
Austin, TX

**Hope Rachel Hetico, RN, MHA, CMP,
CPHQ**
President
Institute of Medical Business Advisors, Inc.
Norcross, GA

**Anne E. Jorgensen, JD**
The Health Care Group
Plymouth Meeting, PA

**Harry L. Leider, MD, MBA, FACPE**
Chief Medical Officer
XLHealth
Baltimore, MD

**David A. Mackoul, MD, MS, FAAP, DFACMQ**
CEO
Mackoul Pediatrics
Cape Coral, FL

**Vittorio Maio, PharmD, MS, MSPH**
Assistant Professor
Department of Health Policy
Jefferson Medical College
Philadelphia, PA

**David Edward Marcinko, DPM, MBA, CFP, CMP**
Academic Provost
Institute of Medical Business Advisors, Inc.
Norcross, GA

**Alan P. Marco, MD, MMM, CPE, FACPE**
Professor and Chairman of Anesthesiology
University of Toledo College of Medicine
Toledo, OH

**David B. Nash, MD, MBA, FACP**
Chairman
Department of Health Policy
Jefferson Medical College
Philadelphia, PA

**Laurie Russell, MS, RN, CCM**
Senior Director of Health Solutions
XLHealth
Baltimore, MD

**Christopher N. Sciamanna, MD, MPH**
Associate Professor
Department of Health Policy
Jefferson Medical College
Philadelphia, PA

**Sara L. Thier, MPH**
Project Director
Department of Health Policy
Jefferson Medical College
Philadelphia, PA

**Christine B. Turley, MD**
Vice Chair for Clinical Services
University of Texas Medical Branch
Galveston, TX

**George P. Valko, MD**
Clinical Assistant Professor and Vice-Chair
for Clinical Programs
Department of Family and Community
Medicine
Jefferson Medical College
Philadelphia, PA

**Karisa Walker**
Medical Student
Jefferson Medical College
Philadelphia, PA

**Raymond L. Wedgeworth, MA**
Director of Reporting and Outcomes
XLHealth
Baltimore, MD

**Stephen E. Whitney, MD, MBA, BCM**
Assistant Professor of Pediatrics
Baylor College of Medicine
Houston, TX

**Jerald L. Zarin, MD, MBA, FAAP**
Regional Medical Director
Blue Cross Blue Shield of Texas
Houston, TX

# Introduction

## David B. Nash, MD, MBA, FACP and Karisa Walker

Many of today's practicing physicians can easily remember when public trust was high, doctor knew best, and independent decision making was the rule of the profession. The majority of physicians were generalists, and most medical students chose to follow in their footsteps. A physician could care for multiple generations of the same family, and relationships were close. This was the "Golden Age" of medicine, but times have changed. Over the past several years, information technology and managed care have transformed the way care is provided. These changes and more are shaping the medical practice in the 21st century.

In this introduction, we set the context of the book as a whole. We describe today's medical students, the issues that affect them, and what they need to know to confront these issues. A few organizations are already making strides, on all levels of medical education and practice, toward improving the current medical climate; these will be presented as well. This introduction is not so much a guide to the book but a portal through which to approach its contents.

We begin by addressing the unique attributes of today's medical students. Similar to their predecessors, they are smart, motivated, and altruistic. But unlike older physicians, they have been warned to stay away from the profession, face a poorly-functioning medical system, and know they will likely graduate with a large financial debt.

People choosing medicine today are not much different than their predecessors. They are well-educated individuals who nimbly jump through the hoops of undergraduate preparation, MCATs, and admissions interviews to become part of their medical school class. Beginning at matriculation, they throw themselves through four years of grueling undergraduate medical education, and up to seven (or more) years of residency and fellowship, not to mention the Board examinations, to finally practice as fully-qualified physicians. Simply navigating this daunting series of obstacles is enough to prove that motivation to enter the medical profession is strong. What is motivating young people to choose medicine?

In the 2005 AAMC survey of entering first-year students, more than 90% cited the opportunity to make a difference in the lives of others as a "very important" factor in choosing a medical career.[1] More than half of the students also cited opportunities for continuing patient contact, intellectual challenge, critical thinking, educating others about healthy living, and social responsibility as equally important.[1]

In contrast, fewer than 12% of students felt that prestige and income were "very important."[1] It seems that tomorrow's physicians are an altruistic, intellectual group, much the same as those who came before them.

Although there are many similarities between the physicians of yesterday and those of tomorrow, the path to a medical career has acquired additional obstacles. Students beginning their medical education in the 21st century are inundated with ominous warnings from physicians, are well aware that the health care system is failing, and face debt so extensive that it may impact their choice of specialty. Medical students receive little encouragement from practicing physicians to enter medicine. Instead of congratulating them on their goals, physicians give potential students copies of recent studies of career dissatisfaction. Physicians are clearly not pleased and warn others against the toils of this long and apparently undesirable road. Those students who were not put off by these warnings ventured on and perhaps made it to medical school, only to hear the same thing from attending physicians. The clear message to potential and current students is, "Get out now."

Another factor affecting today's medical student is an acute awareness of system-wide dysfunction in the medical field. Both the academic press and mass media report problems, from decreasing compensation to patient dissatisfaction. It has been said that when something goes wrong in medicine, the "ABP reaction" ensues, in which the patient seeks to "accuse, blame and punish" the closest target (usually the physician), even though the fault does not lie with one specific person.[2] Although this scapegoating may seem like problem-solving, it takes sophisticated root-cause analysis to detect where the problems in medicine actually originate. Poor-quality physicians are out there, but their presence alone does not explain the failing system. According to a growing body of literature, it is flawed systems involving a "cascade of poor or poorly executed procedures, policies, technologies and training" that are causing the dysfunction.[2] Far more than the previous generation, medical students today are challenged with sorting out the chaos, or at least being able to function within it.

Medical education has always been expensive, but in recent years the indebtedness of medical school graduates has risen to astronomical proportions. The median debt for a public medical school graduate was $100,000 in 2003, $135,000 for graduates of private schools.[3] The proportion of students carrying more than $200,000 in educational loans increased from 6.3% to 7.8% between 2003 and 2005.[4] With tuition and fees at some private schools topping $40,000 annually (not including living expenses, books, supplies, or transportation), it adds up quickly, and there is not much that even the most frugal students can do to avoid it. Most take on this burden unflinchingly, but heavy debts have deep implications for the future physician population. One study asserts that "there was an inverse relationship between the level of total educational debt and the intention to enter primary care, with the most marked effect noted for students owing more than $150,000 at graduation."[5] Students may feel they do not have the option of choosing a lower-paying specialty if they expect to repay the debt from their training. With an anticipated shortage of primary care physicians, the indebtedness issue is one that the government and health care industry cannot afford to ignore.

These are just a few of the many factors that make today's aspiring physician unique. They affect those aspiring physicians that never see a medical school classroom, too, perhaps explaining in part the drop in medical school applicants (37,364 in 2005 compared with 46,586 in 1995).[6] It is difficult to tell, but these students may well have been frightened away by cynicism, negative press, and potential debt. Still, many students persist, and this work will be a guidepost to help them navigate the shifting waters of health care in pursuit of a successful, fulfilling career.

## Changing environment

Although students are generally aware that medicine is in a state of flux, they may not be intimately familiar with the specificity and scope of the changes. In 1993, in the second edition of *Future Practice Alternatives in Medicine*, one of us (DBN) outlined our views on the changing environment of modern medicine. I saw that in the 21st century, medicine would be shaped by profound changes in the patient-doctor relationship, technology, and shifts in control and financing of health care.[7] These predictions have held true, and have profound effects on today's practice environment. Other issues, namely teamwork among health care professionals and quality control, have evolved more recently and strongly influence the profession. In the following six sections, we draw attention to how changes in the patient-doctor relationship, medical record-keeping, Medicare, managed care, "turf wars," and quality control are shaping the future of medicine.

### The Patient-doctor Relationship

Medical information is available everywhere, from books to magazines to Internet blogs. As in the past, sensational media reports (to the tune of "the miracle treatment your doctor is keeping from you!") and convincing advertising ("be sure to ask YOUR doctor about our medication!") contribute to patients' medical knowledge. More recently, patients have gained access to a substantial quantity of Internet sources, some containing high-quality, reviewed articles, and others built on unsubstantiated misinformation. For better or for worse, for many patients these have replaced the primary care physician as the first source of medical information. They educate (and sometimes misinform) patients about conditions and symptoms, and even recommend courses of treatment. Many provide lists of questions for patients to ask during visits. Patients are visibly empowered by this knowledge, and increasingly want to play an active role in their care.

This change has had a palpable effect on office visits. Instead of the physician questioning, examining, and providing treatment, the visit has necessarily become a conference between provider and patient. Time is needed for answering questions, providing clarity, and otherwise shepherding patients through the quagmire of information so they can make informed decisions about their own care. Since some online sources are outdated or inaccurate, physicians sometimes need to re-educate their patients. This process can be difficult, as bad press and other factors have cooled relationships and damaged trust between physicians and patients; providers must combat this mistrust in order to provide care. One way of addressing this is a focus on patient-centered care, one of the six "aims for improvement" called for in the Institute of Medicine's 2001 report titled *Crossing the Quality Chasm*.[8] Cultivating skills for this type of patient-doctor interaction is a critical challenge the profession now faces.

Information technology has surely changed the face of the patient in the United States, but to a larger extent, so has cultural diversity. Some realistically suggest that during the practicing lifetime of today's medical students, ethnic and racial minority groups will become the majority of the US population.[9] The current medical workforce is not meeting the needs of our diverse population, evidenced by health disparities between Caucasians and ethnic and racial minorities, men and women, the wealthy and the poor.[10] Without improvements in these areas, we risk short-changing an even larger percentage of the population than we do now. Efforts to recruit underrepresented minorities to medical school, in hopes that they will someday treat the communities they came from, have fallen short of their goals to increase the number of minority students to a level commensurate with that of their group's percentage of the US population.[11, 12] The 21ˢᵗ century physician, regardless of demographics, is challenged with the task of learning cultural competence, which entails a variety of new skills, such as culturally-sensitive interviewing, simultaneous interpreters, and cultural and religious community leaders in order to provide quality care to their patients. These skills are critical to delivering appropriate care to all our citizens.

The bottom line here is that these educated, diverse patients have become healthcare consumers. In the foreword to the 2000 book *Connecting with the New Healthcare Consumer*, Michael L. Millenson suggests that "focus on the patient experience is…what ultimately will determine the success of the health care consumer connection."[13] Students must learn how to accomplish this to achieve future success in treating their patients.

## Electronic Medical Records

Electronic medical records (EMRs) are an increasingly important method of patient-record keeping. The current encounter-based systems can cause discontinuous patient care and underuse of available information, leading to suboptimal patient care.[14] Sorting through stacks of manila folders and pages of illegible handwriting adds hassle, and potentially error, to medical treatment. Use of an EMR solves this problem by keeping a patient's records organized and accessible. Some programs even allow physicians to manipulate chart data, aiding in diagnosis, disease management, and comparison among similar cases. Many medical trainees are exposed to EMR in some way during their training. A recent poll of over 1,000 medical students, the *Future Physicians of America* survey, found that 90% of current students believe that EMRs will be fully adopted in 10 years (with the contribution of government funds); more than half believe it will "improve medical errors and increase patient safety."[15] Students are recognizing the value of EMR, but they need to know more. Familiarity with their use is key, along with the ability to implement EMR systems and safeguard the patient information within them.

## Medicare

Medicare is the largest single payor in the world; it is responsible for the largest segment of all health care dollars spent in the United States. Due to the growth of Medicare, patients are no longer the direct payors; third parties like Medicare are. This was not unforeseen. In 1987, one of us (DBN) suggested that payors would gain control over health care to the extent that physician services would be controlled by non-physicians.[7] This is the reality of medicine today. Residents in particular are dependent on Medicare dollars for their salaries, and most practicing physicians will see Medicare patients throughout their careers. Because of complicated (and often inadequate) reimbursement, many current physicians have become soured on Medicare and they transmit this negative attitude to their students. They have experienced the transition from independence and autonomy to accountability and quality measurement, and are finding their careers less fulfilling. This explains the ominous warnings to students mentioned earlier. Since involvement in Medicare is a reality for the 21st century physician, students need to move beyond criticism to an understanding of what it means to practice in a third-party payor system.

## Managed Care

Insurance companies are another group of third-party payors. In the 1990s, managed care was able to contain skyrocketing health care costs by controlling payment for physician services. With the advent of the turn of the century, however, managed care has been unable to keep pace with rising expenses and is no longer the leveling factor it once was. Whereas physicians used to be able to practice as they pleased, only lightly regulated by professional organizations, they are now held accountable for using evidence-based medicine, controlling costs, and public reporting of their outcomes. In some cases, pay for performance is becoming the dominant method of payment. In order to build successful practices, 21st century physicians will need to understand the machinations of managed care.

## Turf Wars

With the rising levels of costs and complexities, new non-physician, health care professionals are gaining more responsibilities and, in some cases, replacing physicians.[16] The expansion of these positions has led to posturing and bickering between physician groups and allied health professionals. These battles have been waging for years, but as insurers have become more involved, the discord has grown more intense. Payors are inclined to utilize these professionals, aware that they are less expensive to employ and more flexible about practice environment than primary care physicians.[16] Health professionals are now able to provide services once only offered by physicians, from writing prescriptions to performing laser eye surgery. For example, in a few states PhD-trained psychologists have been granted the right to prescribe psychotropic medications. Psychologists, "who tout PhDs and many years of training, say they're better equipped than an internist or OB-GYN to prescribe drugs for emotional conditions," although psychiatrists disagree, claiming that what is needed instead is more psychiatrists.[16] Although psychiatrists claim it is unsafe for psychologists to prescribe medication, some others suggest that it is a political and economic issue, as studies show these allied health professionals are capable providers.[16] Physicians do not want to be undercut by alternative providers in a climate that micromanages and limits the care they provide.

As these allied health professions have experienced widespread growth in recent years, the ability of all health personnel to work collaboratively has not evolved in kind. Instead, the marketplace is characterized by "a loosely allied group of independent, unrelated practitioners drawn together in a defensive huddle to meet the needs of insurance contracting and managed care."[17] Professionals who should be working together to serve patients are instead locking ideological horns. Each health care worker has unique skills and strengths, and when those contributions are adequately orchestrated, teamwork can produce excellent outcomes. One barrier to developing high-quality medical teams is the practice of teaching medical students and other students in the health professions separately, providing little opportunity to build camaraderie in the earliest years. It is not reasonable to expect group cohesion when these professions have no experience working together.

As managed care strengthens its influence and the costs of medical care continue to rise, it will become increasingly important for these assorted professionals to find a way to get along and work together. It has been repeatedly demonstrated that a team approach provides an excellent backdrop for providing safe, quality patient care;[18, 19] in a climate of high accountability, this approach makes sense. The Institute of Medicine (IOM) recommends emphasizing interdisciplinary teamwork during medical training to improve patient safety.[20] The balance among these professionals will surely be at the forefront of health care policy in the 21st century.

## Quality

Preventable error causes more deaths in the United States than AIDS, motor vehicle accidents, or breast cancer.[20] The 2001 Institute of Medicine report *To Err is Human* brought to the fore this unflattering statistic. The notion that patients may be at risk while under a physician's care has been a challenging model for health care providers. It is paradoxical at the deepest level: those who have taken an oath to beneficence are harming the very same people they are trying to heal. A major factor contributing to these errors is that physicians as a whole are not using the science we know.[21] The IOM report and a growing literature addressing medical error have fueled momentum toward improving quality in health care. Physicians are being held directly accountable for the work they perform, now more than ever before.[9] At the patient level, many consumers lack the skills and resources to adequately assess the quality of their physicians, precipitating a need for objective quality measurement.[13] On the payor level, insurance companies and the government are compensating physicians for their services; they demand information about what they are getting in return.

Education about quality is somewhat lacking. As of 2005, 38.9% of medical school graduates felt they had inadequate training in quality assurance.[4] This statistic is troubling, as it has direct implications for the safety of the public. It should be a top priority for medical trainees to learn about quality and how it affects the care they provide. Physicians may soon find their compensation based on a pay-for-performance system, and they will require a working knowledge of quality to be able to succeed in their chosen careers.

## Changing skill set

Each of the five areas of medical practice described is a strong force shaping health care delivery in the 21ˢᵗ century, but knowing about these issues is only half the battle. Students need to develop new attitudes and skills to confront these challenges. In the following section, we suggest a set of knowledge and skills that will assist tomorrow's physician in this process. The Commonwealth Fund, Centers for Medicare and Medicaid Services (CMS) and the Accreditation Council for Graduate Medical Education (ACGME) all echo similar ideas for addressing the future of health care. In response to these ideas, we suggest the following set of skills to help medical trainees meet the challenges of 21ˢᵗ century practice:

1. business savvy, including knowing how to use microeconomic analyses to effectively finance a practice;[9]

2. a working knowledge of "quality management science;"[9, 22]

3. interdisciplinary cooperation and teamwork experience, to mirror what they will encounter in practice;[9, 23]

4. an awareness of how Medicare and managed care organizations operate;[22, 23] and

5. patient-centered skills, such as cultural sensitivity and active listening.[9, 22, 23]

These skills will allow tomorrow's physicians to hit the ground running when they begin practice. Trial-by-fire training during residency and early practice will not be enough to adequately cultivate these skills; it may take years for them to be adequately refined and of practical use. To ensure these skills are well-developed before new physicians begin practice, instruction and experience in these areas should be provided during each stage of medical education. Lectures on all of these topics can be incorporated into the preclinical curriculum, emphases on best practices can be made during students' initial clinical clerkship experiences, and the skills learned during the undergraduate years can be applied and refined during internship and residency. As others have already suggested, quality education and quality patient care are linked, so changes to education must come in order to improve patient care.[24, 25] Some organizations are already working on incorporating these ideas into medical education and practice; four examples are provided here.

### UME: MD/MBA Combined Degree Programs

Of the 125 accredited U.S. medical schools, 47 offer a combined MD/MBA degree program. In its 2002 report titled *Training Tomorrow's Doctors*, the Commonwealth Fund suggests that to meet the challenge of the evolving health care profession, academic health centers:

"…must convey both concrete skills and an appropriate set of expectations and attitudes. Among the concrete skills that future physicians will need are an ability to work in teams with other physicians and non-physician health professionals; an understanding of how quality of care is defined, measured, and improved; familiarity with certain basic economic constructs such as cost-effectiveness and cost-benefit analysis; and some familiarity with the way health care organizations are managed and the behaviors that are best suited to achieving desired goals within such organizations."[9]

These types of skills can be acquired via formal business training.

For the physician practicing solo or in a small group, business skills are useful in managing a practice. A physician with business knowledge can lead the practice by budgeting, managing employees, and negotiating with managed care. Knowing how to do these things well will logically increase the efficiency of the practice and lead to better time-management and patient care, and perhaps improve compensation.

Business knowledge will also be helpful in the hospital setting in chairing a department, developing internal policy, and identifying and rectifying troubled systems. Physicians with this training are better equipped to navigate health care law, insurance and all its ramifications, and practice management. The MBA degree also enables MDs to take on roles outside traditional practice to assume a definitive leadership role in health care. Physicians with MBAs are well-positioned to become hospital administrators, heads of specialty organizations, drug company executives, and other yet-to-be-defined leadership roles.

Allowing physicians to take greater control of the profession may hopefully lead to a better practice environment. Dr. Joel I. Shalowitz suggests that these physician-executives will be able to lobby for appropriate use of proven technology, develop cost-effective practices, engender realistic expectations from health care consumers, improve quality and safety, and rein in the power of "piecemeal" managed care.[26] MD/MBAs possess the skills and knowledge to manage effectively without losing track of patient care and can serve as a powerful arbitrator among government, medicine, and industry to shepherd the profession to a better future.

### GME: Achieving Competence Today

The Achieving Competence Today (ACT) program in Systems and Practice Improvement, launched in 2003 by Partnerships for Quality Education and funded by the Robert Wood Johnson Foundation, was a method of bringing health policy education to residents. The program involved four weeks of coursework, in which two residents and a faculty mentor learned curriculum modules. The team then reviewed the modules and developed a plan to teach them to other residents. Later in the year, the initial two-resident team began work on proposing institutional curriculum changes, and then transferred the job to new residents the following year. This program not only had the potential to educate residents, but also exact change in academic medical centers to improve existing curricula.

### AMCs: Internal Review

Not all the positive changes occurring are happening via external programs. Some institutions, such as Johns Hopkins University, have taken to an internal auditing and improvement process to improve their systems. Via their new Center for Innovation in Quality Patient Care, they have improved quality in their ICUs and other wards by simply changing their behavior patterns and identifying "bottlenecks to change" throughout the hospital.[2] As a result, they have demonstrated that a large, established institution can break down resistance to innovation and improve patient care on its own. Students working in centers such as Hopkins will be able to glean knowledge about quality improvement as they complete their rotations and residencies.

### Profession: Defining What Works

At the profession-wide level, researchers are devising methods to help groups of physicians improve the quality of the care they provide. Drs. Shortell, Schmittdiel and Wang propose a "scorecard" for determining the performance of medical groups, based on "quality of care, financial performance, and organizational learning capability...in relation to environmental forces, resource acquisition and resource deployment factors, and a quality-centered culture."[27] Their work suggests that although few groups are high-performers in multiple areas, "external environmental and internal organizational factors" and "quality-centered culture outside reporting of results" are key factors in determining the performance of the group.[27] They suggest a cultural shift may then be the most effective way to improve the care physicians provide; this is something that will hopefully be accomplished as today's medical students enter the medical workforce.

## Conclusion

Medical students today require a new road map. In this introduction, we addressed the unique challenges facing the current generation of medical students and trainees as they enter their careers. The skills suggested here, along with examples of current improvement efforts, provide a jumping-off point from which to approach the ensuing chapters. The expert authors of the chapters that follow provide the most currently available information in their respective areas. This compilation of diverse topics covers information likely to be missing, at least in part, from any current medical school curriculum. The information in this volume should prove invaluable to those who carry the responsibility of not only surviving but succeeding in 21$^{st}$ century health care.

## Suggested Readings/Websites

Institute of Medicine – http://www.iom.edu/

National Association of MD/MBA Students – http://www.md-mba.org/

Association of American Medical Colleges – http://www.aamc.org/

Centers for Medicare/Medicaid Services – http://www.cms.hhs.gov/

Medscape Med Students – http://www.medscape.com/medicalstudents/

## References

1. Association of American Medical Colleges. Matriculating Student Questionnaire: 2005 All-schools report. Available at: http://www.aamc.org/data/msq/allschoolsreports/msq2005.pdf. Accessed June 20, 2006.

2. Miller ED. Good outcomes take good systems. Fall 2002. Available at: http://www.hopkinsmedicine.org/hmn/F02/postop.html. Accessed June 20, 2006.

3. Jolly P. Medical school tuition and young physicians' indebtedness. *Health Affairs* 2005;24:527-535.

4. Association of American Medical Colleges. Medical School Graduation Questionnaire: All-schools report. 2005. Available at: http://www.aamc.org/data/gq/allschoolsreports/2005.pdf. Accessed June 20, 2006.

5. Rosenblatt RA, Andrilla CH. The impact of U.S. medical students' debt on their choice of primary care careers: An analysis of data from the 2002 medical school graduation questionnaire. *Acad Med.* 2005;80:815-819.

6. Association of American Medical Colleges. FACTS: Applicants, accepted applicants, and matriculants by sex, 1994-2005. Available at: http://www.aamc.org/data/facts/2005/2005summary.htm. Accessed June 20, 2006.

7. Nash DB, ed. *Future Practice Alternatives in Healthcare*. Second ed. New York: Igaku-Shoin; 1993.

8. Committee on Quality Health Care in America, Institute of Medicine. *Crossing the Quality Chasm: A New Health System for the 21$^{st}$ Century*. Washington D.C.: National Academies Press; 2001.

9. The Commonwealth Fund Task Force on Academic Health Centers. Training tomorrow's doctors: The medical education mission of academic health centers. April 2002. Available at http://www.cmwf.org/usr_doc/ahc_trainingdoctors_516.pdf. Accessed June 20, 2006.

10. Braveman P. Health disparities and health equity: Concepts and measurement. *Annu Rev Public Health.* 2006;27:167-194.

11. Cohen JJ. Increasing diversity in the medical workforce is one solid way to prevent disparities in healthcare. *Med Gen Med.* 2005;7:26.

12. Cohen JJ. The consequences of premature abandonment of affirmative action in medical school admissions. *JAMA.* 2003;289:1143-1149.

13. Nash DB, Manfredi MP, Bozarth B, Howell S, eds. *Connecting with the New Healthcare Consumer: Defining Your Strategy.* New York, NY: McGraw-Hill; 2000.

14. Gittell JH, Fairfield KM, Bierbaum B, et al. Impact of relational coordination on quality of care, postoperative pain and functioning, and length of stay: A nine-hospital study of surgical patients. *Med Care.* 2000;38:807-819.

15. PRNewswire. Medical students diagnose the healthcare industry: Survey results give insight to future physicians' opinions. Available at: http://sev.prnewswire.com/health-care-hospitals/20060412/SFW01712042006-1.html. Accessed June 21, 2006.

16. Gearon CJ. Medicine's turf wars. *US News & World Report.* 2005;138:57-64.

17. Healy B. Teaming up. *US News & World Report.* 2005;138:72-74.

18. Safran DG. Defining the future of primary care: What can we learn from patients? *Ann Intern Med.* 2003;138:248-255.

19. Baker DP, Salas E, King H, Battles J, Barach P. The role of teamwork in the professional education of physicians: Current status and assessment recommendations. *Jt Comm J Qual Patient Saf.* 2005;31:185-202.

20. Kohn JC, Donaldson M, eds. *To Err is Human: Building a Safer Health System.* Washington, DC: National Academies Press; 2000.

21. Reinertsen JL. Zen and the art of physician autonomy maintenance. *Ann Intern Med.* 2003;138:992-995.

22. The Centers for Medicare and Medicaid Services. Quality improvement roadmap. Available at: http://www.cms.hhs.gov/CouncilonTechInnov/downloads/qualityroadmap.pdf. Accessed July 10, 2006.

23. Accreditation Council for Graduate Medical Education. Outcome project: General competencies. Available at: http://www.acgme.org/outcome/comp/comFull.asp#4. Accessed July 3, 2006.

24. Weinberger SE, Smith LG, Collier VU, Education Committee of the American College of Physicians. Redesigning training for internal medicine. *Ann Intern Med.* 2006;144:927-932.

25. Association of Program Directors in Internal Medicine, Fitzgibbons JP, Bordley DR, Berkowitz LR, Miller BW, Henderson MC. Redesigning residency education in internal medicine: A position paper from the association of program directors in internal medicine. *Ann Intern Med.* 2006;144:920-926.

26. Lazarus A, ed. *MD/MBA: Physicians on the New Frontier of Medical Management.* Tampa, FL: ACPE; 1998.

27. Shortell SM, Schmittdiel J, Wang MC, et al. An empirical assessment of high-performing medical groups: Results from a national study. *Med Care Res Rev.* 2005;62:407-434.

## Dedication

*To the long line of white coats that have preceded us, we owe much.*

*To the long line of white coats to follow,*
*we wish you all the best on your journey.*

# Section 1
# Clinical Management

# Chapter 1

## Quality of Care: Terms, Tools, and Techniques

Neil I. Goldfarb

### Executive Summary

The need to improve quality of health care in the United States has been documented in many studies and policy reports, especially within the past five years. Despite recognizing the problem, providers and the health care system have been slow to respond. There are many reasons for this stasis, including: lack of knowledge about how to improve; lack of adequate resources and infrastructure (including information technology); lack of clear evidence-based guidelines; lack of standardized quality measures; and general absence of a systems approach to improvement.

Performance measurement is the cornerstone of performance improvement. Donabedian's classic quality tripod identifies three dimensions for measurement: *structure*, the basic "bricks and mortar" for delivering care; *process*, the way in which care is delivered; and *outcome*, the result of care. Outcomes can be further classified into *clinical outcomes*, such as measures of morbidity, mortality, and physiologic markers; *humanistic outcomes* such as quality of life, pain level, and emotional status; and *economic outcomes*, including the direct cost of providing care and the indirect cost of lost productivity.

Most performance measures being used today to assess provider performance are process measures (such as HbA1c testing for diabetes), although increasingly outcomes (such as HbA1c level) also are being examined. Physicians in practice need to know about these measures for a variety of reasons: they are good markers for actual quality of care delivered, and can be used to self-assess and self-improve performance; they increasingly are being measured and publicly reported on, at the individual provider level; they are increasingly being linked to financial reimbursement through "pay for performance" systems; and, health benefit purchasers, including the government and employers, increasingly are holding providers accountable for the quality of care they deliver.

In light of the growing emphasis on quality measurement, reporting, and reimbursement, practicing physicians need to incorporate performance assessment and improvement into their practice. This may start with accessing education on performance measurement and improvement tools, which are not well-addressed in most academic programs. A wealth of information is available on the Internet and through sources for continuing medical education. At the heart of delivering quality care is understanding the precepts of evidence-based medicine and the appropriate use of care guidelines, and incorporating this information into the daily routine.

## Learning objectives

- To understand that quality of care in the United States needs to be improved

- To recognize that national movements such as public reporting, pay for performance (P4P), and consumer-directed health care are seeking to increase physician accountability and performance

- To learn specific strategies that physicians can incorporate into practice in order to measure and improve the quality of care they provide

- To become familiar with resources that are available to physicians seeking to improve quality

## Keywords

accountability; health outcomes; pay for performance (P4P); performance measurement; quality of care; severity-adjustment;

## Introduction

Quality of care in the United States is far from optimal. Despite spending more per capita on health care, health outcomes are not measurably better, and in many cases are significantly worse, than for other industrialized nations that spend far less. Increasingly, physicians are being expected to deliver "evidence-based medicine" — care that conforms to guidelines and that is based on research evidence of effectiveness and cost-effectiveness, where such evidence exists. In this chapter, we: 1) review the evidence that quality needs to be improved; 2) consider why these problems exist; 3) examine approaches to measuring and improving quality; 4) review recent trends in improving quality and increasing provider accountability in health care; and, 5) suggest practical strategies for incorporating self-assessment and improvement into routine clinical practice.

## The State of Quality in the United States

By most accounts, quality of care in the United States is sorely in need of improvement. The Institute of Medicine (IOM), in a seminal report on patient safety, *To Err is Human*, reported that 98,000 deaths occur annually due to medical errors.[1] In a follow-up report, *Crossing the Quality Chasm*, the IOM called for sweeping changes in the way care is organized and delivered in order to achieve a system that is safe, effective, patient-centered, timely, efficient, and equitable.[2] The IOM defines quality as "the degree to which health services for individuals and populations increase the likelihood of desired health outcomes and [the degree to which they] are consistent with current professional knowledge."

One recent study, conducted by Elizabeth McGlynn and colleagues at the RAND Corporation, demonstrated that care delivery often is not consistent with professional knowledge.[3] Through review of administrative data and medical records for a large national sample of patients, the investigators found that only 55% of recommended care (care that would adhere to widely-agreed upon evidence-based guidelines) is delivered. Other resources available for tracking care quality echo these findings, for example:

- The work of Dr. John Wennberg and colleagues, presented in The Dartmouth Atlas of Health Care, demonstrates wide unexplained variation in health service utilization and outcomes, between and within geographic regions.[4]

- The National Healthcare Quality Report, compiled by the U.S. Agency for Healthcare Research and Quality (AHRQ), tracks 179 measures of quality, available through a variety of sources. The most recent available report for 2005 shows that while quality is slowly improving along many of the tracked indicators, improvement is variable, and much remains to be done. For example, only 53% of adults with diabetes had an HbA1c test, a retinal exam, and a foot exam in 2002 (up from 48% in 2000).[5]

- A related AHRQ product, the National Healthcare Disparities Report, highlights another significant quality problem – wide disparities in access to and delivery of care exist across socio-demographic groups, including race and ethnicity.[6] Many studies have demonstrated disparities in preventive testing, timeliness of care, and likelihood of receiving interventional services such as surgery.

## Why Isn't Quality Better?

If all of this information is available to demonstrate the need for improvement, why do these problems persist? There are many potential explanations:

- Lack of Knowledge — Medical education has been slow to incorporate principles of evidence-based medicine, and quality assessment and improvement into all levels of the curriculum.

- Lack of Recognition of a Problem — Most providers believe that they already deliver high-quality care and that the findings of a national quality problem reflect other providers' practices but not their own.

- Lack of Agreement — Many providers continue to believe that high-quality care is individualized, and does not rely on "cookbook medicine" (guideline-driven care).

- Lack of Motivation — In a system in which clinical quality is typically not measured, discernible by the average customer, or linked to compensation, providers have little motivation to assess or improve their performance.

- Lack of Infrastructure — Many of the approaches to improvement that are being advocated today, such as routine self-assessment, and use of electronic health records, are time-intensive or require additional financial investment.

- Lack of a Systems Approach — The traditional model of care delivery is fragmented, focuses on acute episodes rather than prevention, discourages inter-disciplinary collaboration and communication, and has numerous other problems which stand in the way of delivering care in a consistent, high-quality manner.

A 2003 national survey of physicians regarding quality of care, conducted by the Commonwealth Fund, confirms that for the most part physicians have yet to engage in measuring quality and using improvement tools.[7]  Only one-third of survey respondents were involved in *any* performance improvement activity in their own practices, only one-third had any data on their own clinical performance, and over two-thirds felt that the public should not have access to data on physician quality. Change is needed.

## Conceptualizing and Measuring Quality

Performance measurement is an essential tool for performance improvement.  By measuring performance, providers, or other stakeholders such as benefit purchasers and insurers, can determine if improvement is needed, and gain insight into which interventions are most likely to be effective.  For example, suppose a primary care provider was interested in knowing how many women over age 50 in her practice had received a mammogram within the past two years.  Reviewing a sample of charts for women in the practice, she found evidence of a recent mammogram for 65% of cases; for 10% of cases a patient refusal of mammography was noted; for 15% of cases a mammogram had been ordered but there was no evidence of results; and for 10% of cases there was no notation regarding mammography orders or results.

The review tells the provider that there's certainly room for improvement, and that different interventions may be needed — e.g., some additional patient education, and perhaps a tickler system to remind the provider or the patient when a mammogram is due.

To inform the discussion about measuring performance, let's start with some conceptual definitions. Avedis Donabedian, the father of modern quality measurement, defined the quality tripod as structure, process, and outcome.[8] *Structure* refers to the basic building blocks of delivering quality, such as having a clean facility, having adequate staffing, appropriate access to technology, etc. *Process* refers to the manner in which care is delivered, e.g., children are immunized on schedule, an annual diabetic retinal exam is performed. *Outcome* is the result of care. Outcomes generally can be classified as clinical (morbidity, mortality), humanistic (quality of life, pain, emotional status), or economic (utilization, dollars). Other typologies also shed light on ways to look at and measure quality:

- **Clinical vs. Service Quality:** Clinical quality is concerned with the actual delivery of clinical services, in accordance with evidence-based guidelines and standards, whereas service quality is concerned with the way in which services are delivered, usually from the patient's perspective, e.g., waiting times for appointments, satisfaction with the interaction with the physician and office staff.

- **Overuse, Underuse, and Misuse:** Quality is called into question when services are under-utilized (e.g., children are not immunized on schedule), overused (e.g., unnecessary CT scans are performed), or misused (e.g., a contraindicated drug is prescribed).

These typologies all are useful in helping to identify dimensions for assessing performance.

## Nuts and Bolts of Measurement

While it is unreasonable to think that all physicians will become quality measurement experts, some basic understanding of the issues is necessary in order to review and interpret quality information and determine if action is needed. As an example, suppose that the Medical Director of a health plan in which you participated met with you to review the plan's quality profile of your performance. The Medical Director tells you that you have a high rate of hospitalization for patients with congestive heart failure (CHF), suggesting suboptimal outpatient management. There are many questions that could come to mind, for example: How were patients with CHF identified? Who are you being compared to? Does the analysis adjust for patient age or disease severity? Were the hospitalizations appropriate? Measuring quality is often a complicated affair, so let's review some of the issues in measurement.

Quality measurement is often limited by the amount of information or ease of accessing information. The main sources of data for quality measurement are: administrative records (billing systems and claims data); medical records (paper or electronic charts); and patients (surveys). Although administrative data are the most readily accessible, it is limited to basic information such as diagnosis and procedure codes. Charts are a much richer source of clinical information, but reviewing charts is resource-intensive. The advent of electronic health records may greatly expedite the feasibility and efficiency of clinical quality measurement.

Another issue is the need to severity adjust data, i.e., to recognize that some measures are subject to differences in patient case mix. In our CHF example, you may have a higher hospitalization rate because your patients have more advanced disease than the average population to which you are being compared. Several methods exist for severity adjustment, ranging from basic statistical adjustments for age and gender, to more complex systems such as disease staging, and MediQual risk adjustment.[9] Not all measures need to be severity adjusted. For example, there is generally widespread acceptance that HbA1c should be tested at least annually for all diabetics. So, looking at a population with Type II diabetes, it would be reasonable to expect that all patients in the population would have been tested at least once in the past 12 months, regardless of the severity of their diabetes.

## Sample Quality Measurement Programs

Because of the complexity of measuring quality in a reliable, valid, and feasible manner, many national groups, as well as more localized efforts, have sought to develop standardized approaches to quality measurement. Examples of importance include:

- **JCAHO Core Measures:** The Joint Commission on the Accreditation of Healthcare Organizations (JCAHO) has increasingly been working toward including performance measures in the accreditation processes for hospitals and other health care providers it accredits. The Core Measures project, part of JCAHO's "Agenda for Change," has developed sets of standardized quality measures for several high-volume conditions, such as heart failure, acute myocardial infarction, and community acquired pneumonia.[10] Having hospitals collect and report data in a standardized manner makes it possible to look at any individual hospital's performance in relation to regional and national benchmarks, and to track changes in a hospital's performance over time.

- **HEDIS:** The Health Plan Employer Data and Information Set (HEDIS) is a product of the National Committee for Quality Assurance (NCQA). HEDIS was developed as a set of standardized quality measures at the health plan level. Participating health plans typically select a random sample of members meeting eligibility criteria for a measure (the denominator), and then measure how many members of that sample met the care delivery standard (the numerator). For example, one HEDIS measure looks at cholesterol testing and control for patients with a history of heart disease. The health plan uses administrative (claims and enrollment) data to identify a random sample of patients who have been continuously enrolled in the health plan, and who have had a hospitalization for bypass, angioplasty, or an acute MI. The health plan then examines how many of these patients had a cholesterol test between two months and one year after the hospitalization, and whether their LDLs were less than 100, evidencing good control. Because health plans often don't have sufficiently detailed lab test claims, a chart review within doctors' offices may be needed to obtain the LDL values. This "hybrid" approach to data collection, involving both administrative data and chart reviews, helps to explain why health plans often need access to physicians' records (health plans also typically review charts to assess compliance with charting and documentation standards, to audit accuracy of billing, and to support data collection for other special quality measurement initiatives).

- **Quality Improvement Organizations (QIOs):** The Centers for Medicare and Medicaid Services (CMS) contract with Quality Improvement Organizations (QIOs) around the country to help monitor and improve quality of care under the Medicare and Medicaid programs. Operating under a general guide developed by CMS (the "Scope of Work"), QIOs review quality information and work with providers and other community organizations to develop improvement initiatives. Although the QIO work historically was focused on facility-based care, more recently QIOs have started to assess physician care.

Other groups, such as the Ambulatory Care Quality Alliance (AQA), the Hospital Quality Alliance (HQA), and the National Quality Forum (NQF), as well as professional societies such as the American Medical Association (AMA) and specialty societies, all are engaged in efforts to agree on what needs to be measured, and how it should be measured. As we'll discuss in the next section, physicians need to be aware of these initiatives because they ultimately are expected to impact directly on routine practice and revenue.

## The Increasing National Focus on Quality

The spotlight cast on quality of care by the IOM and other researchers and policy advocates has stimulated a growing movement toward accountability in health care. Purchasers, including the federal and state governments and employers who offer health benefits, have begun to recognize that they are not obtaining value (the relation of quality to cost) for the money they spend on health care. A new generation of "value-based purchasers" is driving the movement to improve quality, through a variety of methods.

Transparency of quality information through public reporting is one approach, predicated on the belief that consumers will make informed care-seeking choices based on quality information. CMS has reported information on nursing home quality for several years on its "Nursing Home Compare" website.[11] The quality ratings come from several sources, including CMS' collection of data on a standardized tool (the MDS), and findings from site inspections conducted by the states. Consumers can go to the website and look at information by nursing home, or for all nursing homes within a geographic region. More recently, CMS has made similar information available on hospital quality based on Medicare data. Reporting at the individual physician level is still several years away, but inevitable.

How consumers use this information, or will use it in the future, is unclear. Several studies suggest that consumers continue to make care-seeking choices based on local word of mouth or convenience. However, more recent findings suggest that when information is packaged clearly, consumers will use it. Furthermore, with the growth of consumerism and consumer-directed health plans, in which consumers have financial incentives to seek higher-quality care, it is expected that the publicly reported information will become increasingly important to consumers.

Transparent information on quality is driving decisions about which providers to include in a health plan's network. Health plans and self-insured employers are expected to become more selective in their contracting decisions, either choosing not to contract with lower-quality providers or to offer consumers incentives (such as lower out-of-pocket payments) to seek care with higher-quality providers. These "tier and steer" approaches could significantly affect income and patient volume for providers who are not in compliance with quality standards and performing at or above benchmarks.

The more concrete form of "pay for performance" is the actual awarding of differing levels of compensation based on quality of care delivered. Pay for performance (P4P) is gaining traction among purchasers and payors, including CMS. Bridges to Excellence (BTE) is one example of a P4P initiative, engineered by a collaborative among employer coalitions, large employers, physician groups, researchers, and others.[12] Under BTE, providers have the opportunity to earn financial rewards for implementing certain practices which have been demonstrated to result in safer, higher-quality care, and for achieving measurable levels of quality for their patients with diabetes or cardiovascular disease. Many insurers also are now rolling out P4P initiatives. CMS has begun to offer bonus payments (1-2% of Medicare compensation) to high-quality hospitals, and is now laying the groundwork through its Physician Voluntary Reporting Program (PVRP) to measure and reward quality for physician services to Medicare members. Although it is not possible to present information on all of the public reporting, recognition and reward, and financial P4P programs, a few others are worth noting:

- NCQA continues to develop a series of physician recognition programs for high-volume chronic conditions.

- The American Board of Internal Medicine (ABIM) has launched a Performance Improvement Module (PIM) project, which offers web-based education and support to providers for assessing and improving their own performance; several insurers have discussed plans to include PIM participation in their P4P initiatives.

- The Leapfrog Group is a purchaser-driven organization seeking to publicly report on hospital compliance with high-quality practices, and to encourage the use of this information in care-purchasing and care-seeking decisions.

- The Institute for Healthcare Improvement (IHI), through its "100,000 Lives" campaign is seeking to encourage hospitals to adapt practices which will promote inpatient quality and safety.

## Strategies for Physicians

As can be seen from many of the examples above, the provider community has not been driving the quality engine (and in some cases has been dragged into the modern era of accountability kicking and screaming). What can you do to more actively engage in addressing the well-documented deficiencies in health care today? Here are a few strategies to consider, for incorporating into routine practice:

1) **Seek education and available resources.** A list of resources to help get you started is included at the end of this chapter. Information on the organizations and initiatives mentioned in this chapter also is available on the Internet. Professional societies, QIOs, and national organizations all have developed educational programs and materials intended to be of help to physicians in measuring and improving their performance.

2) **Practice evidence-based medicine.** Evidence-based guidelines are available in the peer-reviewed literature and through professional organizations. Resources such as the National Guideline Clearinghouse sponsored by AHRQ also exist to help disseminate information.

3) **Self-assess practice.** Consider developing a practice-based quality measurement and improvement initiative (see case study). Tools such as the ABIM's Performance Improvement Modules also are available to help providers design self-assessment and performance improvement programs.

4) **Review and act on feedback reports.** Don't file away those reports without reviewing them. It's appropriate to question the methods used to generate the data, but also consider how you should act assuming the information is correct.

5) **Redesign practices, including adoption of health information technology.** Many believe that Health Information Technology (HIT) (see Chapter 6) will solve many of the health care quality woes we are currently experiencing. Some studies, however, suggest that health information systems may introduce new opportunities for poor quality, or will only be as good as the information that providers enter. Adoption of HIT is only part of an overall systems strategy, modifying care processes and record-keeping to promote an environment of quality.

## Conclusion

It is time for physicians to recognize that quality measurement and improvement are central components of the job. Physicians need to take ownership of the quality problem and reclaim their leadership of the healthcare team, in seeking to address current deficiencies. A wealth of resources is available to support physicians in this endeavor. The era of public accountability and P4P is here, and should be viewed as an opportunity to step up to the plate in improving care.

## Case study

The primary care practice in a large, multi-specialty academic group practice decided to undertake a performance measurement and improvement initiative. The group's leadership recognized the importance of quality from the perspectives of patient care, public relations, and potential increased reimbursement under a pay for performance program. After much discussion, the primary care practice decided to measure hypertension control in its patient population. Information was received from NCQA on the HEDIS measure for "controlling high blood pressure." Because this measure was developed at the health plan level, some modifications to the sampling and measurement methodologies needed to be made, for measurement at the provider group level. A project protocol was developed in consultation with a nurse in the hospital's performance improvement department.

All patients with a diagnosis of hypertension on at least one billed visit during a 12-month period were identified from the practice's billing system. A random sample of 300 patients was selected from this listing. Charts were reviewed to both confirm that the patient carried a diagnosis of hypertension, and to determine if blood pressure was controlled. Control was defined as having a BP $\leq 140/90$ as of the last visit during the calendar year.

The practice found that only 66% of hypertensive patients in the sample had blood pressure controlled. The physicians in the group met to discuss possible improvement strategies. The resulting intervention included: 1) educating all providers in the practice as to hypertension treatment guidelines and the study's baseline findings; 2) developing educational materials on hypertension for patients and providers; and, 3) developing a "discharge instructions" form for patients with hypertension.

After one year, the impact of this intervention was assessed, by repeating the baseline measurement methodology on a newly identified sample (meeting the same criteria as were used for the baseline group, but for the subsequent time period). A control rate of 75% was found on the follow-up; this difference (from 66% at baseline) was statistically significant. This case illustrates that performance measurement and improvement can take place as part of clinical practice.

## Study/discussion questions

1. The United States spends more per capita on health care than any other industrialized nation, but health outcomes such as life expectancy at birth, are much worse in the U.S. than in most of these other nations. Why aren't we seeing more "value" for our spending?

2. How might you, as a practicing physician or physician executive, seek to improve the quality of care you provide to your patients, and the quality of care delivered to patients in general?

3. Besides physicians, who else needs to be involved in measuring and improving quality in health care? How can physicians involve these other stakeholders in quality improvement projects?

4. Pay-for-performance programs are seeking to align financial rewards with results of care. What do you see as some of the challenges in implementing these programs, and how do you think these programs would influence your own clinical decision making?

5. In the hypertension case study (above), improvement in care was seen from baseline to follow-up. Can this improvement be attributed to the intervention? What else might explain these findings? Given the 75% control rate on follow-up, should the interventions be continued? What more would you do?

## Suggested Readings/Websites

A summary of the RAND report on quality can be found at
http://www.rand.org/pubs/research_briefs/RB9053-2

Become familiar with how CMS is making quality information available on the Internet by looking at the CMS Hospital Compare Website as an example:
http://www.hospitalcompare.hhs.gov/hospital/home2.asp

You can do this for nursing homes as well, looking at the CMS Nursing Home Compare website.  http://www.medicare.gov/NHCompare/home.asp

Information on NCQA's accreditation program and HEDIS report is available at http://www.ncqa.org.  You also can look at how information on quality at the health plan level is being reported by NCQA.

As an example of a pay for performance program, look at the Bridges to Excellence web site http://www.bridgestoexcellence.org/

A briefing on Medicare's growing involvement in the pay for performance movement available at:  http://www.cms.hhs.gov/apps/media/press/release.asp?Counter=1343

The 2005 National Quality Report from the Agency for Healthcare Research and Quality is available at http://www.qualitytools.ahrq.gov/qualityreport/2005/browse/browse.aspx?id=7939

Kohn LT, Corrigan JM, Donaldson MS, eds. *To err is human: building a safer health system.* Washington, DC: National Academies Press; 2000.

Committee on Quality of Health Care in America, Institute of Medicine. *Crossing the quality chasm: a new health system for the 21st century.* Washington, DC: National Academies Press; 2001.

## References

1. Kohn LT, Corrigan JM, Donaldson MS, eds. *To Err is Human: Building a Safer Health System.* Washington, DC: National Academies Press; 2000.

2. Committee on Quality of Health Care in America, Institute of Medicine. *Crossing the Quality Chasm: A New Health System for the 21st Century.* Washington, DC: National Academies Press; 2001.

3. McGlynn EA, Asch SM, Adams J, Keesey J, Hicks J, DeCristofaro A, Kerr EA. The quality of health care delivered to adults in the United States. *N Engl J Med.* 2003:348:2635-45.

4. The Dartmouth Atlas of Health Care. Available at: www.dartmouthatlas.org.

5. 2005 National Healthcare Quality Report (NHQR). Available at: www.qualitytools.ahrq.gov/qualityreport/2005. Accessed August 18, 2006.

6. 2005 National Healthcare Disparities Report. Available at: http://www.qualitytools.ahrq.gov/disparitiesreport/2005/browse/browse.aspx. Accessed August 18, 2006.

7. The Commonwealth Fund 2003 National Survey of Physicians and Quality of Care. Available at: www.cmwf.org/surveys/surveys_show.htm?doc_id=278869. Accessed August 18, 2006.

8. Donabedian A. Evaluating the quality of medical care. *Milbank Memorial Fund Quarterly.* 1966:44:166-206.

9. Iezzoni LI, ed. *Risk adjustment for measuring health care outcomes, 3rd edition.* Chicago, IL: Health Administration Press; 2003.

10. Performance Measurement Initiatives. Available at: www.jointcommission.org/performancemeasurement/performancemeasurement. Accessed August 18, 2006.

11. Nursing Home Compare. Available at: www.medicare.gov/NHcompare. Accessed August 18, 2006.

12. Bridges to Excellence. Available at: www.bridgestoexcellence.org. Accessed August 18, 2006.

# Chapter 2

## Ensuring the Safety of Our Patients

Alan P. Marco, MD, MMM, CPE, FACPE and Brian M. Aboff, MD, FACP

### Executive Summary

Health care networks must design systems to reduce medical error and improve the safety of patients. Traditional concepts regarding the causes of medical errors have not led to improvements. The careful use of new approaches, such as systems-based thinking, is needed to make progress in patient safety through error reduction. Several tools exist to help with performance improvement, such as root cause analysis, sentinel event analysis, flowcharts, Pareto charts, fishbone diagrams, and control charts.

Physicians must be leaders in the development of a "culture of safety." Protocols for effective communications, such as the SEGUE process and legible handwriting, are crucial to developing this culture. While technologic advances may help improve safety, encouraging patients to actively participate in their care is something that all physicians can put into practice immediately. Caring for oneself as a physician, such as ensuring to get enough sleep, can also improve patient safety.

Increased awareness of safety issues and involvement of physicians, government agencies, and patients can help to create the culture of safety that will ultimately improve the quality of health care.

### Learning Objectives

1. Review the definitions and prevalence of medical error.

2. Identify models for understanding error and how they apply to current practice.

3. Analyze strategies to reduce error.

4. Identify resources for reducing medical errors.

### Keywords

control charts, culture of safety, medical error, patient safety, root cause analysis, sentinel events.

## Introduction

What is patient safety? As stated in the Institute of Medicine (IOM) report, *To Err is Human: Building a Safer Health System*, patient safety is "freedom from accidental injury."[1] Others define it operationally: patient safety is the concept that patients in health care settings achieve intended outcomes. In order to ensure patient safety, operation systems and processes that minimize the likelihood of errors must be developed. While the ideal goal is to eliminate errors, the reality is that we must develop systems that minimize the chance of an error occurring, and that if one does occur, it is recognized as soon as possible to minimize the impact on the patient. The National Patient Safety Foundation defines medical error as "an unintended health care outcome caused by a defect in the delivery of care to a patient."[2] Errors may be errors of commission (doing the wrong thing), omission (not doing the right thing), or execution (doing the right thing incorrectly).

As a profession, we are just beginning to understand the magnitude of the problem. *To Err is Human* suggested that as many as 98,000 lives are lost each year in the United States as a result of medical errors. Compare this to the lives lost in motor vehicle crashes — approximately 40,000 per year.[3] The American Cancer Society estimates that 40,000 women die each year of breast cancer.[4] Until recently, patient safety has not received the same degree of attention.

## Identifying the Underlying Causes of Medical Error

What are the causes of medical error? Traditionally, we "know" that errors are caused by slovenly, stupid, ill-trained, mean-spirited careless people who don't really care about the people that get hurt. If only Dr. X or Nurse Y cared enough to do a good job, the patient would not have suffered. The only way to stop errors is to root out these bad apples! However, think of the last error that <u>you</u> made — was it because you were stupid, lazy, and uncaring? Not likely, and modern thinking has evolved to understand that people are basically well-intentioned, but often are limited by the system from doing a good job. Sometimes, the adverse event is due to a single, overwhelming error. More commonly, it is due to a series of small errors that by themselves do not cause the patient significant harm but, when added together, cause an adverse event. This model has been termed "organizational accidents" by James Reason.[5] This does not mean that no error is due to personal lapses and that no one should ever be held responsible, but in almost all situations it is multiple flaws in the system that allow the error to occur. This is commonly known as the Swiss cheese model.[6] Every system has barriers to error (slices of cheese). However, these barriers have gaps in them (holes). If the holes line up just so, the error gets through. The idea is to make the holes as small as possible and few enough so that, with multiple layers, the error is unlikely to get through to the patient.

Let's look at an example of a medication error.

> Dr. Smith is on call and gets a call from Bill, the 4 West nurse. "Dr. Smith," Bill says, "I understand you are covering for Dr. Jones? Well, Ms. Englehart is feeling nauseated after her surgery today." "I'll be up to evaluate her shortly," says Dr. Smith. Unfortunately, Dr. Smith is delayed by a call to the Emergency Department and arrives bleary-eyed in the wee hours of the morning to evaluate Ms. Englehart. He scrawls Anzemet 12 mg q6 and crawls off to bed. By this time, the nurses have changed shift and Barb is now taking care of Ms. Englehart. She transcribes the order as Avandamet 1-2 qd and administers the first dose. The following day, the patient is noted to be lethargic and hypoglycemic, and is transferred to the Intermediate Care Unit for evaluation and treatment.

Why did this medical error occur? Surely we don't believe that the doctors and nurses are evil, bad people. The system has broken down and allowed this error to get through the holes in the cheese.

In analyzing adverse events, a common approach is to use root cause analysis (RCA). The approach encourages one to look beyond the superficial, "obvious" causes and get at the root cause. The superficial cause in this case is that the patient received the wrong drug, but the root lies deeper. We must find out what happened, why it happened, and how it happened.[7] RCA is a series of structured questions that lead to the fundamental issues and allows us to develop workable approaches to preventing errors in the future.[8] The general process for RCA is:

1. Define the problem
2. Gather data/evidence.
3. Analyze cause/effect relationships.
4. Identify root causes.
5. Develop solution recommendations.
6. Implement the solutions.

Unfortunately, we in health care frequently think we know the "cause" of a problem (and its solution) long before we know all the facts of the situation. Jumping to conclusions diverts our attention from the real issues and solutions.

Sometimes the issue is serious enough to be termed a sentinel event. The Joint Commission on Accreditation of Healthcare Organizations (JCAHO) defines a sentinel event as "an unexpected occurrence involving death or serious physical or psychological injury, or the risk thereof."[9]   Examples of sentinel events include suicide in a hospitalized patient, wrong-site surgery, medication errors, patient falls resulting in injury and patient death, or injury as a result of the use of restraints.  It is "sentinel" because it is so serious that it serves as an early warning of an underlying problem that warrants immediate investigation.

Let's look at our example above. The obvious "cause" is that the nurse made an error in transcription and gave the wrong medication. But are there other contributing factors? Why did the nurse make the error? Perhaps because Anzemet and Avandamet are sound-alike medications.[10]   The doctor's illegible scrawl certainly contributed to the problem.  If the writing was illegible, why didn't the nurse call for clarification? Was she afraid of being scolded?  All too often there is a problem with the working relationship between doctors and nurses that results in breakdown of communication.  What about the hand-off from one nurse to another? Could there have been a miscommunication about changes in the patient care plan? How about the order itself?  If it wasn't in proper form, the pharmacy should have checked the dose before supplying it. There may also be contributions from resident fatigue, distractions (call to the Emergency Department, other patient issues, chatting at the medication station), or other issues. So, we have identified at least ten potential contributions to the error that would have to be investigated before we "know" what caused the error.

## Charting Systems and Processes

Other tools for performance improvement include data analysis through flowcharts, fishbone diagrams, control charts, Pareto charts, histograms, and others. It is important in current practice to be able to analyze data so that information may be extracted from them. Hospitals and practices typically are awash with data, but information needs to be digested to get the benefit. The old QA (quality assurance) approach of weeding out the bad apples does not shift the performance curve significantly, and health care providers must be ready to look at how their actions affect the system. Careful analysis of the data makes this possible.

Flowcharts are an excellent way to graphically describe a process. The very act of sitting down with the involved parties and plotting out what actually is done, by whom, and when can be very enlightening. In one recent example, a surgeon complained that his pre-operative notes were not getting to the patient's chart despite his giving them to the pre-operative clinic. When he and the manager looked at what was happening and tried to graph it on a flowchart, it rapidly became apparent that he merely handed the note to his clinic staff, and somehow that was supposed to make it appear on the chart. The staff didn't know where to send it nor did they worry about timeliness. Flowcharting brought out these issues.

Fishbone diagrams, also known as Ishikawa diagrams, were invented by Dr. Kaoru Ishikawa, a Japanese quality improvement expert.[11] (Figure 1, below) These provide a visual way of representing cause and effect, and look a bit like the bones of a fish, hence the common appellation of fishbone diagram. Fishbone diagrams are used whenever the team needs to study a problem to determine the root cause or wants to study all the possible reasons why a process is having problems. To construct a diagram, draw a line with the problem as the head of the fish. Label "bones" of the fish according to one of these common systems: the 4 Ms—Methods, Machines, Materials, Manpower; the 4 Ps—Place, Procedure, People, Policies; the 4 Ss—Surroundings, Suppliers, Systems, Skills. Brainstorm to come up with factors affecting each of these, and continue to ask "why" until no more useful information is generated. Next, prioritize the items that are listed as contributing factors.

## Figure 1: Typical Fishbone Diagram

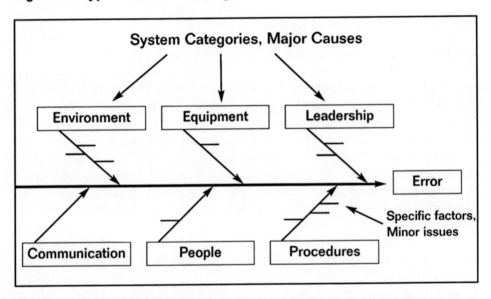

Run charts plot the data points as a function of time, such as average temperature by day of the week. Control charts allow you to see if the changes from one point to another are statistically significant without doing a bunch of calculations (or understanding statistics for that matter!). The limits for control charts are set at three standard deviations above and below the mean, and points that lie outside these limits are said to be "out of control," i.e., they are unpredictable and due to some special cause. Control charts can be constructed easily through simple calculations by hand, or various software products can do it for you. There are four major types of control charts: the x-chart (and related x-bar, r-, and s-charts), the p-chart, the c-chart, and the u-chart. These charts are used when the data being measured meet certain conditions (or attributes). The x-chart is a basic control chart that is used with variable data (measurements), such as weights of candy bars coming out of the mold or number of cases per month. P-charts are used with binomial (go-no go) data, such as percent patients with a screening test completed. When counting the number of defects in a given sample, such as the number of charts missing a signature in a monthly sample of 30 charts, a c-chart is used. When the number in the sample varies (audit all charts weekly, but the number may vary week to week), a u-chart is used. There are many resources available for further information on the use of control charts.[12,13]

The Pareto principle can be stated simply by the aphorism 80% of the problems are caused by 20% of the people. This is actually true (more or less)! If you graph the contributing cause to a problem in descending order, it rapidly becomes apparent which two or three account for most of the problems. This allows you to focus on the ones that will give you the biggest impact.

## Establishing a Culture of Safety

As physicians, what can we do to improve patient safety? First and foremost, we need to help establish a culture of safety. We should be leaders in everything from hand washing to clinical care protocols. Building a culture of safety takes a sustained effort that starts with the institutional leadership.[14] Encouraging open communication is critical. No member of the team (and the importance of "team" cannot be over emphasized) should be afraid to question a decision or raise a point for clarification. Some physicians fear that encouraging these questions will lead to a situation where every order is questioned, which could be a problem in critical situations. However, in practice this does not appear to be the case. When other members of the team are confident in your decision making, they will support your decisions in a crisis. Besides, wouldn't you want someone to point out that the patient is allergic to the medication you just ordered, even if it is an emergency? Fear of the boss can impede the nurse's ability to report errors.[15]

Effective communication with patients is a critical component of the effort to improve safety. When it comes to patient encounters, the SEGUE framework can enhance effective communication, improve patient compliance, and avoid misunderstanding.[16]

S  = Set the stage: Establish an effective rapport with the patient

E  = Elicit patient information

G  = Give information – including your diagnosis and recommended treatment

U  = Understand the patient's perspective and ensure that they understand your recommendations and treatment specifics

E  = End the encounter effectively and ensure adequate follow-up

Legible handwriting is critical. Half of all physicians' orders are illegible,[17] although their handwriting may not be any worse than the general public's.[18] Computerized physician order entry (CPOE) may help,[19] but errors can still be made through physician overrides.[20] Some researchers report an increase in medication errors or failure to improve rates of adverse drug events even after implementation of CPOE.[21,22] Minimizing distractions can also help improve communication and may reduce medication errors. Communication failures can lead to confusion about patient care.[23] Written patient care goals can improve the care of critically-ill patients.[24] Simply ensuring an adequate sign-out to fellow residents and nurses can improve patient care and nurses' understanding of the goals for the patient.[25,26]

Physicians can play a critical role in reducing medication errors. In addition to legible handwriting, all prescriptions should include the patient's name, patient-specific data (e.g., date of birth), the generic or brand name of the drug, strength, dosage form (e.g., po, IV), amount, and explicit directions for use. Avoid abbreviations and phrases such as "use as directed" as they increase the risk for misunderstanding and error. JCAHO has identified a number of commonly used prescription abbreviations that increase the risk for error.[27]

## Table 1: "Do Not Use" abbreviations[i]

| Do Not Use | Potential Problem | Use Instead |
|---|---|---|
| U (for unit) | Mistaken for "0" (zero), the number "4" (four), or "cc" | Write "Unit" |
| QD, Q.D., qd, q.d. | Mistaken for each other | Write "Daily" |
| QOD, Q.O.D., qod | Period after the Q mistaken for "I" and the "O" mistaken for I | Write "every other day" |
| Trailing zero (X.0 mg) | Decimal point missed | Write "X mg" |
| Lack of leading zero (.X mg) | Decimal point missed | Write "0.X mg" |
| MS MSO4 and MgSO4 | Can mean morphine sulfate or magnesium sulfate | Write "morphine sulfate" Write "magnesium sulfate" |
| > (greater than) < (less than) | Misinterpreted as the number "7" (seven) or the letter "L" | Write "greater than" Write "less than" |
| cc | Mistaken for U (units) when poorly written | Write "ml" or milliliters |
| µg (for micrograms) | Mistaken for mg (milligrams) resulting in one thousand-fold overdose | Write "mcg" or micrograms |

[i] Based on the recommendations of the JCAHO and the Institute of Safe Medical Practices

## Using Technology

Technology has helped in the crusade for patient safety. Improvements in monitoring have led to safer medical practices. Anesthesiology as a medical specialty was cited in the Institute of Medicine's report for improving patient safety. The use of such devices as pulse oximeters and end-tidal carbon dioxide monitors has improved patient outcomes (at least as reflected in the American Society of Anesthesiologists Closed Claims project).[28] Simulation may also improve patient safety through the ability to practice uncommon or high-risk situations before they happen to real people. The federal government is looking at funding such studies through the Agency for Healthcare Research and Quality (AHRQ).[29] Information technology may also help improve patient safety by improving communication, providing access to information, requiring information and assisting with calculations, monitoring, decision support, rapid response to and tracking of adverse events.[30] Medication administration may be helped through such technologies as bar codes.[31,32]

## Encouraging Partnerships to Improve Safety

There are other non-technological and inexpensive approaches to improving patient safety. Actively involving the patient, family members and caregivers (as appropriate) can add another layer of checks and balances. For example, in the out-patient setting, a physician's office may routinely contact patients with the results of tests. On occasion, however, test results don't arrive at a physician's office, or are not seen by the physician. Advising the patient to call the physician's office if they have not heard anything within 2-3 weeks after the test helps to ensure that the physician has seen the results. Family members and caregivers can often be helpful. Having a family member present during a doctor-patient appointment can help patients recall information and instructions long after the office visit has ended. When the patient cannot fully participate in his or her care, involving the family can help reconcile medication switches, avoid duplicate medications at home (thus, the implementation of the medication reconciliation record), and other aspects of patient care. For this to actually work there must be good communication between the care providers and the patient and his or her family. By becoming active members of their own health care team, patients (and their families) can promote safety and improve their own outcomes. AHRQ offers useful advice for patients, outlined below.[33]

**What Can You Do? Be Involved in Your Health Care**

- The single most important way you can help to prevent errors is to be an active member of your health care team.

**Medicines**

- Make sure that all of your doctors know about everything you are taking. This includes prescription and over-the-counter medicines, and dietary supplements such as vitamins and herbs.

- Make sure your doctor knows about any allergies and adverse reactions you have had to medicines.

- When your doctor writes you a prescription, make sure you can read it.

- Ask for information about your medicines in terms you can understand—both when your medicines are prescribed and when you receive them.

- When you pick up your medicine from the pharmacy, ask: Is this the medicine that my doctor prescribed?

- If you have any questions about the directions on your medicine labels, ask.

- Ask your pharmacist for the best device to measure your liquid medicine. Also, ask questions if you're not sure how to use it.

- Ask for written information about the side effects your medicine could cause.

**Hospital Stays**

- If you have a choice, choose a hospital at which many patients have the procedure or surgery you need.

- If you are in a hospital, consider asking all health care workers who have direct contact with you whether they have washed their hands.

- When you are being discharged from the hospital, ask your doctor to explain the treatment plan you will use at home.

**Surgery**

- If you are having surgery, make sure that you, your doctor, and your surgeon all agree and are clear on exactly what will be done.

**Other Steps You Can Take**

- Speak up if you have questions or concerns.

- Make sure that someone, such as your personal doctor, is in charge of your care.

- Make sure that all health professionals involved in your care have important health information about you.

- Ask a family member or friend to be there with you and to be your advocate (someone who can help get things done and speak up for you if you can't).

- Know that "more" is not always better.

- If you have a test, don't assume that no news is good news.

- Learn about your condition and treatments by asking your doctor and nurse and by using other reliable sources.

## The National Landscape

Although society's goal of a minimal risk health system has not yet been achieved, significant progress has been made. Several national organizations have taken the lead in promoting patient safety. JCAHO regularly establishes and updates national patient safety goals. These goals include: improving the accuracy of patient identification, improving the effectiveness of communication among caregivers, improving the safety of using medications, reducing the risks of health care associated infections, and reducing the risk of patient harm resulting from falls.[34]   In the hospital and ambulatory surgery center settings, specific protocols to eliminate wrong-site surgery have been put in place.[35] Using these protocols, patient, procedure site, and other interventions (antibiotics, special equipment) can be confirmed before the procedure starts. Even simple steps, such as ensuring proper hand washing, that can be implemented quickly have a significant impact on outcomes.[36] The Institute for Healthcare Improvement (IHI) is also a major catalyst for improving patient safety. Among its initiatives, the organization has promoted the widespread institution of rapid response teams (RRTs). RRTs usually consist of a critical care-trained nurse, a respiratory therapist, and a physician. These teams, which are called not when the patient "codes" but rather when any member of the health care team is concerned that the patient has entered the slippery slope to a code, have been shown to improve hospital-wide measures such as the frequency of cardiac arrests.[37,38] Creation of these teams demonstrates the move to prevention of illness even in acute health care.

Fatigue and lack of sufficient sleep have been linked to increased risk for medical errors. The Accreditation Council on Graduate Medical Education (ACGME) has established duty hour limits to residency training, wherein residents' work hours are limited to 80 hours per week and residents cannot work in the hospital for more than 30 hours continuously. This move has the two-pronged effect of improving both patient and provider safety. Patients of sleep-deprived residents have more complications[39] and the residents are more likely to make errors.[40,41] Reducing work hours, besides improving patient safety, also improves residents' safety. Drowsy driving after extended work periods increases the chance of the provider being involved in a motor vehicle crash.[42] Unfortunately, nothing is in place to protect attending physicians and their patients from the effects of sleep deprivation and fatigue. This may be more of an issue in teaching hospitals, as work traditionally assigned to residents gets picked up by attending staff.[43]

## Conclusion

Patient safety involves a multitude of people and processes. We must simultaneously develop and employ more efficient and effective tools (technology approach) and the culture of safety (people approach). Having the best technology is useless if the people-oriented systems for reporting and studying errors are not effective. In order to successfully improve patient safety, health care systems must systematically study the problem and apply well-developed process-improvement tools. Only by making a concerted, focused effort can safety be improved.

## Case Study

Vic Vicuna, the Vice President of Medical Affairs at Community General Medical Center, had a problem. Two of the experienced medical staff were in his office with a complaint. "Bob," said Dr. Leslie Longshanks, "we have a real problem up on 4 North. I ordered blood on my patient on rounds yesterday morning and the transfusion wasn't given until 10:00 this morning!" Dr. Pat Paternoster chimed in, "Yes, and I had the same problem last week!" Vic knew what was coming next and silently winced in anticipation. Leslie shouted "You've got to fire the nurse who was supposed to be taking care of my patient. He's obviously to stupid or uncaring to work here!" Pat agreed, "Transfusion delays can kill our patients. We have to get this fixed today. The manager may need to be replaced if she can't run the floor efficiently."

Four North had had a series of turnovers in the nursing staff, but had recently been brought up to full strength. Could it be that the nurses there were too inexperienced? Molly Malone was a good nurse manager. She had years of experience and when she heard about the problem, she was livid. "I'll schedule some in-services for the staff, but if it was the same nurse for both cases, she (or he) is out of here!" she said loudly. Vicuna chewed on this thought for a moment. It was unlikely that the nurses on 4 North were uncaring louts. Perhaps the problem is more complex. He came up with the following questions that needed answers before deciding what to do next.

1. Were there any extenuating circumstances that delayed a cross-match (such as antibody incompatibility)?

2. Are there other potential reasons for delays? Which one should we tackle first? Perhaps a Pareto Chart would be useful.

3. How are blood orders handled? Is it a different path than medication orders? Would a flowchart to describe the process help?

4. How does the ward know that blood is ready? Does the Blood Bank call, or do they check the computer for results? Can a message be automatically sent to the ward when the blood is ready? Should this be for all cross-matches or only the one where transfusions are actually ordered?

5. How do the ward clerk and nurses communicate that a transfusion has been ordered, especially if there is a change of shifts?

6. How will we measure the magnitude of the problem, and whether or not our actions have had an effect? Would techniques of Statistical Process Control be useful here?

## Study/Discussion questions:

1. What are some barriers to the successful implementation of a patient safety program?

2. How can good communication (doctor-nurse, nurse-doctor, nurse-nurse, doctor-doctor) help create a culture of safety?

3. How can Statistical Process Control (SPC), an industrial concept, be applied to health care?

4. Many organizations are promoting patient safety. Which of their proposals can be implemented on the local level?

## Suggested Readings/Websites

Resources for information about patient safety

Anesthesia Patient Safety Foundation (APSF): www.apsf.org/

Institute for Healthcare Improvement (IHI) (100,000 Lives campaign): www.ihi.org/ihi

Institute for Safe Medical Practice: www.ismp.org/

Joint Commission on Accreditation of Healthcare Organizations (JCAHO): www.jcaho.org

Physician Consortium for Performance Improvement: www.ama-assn.org/ama/pub/category/2946.html

Introduction to Physician Performance Measurement: www.ama-assn.org/ama/upload/mm/370/introperfmeasurement.pdf

Principles of Performance Measurement: www.ama-assn.org/ama1/pub/upload/mm/370/principlesperfmeas.pdf

*Advances in Patient Safety: From Research to Implementation.* Volumes 1-4, AHRQ Publication Nos. 050021 (1-4). February 2005. Agency for Healthcare Research and Quality, Rockville, MD. http://www.ahrq.gov/qual/advances/

*Crossing the Quality Chasm: A New Health Care System for the 21st Century.* Institute of Medicine, Washington, D.C. (USA): National Academies Press; 2001.

*Patient Safety: Achieving a New Standard of Care.* Institute of Medicine, Washington, D.C. (USA); National Academies Press; 2003.

Lighter DE, Fair DC. *Principles and Methods of Quality Management on Healthcare.* Gaithersburg, MD: Aspen Publishers Inc.; 2000.

Wheeler DJ. *Making Sense of Data 2003.* Knoxville, TN:SPC Press; 2003.

Wheeler DJ and Chambers DS. *Understanding Statistical Process Control,* 2nd ed. Knoxville, TN: SPC Press; 1992.

Brassard M, Ritter D. *The Memory Jogger II.* Salem, NH: GOAL/QPC; 1994.

## References

1. Kohn LT, Corrigan JM, Donaldson MS, eds. *To Err is Human: Building a Safer Health Care System.* Institute of Medicine. Washington, DC: National Academies Press; 2000.

2. National Patient Safety Foundation. Available at: http://www.npsf.org/html/about_npsf.html. Accessed June 12, 2006.

3. Bureau of Transportation Statistics Table 2-1: Transportation Fatalities by Mode Available at: http://www.bts.gov/publications/national_transportation_statistics/html/table_02_01.html. Accessed June 12, 2006.

4. American Cancer Society. Breast Cancer Facts and Figures, 2005-2006. Available at: http://www.cancer.org/downloads/STT/CAFF2005BrF.pdf. Accessed June 12, 2006.

5. Reason J. *Managing the risk of organizational accidents*. Aldershot, United Kingdom: Ashgate Publishing Ltd; 1997.

6. Reason J. Human error: models and management. *BMJ*. 2000;320:768-770.

7. Rooney JJ, Vanden Heuvel LN. Root Cause Analysis for Beginners. Available at: http://www.asq.org/pub/qualityprogress/past/0704/qp0704rooney.pdf. Accessed June 13, 2006.

8. U.S. Department of Energy. Root Cause Analysis Guidance Document, February 1992. Available at: http://www.eh.doe.gov/techstds/standard/nst1004/nst1004.pdf. Accessed June 13, 2006.

9. Joint Commission International Center for Patient Safety. Sentinel Event Policy and Procedures Available at: http://www.jcipatientsafety.org/show.asp?durki=9749&site=165&return=9808. Acessed June 13, 2006.

10. Institute for Safe Medical Practices. List of Confused Drug Names. Available at: http://www.ismp.org/Tools/confuseddrugnames.pdf. Accessed June 15, 2006

11. Ishikawa Diagram. Available at: http://mot.vuse.vanderbilt.edu/mt322/Ishikawa.htm. Accessed September 18, 2006.

12. The Balanced Scorecard Institute. Module 10. Control Chart. Available at: http://www.balancedscorecard.org/files/control.pdf. Accessed August 9, 2006.

13. An Introduction to SPC. http://lorien.ncl.ac.uk/ming/spc/spc1.htm Accessed August 8, 2006.

14. Pierce GW. National Patient Safety Foundation. Building the Foundation for a Culture of Safety. Focus on Patient Safety. 2005;8(2). Available at: http://www.npsf.org/download/Focus2005Vol8No2.pdf. Accessed June 18, 2006.

15. Mayo AM, Duncan D. Nurse perceptions of medication errors: What we need to know for patient safety. *J Nurs Care Qual*. 2004;19:209-217.

16. Makoul G. The SEGUE Framework for teaching and assessing communication skills. *Patient Educ Couns*. 2001;45:23-34.

17. Anonymous. A study of physicians' handwriting as a time waster. *JAMA*. 1979;242:2429-2430.

18. Berwick DM, Winickoff DE. The truth about doctor's handwriting: A prospective study. *BMJ*. 1996;313:1657-1658.

19. Upperman JS, Staley P, Friend K, et al. The impact of hospital wide computerized physician order entry on medical errors in a pediatric hospital. *J Pediatr Surg*. 2005;40:57-59.

20. van der Sijs H, Aarts J, Vulto A, Berg M. Overriding of drug safety alerts in computerized physician order entry. *J Am Med Inform Assoc*. 2006;13:138-147.

21. Han YY, Carcillo JA, Venkataraman ST, et al. Unexpected increased mortality after implementation of a commercially sold computerized physician order entry system. *Pediatrics*. 2005;116:1506-1512.

22. Nebeker JR, Hoffman JM, Weir CR, Bennett CL, Hurdle JF. High rates of adverse drug events in a highly computerized hospital. *Arch Intern Med*. 2005;165: 1111-1116.

23. Arora V, Johnson J, Lovinger D, Humphrey H J, Meltzer DO. Communication failures in patient sign-out and suggestions for improvement: a critical incident analysis. *Qual Saf Health Care*. 2005;14:401-407.

24. Pronovost P, Berenholtz S, Dorman T, Lipsett PA, Simmonds T, Haraden C. Improving communication in the ICU using daily goals. *J Crit Care*. 2003;18:71-75.

25. Sidlow R, Katz-Sidlow RJ. Using a computerized sign-out system to improve physician-nurse communication. *Jt Comm J Qual Patient Saf*. 2006;32:32-36.

26. Computer system helps nurses in care delivery. *Healthcare Benchmarks Quality Improv*. 2006;13:28-30.

27. Joint Commission on Accreditation of Healthcare Organizations. Available at: http://www.jointcommission.org/NR/rdonlyres/2329F8F5-6EC5-4E21-B932-54B2B7D53F00/0/06_dnu_list.pdf. Accessed June 19, 2006.

28. American Society of Anesthesiologists. Available at: www.asaclosedclaims.org. Accessed August 31, 2006.

29. National Institutes of Health. Available at: http://grants.nih.gov/grants/guide/rfa-files/RFA-HS-06-030.html. Accessed June 18, 2006.

30. Bates DW, Gawande AA. Improving safety with information technology. *New Engl J Med*. 2003;348:2526-2534.

31. Zebra Technologies. Available at: https://www.zebra.com/id/zebra/na/en/documentlibrary/whitepapers/its_all_wrist.DownloadFile.File.tmp/WP_wristband.pdf. Accessed June 18, 2006.

32. Kaushal R, Barker KN, Bates DW. How can information technology improve patient safety and reduce medication errors in children's health care? *Arch Pediatr Adolesc Med*. 2001;155:1002-1007.

33. Agency for Healthcare Research and Quality. Patient Fact Sheet: 20 Tips to Help Prevent Medical Errors. Available at: http://www.ahrq.gov/consumer/20tips.htm. Accessed August 9, 2006.

34. JCAHO. National Patient Safety Goals. Available at: http://www.jointcommission.org/PatientSafety/NationalPatientSafetyGoals/ Accessed June 26, 2006.

35. JCAHO. Universal Protocol for Preventing Wrong, Site, Wrong Procedure, Wrong Person Survery. Available at: http://www.jointcommission.org/NR/rdonlyres/E3C600EB-043B-4E86-B04E-CA4A89AD5433/0/universal_protocol.pdf. Accessed June 18, 2006.

36. Centers for Disease Control and Prevention. Guidelines for Hand Hygiene in Health-Care Settings. Morbidity and Mortality Weekly. October 25, 2002. Available at: http://www.cdc.gov/mmwr/PDF/rr/rr5116.pdf. Accessed June 18, 2006.

37. Rapid response team reduces cardiac and respiratory arrests. *Perform Improv Advis.* 2005;9:25-27.

38. Bellomo R, Goldsmith D, Uchino S, et al. A prospective before-and-after trial of a medical emergency team. *Med J Aust.* 2003;179:283-287.

39. Haynes DF, Schwedler M, Dyslin DC, Rice JC, Kerstein MD. Are postoperative complications related to resident sleep deprivation? *South Med J.* 1995;88:283-289.

40. Taffinder NJ, McManus IC, Gul Y, Russell RC, Darzi A. Effect of sleep deprivation on surgeons' dexterity on laparoscopy simulator. *Lancet.* 1998;352:1191.

41. Landrigan CP, et al. Effect of reducing interns' work hours on serious medical errors in intensive care units. *N Engl J Med.* 2004;351:1838-1848

42. Barger L, Cade B, Ayas N, et al. Extended work shifts and the risk of motor vehicle crashes among interns. *N Engl J Med.* 2005;352(2):125-134.

43. Coverdill JE, Finlay W, Adrales GL, et al. Duty-hour restrictions and the work of surgical faculty: results of a multi-institutional study. *Acad Med.* 2006;81(1):50-56.

# Chapter 3

## Preparing for Pay for Performance

David A. MacKoul, MD, MS, FAAP, DFACMQ

### Executive Summary

Pay for performance initiatives are driving the change towards a quality-based, patient-centered health care system. Though important, pay for performance should not be the sole model upon which your delivery system design is based. Pay for performance will change and adapt to health care's numerous stakeholders. Your organization must also be agile to keep pace with medical, organizational, and economic innovations. A health care system that focuses on the patient while delivering evidence-based care whenever possible will increase value to the patient, payors, and providers.

This chapter will discuss key concepts that will help your organization develop the skills necessary to prepare for success in a quality-based, patient-centered reimbursement world. These concepts include:

1. Patient-focused care;

2. Evidence-based practice;

3. Safety;

4. Staff satisfaction;

5. Continuous change; and

6. Institute of Medicine aims for care.

Your organizational culture must embrace and implement these concepts, with regular reevaluations to ensure continuous quality improvement. If successfully implemented and monitored, you will increase your chance of success regardless of current payment systems.

**Learning Objectives**

1. Identify and apply principles of patient-centered care.

2. Identify and apply evidence-based care.

3. Identify and apply Institute of Medicine six aims of care.

4. Develop organizational culture that supports 1, 2 & 3.

**Keywords**

clinical practice guidelines (CPG); continuous change; evidence-based care; patient-centered care; pay for performance; staff satisfaction

## Introduction

This chapter is really about preparing for success in the delivery of medical care. Pay for performance forces us to consider how care is delivered and how best to improve the quality and delivery of that care. Key points and concepts include:

1. Patient-focused care, which demands attention not only to quality but service and access to care.

2. Evidence-based practice is not merely desirable but expected and defines quality of care as it applies to the patient.

3. Safety of care is more important than ever since poor safety negatively impacts quality, cost, delivery, and access to care. In addition, poor safety displays lack of patient focus.

4. Staff satisfaction is necessary to achieve all of the above.

5. Successful organizations will achieve these goals while continuously adapting to the changing health care environment.

If thoughtfully applied and constantly monitored in a patient-centered environment, these key points and concepts will increase the chance of success in any health care or payment program. Pay for performance should be thought of as a first step in American health care's journey toward quality-based, patient-centered reimbursement. Indeed, Doran et al,[1] have shown pay for performance programs in the United Kingdom that adequately reimburse providers for high levels of achievement have also demonstrated measurable success in improving the quality of care. The debate now surrounds whether these gains are real, or could be due to standards being set too low or rigging of the system. In addition, reimbursement for quality gains in the United Kingdom is much higher than that set for the United States. Whether such results will be obtained in the United States with lower reimbursement levels, and whether Americans are willing to pay for quality gains, remains to be seen.[2]

Understanding the six Institute of Medicine (IOM) aims for care.[3] The six aims for care set the groundwork for success. They include:

a. Effective

b. Efficient

c. Safe

d. Timely

e. Patient-centered

f. Equitable

We will review each of these aims as the chapter unfolds. It is important to realize that little if any research exists to support success in preparation for pay for performance. Therefore, discussion will focus on application of existing government and employer demands that have and will be made upon the practitioner, almost all of which revolve around the aims for care. These demands, coupled with the six IOM aims for care, will result in development of or changes to existing business plans. This is a useful and necessary analogy. Business plans are local and specific and don't require evidence-based data to develop and apply. The business plan for a medical group involves identifying your customers (including the patient, your most important customer) and developing systems to deliver medical care based upon the patient's needs and demands. It is important to understand why the patient is described as a customer in this context. Physicians develop professional relationships based upon trust and mutual respect to deliver medical care services to maintain and heal the patient and his or her family members. Businesses develop relationships with customers based upon price, product and service. Although health care services delivered to the patient are more personal and complex than traditional business goods and services delivered to the customer, if your business plan does not center on the patient nor address each of the aims, you lower your chance of success.

Central to success is the notion of patient-centered care. Not too long ago, care centered on the provider, institution, employer sponsor, etc.; nowhere was the patient included. As the cost of health care increased and patient safety failures became public knowledge, the patient, employer sponsors, and the government became more vocal and demanded a stake in health care administration. It soon became apparent that to deliver the aims for care efficiently, the care delivery system had to revolve around the patient's demands. What were those demands? Were they reasonable? Were they based upon quality of care or convenience? Who defined quality? The questions seemed endless, so perhaps it was better to ask how to proceed. To be patient-centered, you need to understand your practice environment and your patient's needs. This will require an evaluation of your care delivery system's strengths and weaknesses.

## Create or redefine your organizational culture around the IOM aims of care

This can only be accomplished by taking a critical look at your culture's beliefs to determine whether they revolve around the IOM aims. As noted above, patient-centered care is a cornerstone to your success. All business decisions must revolve around the patient's needs, coupled with providing evidence-based scientifically valid health care in a safe environment, making efficient use of the provider's and patient's time. All patients are treated equally, without regard for their insurance status. Most institutions fail this test. Business decisions usually place profit considerations on an equal footing with patient care decisions. This is not patient-centered care. When determining when and how to provide care, your first consideration should be how patients are accessing your system. This is critical, since without access your system is of no value and can't deliver evidence-based care in a timely and efficient manner. Patient-centered means the patient is seen when he or she wants to be seen, on the same day if possible.

Consider the potential economic value of seeing patients on demand. Revenue and patient satisfaction increase, liability decreases, your reputation benefits, and your time is used more efficiently. The bottom line benefits since costs of operation remain the same (your hours and costs per day don't change if you see 10, 20 or 40 patients), your salary increases, and practice growth helps to guarantee future revenue stability.

By using your nursing staff to gather appropriate information, you can spend more time diagnosing, treating, and explaining the disease, treatments, and expected outcomes. Patient satisfaction is likely to increase and the amount of time spent with each patient should stabilize (and may actually decrease) since non-diagnostic, bureaucratic and administrative matters are handled by support personnel.

Everything described is in line with the IOM aims of care and many providers have utilized this care delivery approach long before the IOM delivered its message. All members of the care delivery team, from front office, nursing, provider, billing, and management staff must hold patient-centered care as the absolute gold standard around which all decisions revolve. This can only happen if your organizational culture supports this standard with words and actions. Organizational cultures and characteristics can have a negative impact on quality of care delivered.[4] Aligning your organization's culture with patient-centered care is your first step to success.

## Define goals

Since the patient is in control, it's important to define what the patient wants and then to act on that information. Our practice evaluation revealed that our patients valued continuity of care that was delivered in a timely fashion, was appropriate to the situation at hand (many check the Internet to ensure treatment is in line with their diagnosis), and fully explained (including diagnosis, treatment, course of illness, and complications of treatment and illness) in terms they could easily understand. They wanted to know what to expect. Our patients defined these elements of care as valuable. If you ask your own patients, you'll most likely find that they feel the same. Let's break down each of these elements of care further.

Continuity of care means the patient sees the same doctor almost all the time. Our patients came to our practice because this element was very important to them. In addition, continuity of care increases quality and efficiency of care.[5] Initially, as the patient acclimates to the practice, time is spent discussing important aspects of care, for example, antibiotics are not prescribed for the common cold. After several such episodes, a diagnosis of common cold no longer elicits the request for antibiotics. Eventually the patient may no longer demand a visit, since past experience reveals a continuous and consistent pattern of reassurance and guidance as the principal treatment for this diagnosis. While it's true that extra time is taken in the beginning of the patient's history with the practice, educational efforts in the office regarding the common cold yield patient comfort with the illness and, most importantly, the knowledge that access to care will be provided in a timely fashion when the illness course deviates from the norm. This helps to develop a sense of teamwork with your patient, and team members stick together. Eventually, you will also increase the time you are available for other patients, further increasing access and efficiency of time use. Quality of care is advanced individually for the patient and for the community, as adherence to reassurance and guidance for the common cold should reduce the number of unnecessary antibiotic prescriptions, which in turn will decrease the emergence of multiple drug-resistant bacteria and reduce the overall cost of unnecessary care. Most important of all is the development of a personal relationship with your patients that is framed in a professional setting and anchored by trust. The provider is trusted by the patient to discuss difficult and personal issues such as non-adherence to medical advice, living will, end-of-life care, errors in diagnosis and delivery of care. This allows the provider to quickly focus the patient on the problem and to discuss resolutions. Care becomes more effective, since patients who are more comfortable and confident are also more likely to follow your advice. Safety is likely to improve, since errors in diagnosis or treatment will be quickly brought to attention. Continuity of care is truly the foundation upon which patient-centered care will succeed.

Appropriate care is individualized and aligned with scientifically valid, evidence-based clinical practice guidelines (CPGs). Unfortunately, the evidence base for many CPGs may be flawed due to conflict of interest[6] and unproven interventions.[7] Also, The National Guideline Clearinghouse (http://www.guideline.gov/) listed more than 2, 000 active CPGs in September 2006, many covering the same disease. Accessing the appropriate document at the appropriate time may be impossible at the point of care. In addition, the application of CPGs by physicians in the office setting is limited and poorly understood.[8] Despite all this, CPGs have demonstrated benefits in patient outcomes for the management of single disease entities such as diabetes, hypertension, asthma, etc.[9] Still, not all CPGs should be applied equally to all patients. Recent studies by Boyd et al, have suggested that application of current CPGs may have undesirable effects, reducing the quality of care in older patients with multiple co-morbid diseases.[10] As noted by O'Connor in an accompanying editorial,[11]

> "Despite their limitations, evidence-based CPGs remain an important and necessary tool in the effort to improve health care quality. Strategies to address the limitations of current CPGs need to be developed and implemented, including providing recommendations based on level of evidence for particular patient groups and considering the potential economic and personal burden on the patient and caregiver as well as potential interactions with co-morbid conditions....Encouraging customization of care in complex clinical scenarios respects the individuality of patients and the professional judgment of highly skilled physicians and minimizes the problem of overtreating patients most susceptible to drug interactions, drug adverse effects, and medical error... Physicians and designers of CPGs owe it to themselves and their patients to consider these issues carefully and to craft CPGs and pay-for-performance accountability measures that will reinforce excellent clinical care while being mindful of resource use and being respectful of patient preferences and priorities."

You may be wondering how best to proceed. First, choose guidelines that have been shown to improve patient outcomes, such as National Heart, Lung and Blood Institute (NHLBI) asthma guidelines. Next, apply the guidelines in a patient-spe-

cific manner. Maintain continuity of care; only the primary care provider in con-
cert with the patient as a team can choose which course of treatment can optimize
outcomes, reduce unnecessary care, and improve patient compliance. Finally, keep
yourself and your support staff up to date on medical advances. As we will discuss
later, it is your support staff that will ensure your care is timely and appropriate.

Timely care can be defined in two ways. First, as it applies to delivering appropriate care to the appropriate patient at the appropriate time (emergent care is provided immediately). Second, as it applies to consideration of the patient's time
(scheduled appointments are seen on time and urgent care appointments are notified regarding expected wait times). To succeed in pay for performance, both
aspects must be taken into account.

Clearly, this situation revolves around scheduling and work flow. The provider
must determine the minimum number of patients that must be seen to meet ongoing expenses. You will need to understand how to read a profit and loss statement
(P&L) and a balance sheet. If you don't have the time or inclination to do so, hire
someone to do this for you. No matter how aligned your organization is with the
IOM aims, you can't deliver if your business platform fails. Next, determine how
many additional patients you are able to see to provide ready access to your organization. Third, determine the maximum number of patients you are able to see com-
fortably. Understand that fewer patients mean less income for all involved, starting
with the provider who sets the patient visit scale. Pay for performance will measure
patient data that includes access and satisfaction ratings. The fewer patients you
allow to be scheduled, the lower your accessibility rating, and most likely the lower
your patient satisfaction scores, which will result in lower reimbursements to your
organization. These data may also be publicly reported, which may impact future
revenue streams. Access can affect quality, since too few, or too many, patient visits results in missed opportunities for early diagnosis and treatment.

With these basic thoughts in mind, you are now ready to set your schedule for efficient use of time. Providers are highly skilled and highly paid members of the team,
whose time should not be spent filling out forms or gathering basic data. These
tasks are critically important to providing high-quality care but don't require a medical degree to accomplish, and can potentially cost the practice a tremendous
amount of revenue. As an example, if a provider spends two minutes with each
patient collecting basic history and plans to see 30 patients per day, this task represents 60 minutes of patient interaction time per day. At 30 minutes per urgent visit,
this represents two patient visits per day, 10 per week, 40 per month, and 480 per
year. At $65 per urgent visit, the provider would lose $31,200 of potential revenue,
along with valuable patient access time, collecting data that could be gathered by
the nursing staff.

The above example illustrates the importance of work flow and staff satisfaction. The physician knows what general information is required, and can easily outline for the clerical and nursing staff what needs to be collected, where it should be documented, and why it is important. Understanding the task and its effect on the outcome of care creates buy-in to the concept of team care. It also makes staff members value their positions and take pride in the execution of their work. Management staff must also contribute since they handle all business, legal, and regulatory issues and must inform clerical, nursing, and provider staff as to their requirements. To prevent the rigid division of work, all staff members in their departments should be cross-trained to allow for efficiency of work and patient flow. Nothing destroys efficiency like waiting for a team member to execute a function when other members are idle!

With knowledge of these requirements, the clerical and nursing staff can create a schedule that will allow for maximum patient flow, with minimum wait time for urgent care visits. The provider should allow development of the schedule to be the priority task of clerical and nursing staff, since it is their responsibility to ensure optimal patient flow. Once created, the process needs to be monitored and changed as needed. Through this effort, you can achieve maximum use of provider time, increase access to medical care and decrease patient wait times. These efficiencies, in turn, improve patient satisfaction. In addition, by successfully implementing an efficient schedule, service, and value are improved. Patients value their time and yours; by efficiently utilizing your time, you reduce wait times and also demonstrate respect for your patients' time demands. Patients notice this concern and satisfaction increases.

## Staff Satisfaction

Patients will consider a practice based upon the reputation of the provider; patients will stay or leave based upon their interaction with the staff. Consider your schedule; if not properly implemented and monitored, patient wait times increase, and access and satisfaction decrease, all without the knowledge of provider or management staff. The team has failed because the focus was not the patient and monitoring was not performed. Staff buy-in to patient-centered care will decrease the chances of this type of failure, and buy-in will only occur if staff work is highly valued.

First, remember that all members of the care team are considered change agents. Do not micromanage. Your clerical staff is much better at identifying active insurance status than nursing or provider staff. If they identify a more efficient way to complete their task, and there is no interference with organizational cultural goals, listen and implement their suggestion as long as it is reasonable and feasible. If implementation is not possible, explain why and ask for suggestions regarding problem resolutions. Involve your staff, and they will involve themselves in the delivery of efficient medical care.

Second, setting high standards of patient care raises the bar for staff performance. The staff knows they are held to a higher standard and they respond appropriately. This behavior is easily and readily noted by patients throughout the organization, resulting in improved service for all patient demands, whether medical or non-medical. If your organization is patient-centered, and access to health care is regulated through the patient schedule that has been created and is maintained by your staff, your staff must be an integral part of the health care team. They must readily and easily critique themselves and the team in order to exceed the high standards asked of them. In line with your organizational culture, all eyes must be focused on the patient and his needs.

One last item to consider is staff pay. If you value your employees' efforts and output, you must pay them well. If you intend to be the best in your location, and wish patient report cards and pay for performance reports to reflect the same, remember it is the combined efforts of you and your employees that cultivate positive patient perceptions of service and value. Therefore, pay should be in line with the high standards you set. Your employees will develop loyalty for you and their organization through job satisfaction and pay performance. Your employees are also your customers and must be treated well.

## Payor Satisfaction

What we have discussed revolves around the patient, specifically the patient-provider interaction. After all, what do ready access, dedicated staff, and efficient use of time accomplish if the core of your service does not fulfill patient and payor needs? The payor must be brought into the equation because payors, not patients, demand pay for performance reimbursement. Recall our initial discussion that pay for performance seems to improve quality, but at a cost. Early results from pay for performance programs are inconclusive and years of research and observational studies may further alter pay for performance mechanics, but let's assume pay for performance is here to stay. Accordingly, what are the basic goals at the level of the patient-provider interaction? Let's start with the patient. Patients want to tell their story and have someone listen respectfully. This is basic medical history-taking skills, but "no one listened to me" is a common complaint among patients. Even if the patient's story and physical exam findings are divergent, be respectful and explain the disconnect and how you plan to help the patient. Nothing destroys the patient-provider interaction more quickly and thoroughly (thereby creating negative patient perceptions of care and service) than dismissal of patient concerns as trivial. A common response is "this will take too long and I have lots of patients to see." If you actually time your patient's story you will find most patients talk for no more than two minutes! It's our perception of time, not the actual time spent listening, that is concerning! So do yourself, your patients, your staff, and your organization a favor: sit down, shut up, and listen.

Payors want resources spent on evidence-based medicine. The British experience[1] has shown, at least initially, that pay for performance improves outcomes and increases salaries and taxes. It is unclear if this is due to true improvement, exclusions of difficult patients, standards that have been set too low or gaming the system. In any event, the results are interesting and require further study. In the meantime, American health care will be expected to reach standards of care in exchange for higher reimbursements. Payors, especially the federal government, will bear the brunt of the cost. It will be interesting to see if bonuses for reaching standards will continue, come at the expense of other providers, and be tolerated by citizens through higher taxes. Whatever outcome and reimbursement design the government utilizes, standards of care defined by clinical practice guidelines will be the foundation of current and future forms of pay for performance. Therefore, it is necessary to incorporate evidence-based care into daily routines at the provider-patient level.

As you by now have surmised, change is continuous and pervasive. Whatever new approach is introduced (and there will be many), make a change only for the sake of improvement. Hopefully you agree that reimbursement will be tied to quality care, service, access, efficiency, and safety—all wrapped around the patient's needs. Choose only change that improves these aims and does not disrupt patient-centered care. When you do change, change quickly and monitor your progress. If you make a poor choice, admit it, reverse or change course again, and continue to monitor. Since medical care is a team sport, change only after you receive input from your team members.

Efficiency, or maximizing resource utilization to capture maximum revenue, has always been a taboo subject in health care. To discuss reducing expenses was equivalent to reducing quality. Unfortunately, many organizations have given credence to this statement. As mentioned earlier, their focus is profit maximization, not patient-centered care. I feel strongly about and have practiced patient-centered care with success and a healthy profit margin. There is nothing wrong with making a profit, as long as the patient is your focus. If you practice patient-centered care and make a profit, celebrate and shout from the roof tops! It is also your responsibility to your patients to reduce unnecessary expenses. Money for health care is finite. If we spend it on unproven or useless interventions, that is less money for worthwhile, proven interventions. Many mandated interventions are politically motivated and waste money. Just as the government demands evidence-based care from providers, medical providers need to demand from the government and private payors evidence-based justification for reimbursement of unproven interventions. With scarce resources, the time has come to consider all our expenses on equal footing and demand all providers, mainstream or alternative, deliver evidence-based, scientifically-valid health care.

Efficiency also involves controlling expenses in your organization. Waste at the management, clerical, nursing, or provider level will decrease available resources. If a service does not positively impact the quality, delivery, or access to health care, it should be subject to rigorous evaluation. To accomplish this task, you must be able to understand the profit and loss statement and the general ledger. If you are unable or unwilling to spend the time to do so, hire a good bookkeeper and accountant and ask them to monitor expenses for you. Otherwise, you will have no idea where and how you spend your money, with potentially devastating results.

One of your biggest expenses is staff salaries and benefits. This is usually larger than provider salaries and on par with medicinal expenses. This is how it should be. Your staff will affect your ability to retain and recruit patients, and represent one of your greatest assets. They must be part of the team to increase success in the delivery of high-quality evidence-based care with excellent patient satisfaction, and will increase value to the organization if well paid. Staff soon realize that money wasted is money out of their pockets, especially if the organization is committed to sharing the wealth of the group's success. They will ensure and demand any change be carefully designed and implemented since it is their workload that is affected; upset patients complain to staff members most often. By obtaining multiple inputs on any anticipated change you increase your chances of doing things right the first time. Remember, the provider is an excellent provider but probably a poor receptionist. Respect your fellow team members' efforts, expertise, and responsibilities. Ask for their input; thank them for good ideas, explain your reasons for rejecting bad ideas, encourage self-critique and critical thinking and your unnecessary expenses should disappear.

A major tool that helps support organizational goals, improves quality monitoring, and increases your chance for improvement is the electronic medical record (EMR). Complete discussion of the EMR is beyond the scope of this chapter, but is explored in more detail in Chapter 6. In summary, the EMR should be thought of as a tool; it is not a change agent nor will it lead to improved quality if improperly applied.

Without it, monitoring your progress is cumbersome and expensive. EMRs are costly and you must understand how to use them appropriately An EMR should only be implemented after a thorough discussion regarding the return on investment, especially relating to patient quality and satisfaction. Through this exercise, you will develop a set of requirements the EMR must be capable of performing and may proceed with caution.

## Conclusion

You have all the tools needed to begin preparing for pay for performance. Your organizational culture is patient-centered. You measure quality in conjunction with CPGs. You are executing your plan in line with the IOM aims of care. You efficiently and effectively utilize resources to deliver your services in a timely, equitable and safe manner. Your EMR is ready to help document your experience and monitor your progress. It's time to put it all to work. Expect to make errors, but with your staff an integral part of the team, these errors will be identified quickly. Discuss and eliminate root causes of error and remeasure to ensure success and guard against secondary errors. Embrace every error as a learning opportunity. Learn from your mistakes and you won't make them again. Monitor and celebrate the successes you worked hard to achieve. Don't feel embarrassed about leveraging payors, politicians, and even patients with your success. Only you can prove how good you are, so let people know and demand appropriate reimbursement for your services. Valid evidence-based data outlining high-quality, service-oriented, patient-centered health care are the future.

## Case Study

As all pediatricians know, the respiratory season is busy. Patient wait times can increase along with patient and staff frustrations. Our practice was no exception. However, in our drive to provide patient-centered care we explored the root cause of increased wait times in the office. For a period of one month, all patient appointment times were compared with the following:

1. When the patient signed into the office;

2. When the patient was brought to triage by nursing staff;

3. When the patient was placed into the exam room;

4. When the patient was seen by the physician;

5. When nursing staff performed necessary tests, procedures, etc., if any;

6. When the patient signed out of the office.

To avoid geographical, economic, and travel time bias, three offices in separate cities were evaluated. Several areas of concern were identified and discussed with all staff members, including providers. First, all patients waited in the reception area on average 15 minutes beyond their appointment times due to insurance status issues on a minority of patients (less than 20% overall). Second, patients were brought to the exam rooms by time of sign-in, not appointment time. Third, delays in placing patients in exam rooms correlated with high patient volume. Fourth, walk-in patients were seen without regard to scheduled patient times.

Clerical, nursing, provider and management staff discussed reducing patient wait times based upon these data. Conclusions were reached and implemented. First, all patient insurance status was verified 24 hours prior to the appointment; any difficulties were discussed with the patient prior to the visit. This reduced reception wait times to 5 minutes beyond sign-in or appointment times. Second, a schedule of patient appointment and sign-in times was posted by the chart area. All nursing staff checked the scheduled and sign-in times to ensure on-time patients were seen on time. Every effort was made to see scheduled patients on time. Third, when all exam rooms were full, nursing staff performed necessary triage on patients waiting to be seen and asked these triaged patients to wait for the next available exam room. This resulted in immediate turnover of exam rooms, further reducing patient wait time and greatly improving efficiency of exam room use. Fourth, all walk-in patients were told of possible wait times; this created reasonable expectations, thereby reducing patient frustration. Interestingly, we also noted a 50% decrease in walk-in patients without a concomitant increase in ER or urgent care use (through evaluation of provider identifiers provided by third-party payors for our patients) and without a decrease in patients seen in the office. Scheduled patients were seen within 5 – 10 minutes of their appointment times and same day/walk-in patients were seen within 60 minutes of their appointment times. Patient volume in the office increased by 20%. Evaluation of patient satisfaction with our new patient scheduling and flow system is improved and ongoing.

## Study/Discussion Questions

1. Are we patient-focused?

2. Do we succeed in implementing the Institute of Medicine's aims for care?

3. What are our organizational values and culture and do they support the above?

4. Do all members of our health care delivery team have a say in evaluating, analyzing, implementing change, and monitoring our progress?

## Suggested Readings/Websites

1. Lighter DE, Fair DC. *Principles and Methods of Quality Management in Health Care.* Gaithersburg, Maryland: Aspen; 2000.

2. Couch JB. *Health Care Quality Management for the 21st Century.* Tampa, Florida: American College of Physician Executives; 1991.

3. Chassin MR, Galvin RW. The urgent need to improve health care quality. Institute of Medicine National Roundtable on Health Care Quality (review: 41 refs). JAMA. 1998; 280(11):1000-1005.

4. Committee on Quality of Health Care in America, Institute of Medicine. Kohn LT, Corrigan JM, Donaldson MS (eds). *To Err is Human: Building a Safer Health System.* Washington, DC: National Academies Press; 2000.
Available at: http//books.nap.edu/books/0309068371/html/index.html.

5. Committee on Quality of Health Care in America, Institute of Medicine. *Crossing the Quality Chasm: A New Health System for the 21st Century.* Washington, DC: National Academies Press; 2001.
Available at: http://books.nap.edu/books/0309072808/html/index.html.

6. *Core Curriculum for Medical Quality Management.* American College of Medical Quality; 2005.

7. Web Sites for Health Care Quality. *Core Curriculum for Medical Quality Management.* American College of Medical Quality; 2005:65.

## References

1. Doran T, Fullwood C, Gravelle H, et al. Pay-for-performance programs in family practices in the United Kingdom. *N Engl J Med.* 2006;355:375-384.

2. Epstein A. Pay for performance in the United States and abroad. *N Engl J Med.* 2006:355:406-408.

3. Committee on Quality of Health Care in America, Institute of Medicine. *Crossing the Quality Chasm: A New Health System for the 21st Century.* Washington, DC: National Academies Press; 2001.

4. Randolph G, Fried B, Loeding L, Margolis P, Lannon C. Organizational characteristics and preventive service delivery in private practices: a peek inside the "black box" of private practices caring for children. *Pediatrics.* 2005:115:1704-1710.

5. Tinetti ME, Bogardus ST Jr, Agostini JV. Potential pitfalls of disease-specific guidelines for patients with multiple conditions. *N Engl J Med.* 2004;351:2870-2874.

6. Bekelman JE, Li Y, Gross CP. Scope and impact of financial conflicts of interest in biomedical research: a systematic review. JAMA. 2003;289:454-465.

7. Rossouw JE, Anderson GL, Prentice Rl, et al. Risks and benefits of estrogen plus progestin in healthy postmenopausal women: principal results from the Women's Health Initiative randomized controlled trial. JAMA. 2002;288:321-333.

8. O'Connor PJ. Overcome clinical inertia to control systolic blood pressure. *Arch Intern Med.* 2003;163:2677-2678.

9. Barton S. *Clinical Evidence.* London, England: BMJ Publishing Group; 2004.

10. Boyd CM, Darer J, Boult C, Fried LP, Boult L, Wu AW. Clinical practice guidelines and quality of care for older patients with multiple comorbid diseases: implications for pay for performace. JAMA. 2005;294:716-724.

11. O'Connor PJ. Adding value to evidence-based clinical guidelines. JAMA. 2005;294:741-743.

# Chapter 4

## Achieving Positive Patient-Physician Relationships: The Importance of Patient-Centeredness

Sara L. Thier, MPH and Christopher N. Sciamanna, MD, MPH

### Executive Summary

Creating a patient-centered practice will support the development of a positive physician-patient relationship. The Institute of Medicine (IOM) defines patient-centered care as: "Providing care that is respectful of and responsive to individual patient preferences, needs and values and ensuring that patient values guide all clinical decisions."[1] There are several factors that contribute to providing patient-centered care. Knowing your population's demographics is important for ensuring cultural sensitivity. Understanding patients' expectations and promoting shared decision making are just two of several ways to develop a trusting relationship between a physician and patient, which can lead to improved compliance and health outcomes. Appropriate, timely and supportive communication is paramount in creating a patient-centered practice. Thoughtful attention to potential challenges such as patients' health literacy, readily available patient education materials and resources, communication to facilitate transitions and assure continuity of care, and the integration of technology can improve the overall quality of care as well as increase patient satisfaction. Finally, measuring patient satisfaction and being responsive to issues that are raised is essential to maintaining true patient-centeredness.

### Learning Objectives

1. Describe how creating a patient-centered practice can improve your relationship with your consumers.

2. Review strategies that can be implemented to create a patient-centered practice.

3. Understand how soliciting, reviewing and using patient satisfaction data to make appropriate changes to process and practice can improve your relationships with your patients.

## Keywords

active listening; cultural competency; cultural sensitivity; health literacy; patient-centeredness; patient-centered care; patient-centered practice; patient expectations; patient satisfaction; shared decision-making; Trust

## Introduction

Research has shown that a positive patient-physician relationship can result in an increase in patient adherence to treatment recommendations and lead to more positive health outcomes.[2] One strategy to facilitate the development of positive relationships is to integrate patient-centered practices. The Institute of Medicine (IOM) defines patient-centered care as: "Providing care that is respectful of and responsive to individual patient preferences, needs and values and ensuring that patient values guide all clinical decisions."[1]

### Nine Steps in Patient-centered Care

These steps were designed for the training of and use by Veterans Administration physicians in providing care to Gulf War veterans.[3] The IOM stressed that physicians should be allowed ample time with each patient to follow through with each step. Though created for a distinct population, this model can be useful for all physicians striving to provide patient-centered care.

1. The patient must express all of his or her concerns during the clinical encounter.

2. The physician addresses all of the patient's concerns.

3. The physician and the patient share models of disease and symptoms.

4. The physician and patient must share goals for treatment.

5. The physician and the patient should agree on treatment goals, state them explicitly, and set priorities.

6. The physician and the patient should share their respective ideas about the purpose and course of treatments.

7. The physician and patient should identify potential difficulties in the care plan.

8. The physician and the patient should plan how to overcome anticipated compliance difficulties.

9. The physician should provide written information on the disease and treatment regimen.

## Creating a Patient-centered Practice

Practicing patient-centered care requires attention to a variety of practice skills and elements. Most are simple and intuitive; others may take a more conscious effort by you and those you work with to create an environment and develop processes that facilitate appropriate care for each individual patient. There is no ideal way to construct the perfect patient-centered practice. These efforts require adjustments, not only in processes and procedures, but in attitudes and communication methods.

### Know Your Population's Demographics

No two patients are the same; no two communities are the same. Variations in socioeconomic status, education level, race and ethnicity, and cultural and religious beliefs make the provision of care both challenging and exciting. As a physician, it is important to learn about the population to which you will provide care. If you are in private practice, it is imperative to understand the demographics of your community and its residents. Do you provide care in a suburb, where most have commercial insurance coverage and their own transportation? Or is your office situated in the inner city, where people rely on Medicaid and public transportation? Do most of your patients speak English, or do you serve a large immigrant population and need to ensure you have a diverse, multilingual staff?

Recognizing that cultural competency and sensitivity to differences are essential to tailoring care, to truly be a patient-centered practice, all staff must strive to be "respectful of and responsive to the health beliefs and practices, and cultural and linguistic needs of diverse patient populations."[4] A variety of tools are available for measuring and improving cultural competency. These tools include measures on communication (i.e., *I keep in mind that limitations in English proficiency is in no way a reflection of their level of intellectual functioning*) and attitudes (i.e., *I recognize that the meaning or value of medical treatment and health education may vary greatly among cultures*), as well as guides for improving procedures and facility characteristics (i.e., number of multilingual/multicultural staff ratio by culture of staff to clients).[5]

Tapping into community resources for support and guidance is a wonderful way to connect with key opinion and cultural leaders. In areas with great cultural diversity, the health care system may not meet all patients' needs. Adjunct community organizations, such as Alcoholics Anonymous, local senior centers, and support groups for health conditions or emotional needs can help to provide a more complete web of services that can serve patients across social, emotional and medical realms. For this reason, it is important to be aware of local organizations, support groups and events. For example, providing free screenings at local health fairs is an important way to demonstrate your interest in the community and its residents and to connect with other key organizations.

### Knowing and Managing Patient Expectations

Physicians must not assume that all patients come to a doctor's visit with the same expectations or anticipated outcomes. Some may want a physician to make all the decisions; others want to be actively involved in their care choices. A gregarious physician may be ideal for some; others may want someone more straightforward and direct. Some patients are happy with reassurance, while others want a test. Still others may demand a more comprehensive treatment option. It is important to understand each patient's expectations of not only each visit, but of your relationship with them.

It's helpful to use open-ended questions to understand a patient's expectations early in the interaction, rather than waiting until you have your hand on the door and the patient says "but doctor…" Most unmet expectations have to do with symptoms not being addressed,[6] though patients have unrealistic expectations for doctors to perform physical exam maneuvers (e.g., reflex testing) and clinical tests (e.g., urine) for which there is no evidence. It is essential to understand and be able to respond to these expectations.

### Striving Towards Shared Decision Making

Until the more recent past, health care decision making took a more paternalistic form, with the physician making the decisions for care and treatment with little or no input from patients or families.[7] However, as the breadth of literature on informed consent, risk reduction, and treatment options grew, it became clear that patients wanted, and in many cases needed, to be involved in decision making.

This shared decision-making model is essential to creating a patient-centered practice. As we discussed earlier, patients will vary by socioeconomic status, culture, race/ethnicity, health beliefs, and health care coverage. These variances may lead a patient to choose one treatment option over another or, in some cases, to opt for no treatment at all. Instead of physicians being prescriptive, physicians now are learning to seek out all relevant information and work collaboratively with the patient so that together they can arrive at the best choice.[8,9,10]

It is important to gauge each patient's interest in shared decision making. Realize that the patient is an active partner. Though you should avoid making final decisions without the patient's consent and ideas, some patients may want you to be prescriptive and will not be as active a participant in making choices ("Tell me what I need to do, doctor.") Your goal will be to avoid situations where the patient does not go for the test or take the medications that you prescribe, as this causes both patients and doctors to feel awkward during future encounters. Try to get your patient's buy-in for any decision made. More and more, doctors need to be "selling" their patients on treatments and behavior changes, particularly since many pay for performance initiatives hold doctors accountable for patient behaviors. For example, if the patient doesn't go for their colonoscopy, it will look like the doctor never recommended one, since health plans don't ask patients if their doctor recommended the test, but only verify that a claim for the test is submitted.

Open-ended and non-judgmental questions, such as "What do you think about (treatment option)?" can help in this regard. Another useful strategy is to frame the decision as a choice, so that the patient can have a way of expressing that they may not agree with the choice that you propose. An example of this would be "I would recommend that you start a medication for your blood pressure now, but if you would rather wait a month while you try to exercise more and lose a few pounds, that might be reasonable as well. What do you think?" This helps the patient understand your recommendations while still preserving the opportunity to be involved in the decision.

### Practice Environment Processes

Patients are keenly aware of office practices that either enhance efficiency or decrease responsiveness. Chapter 15 covers the ins and outs of open access scheduling. As an example for practice processes, open access, which allows for same-day appointments, demonstrates to your patients that you take their health concerns seriously. Other process changes that can create an efficient and effective practice and increase patient satisfaction include group visits and other practice innovations. The literature on group visits (which can be a scheduled or more of an informal, support group-type format) is inconclusive about their effects on health outcomes. Yet, in terms of the patient satisfaction of those who participate, it has a positive effect.[11]

Whether you are considering an office practice, a specialty clinic, or a hospital ward, the key is to focus processes and organizational management in a manner that is consumer-centric. What does the consumer need, want, or require, and how can you design your environment and lead your team to meet these needs?

### Developing Trust: Why it is Important

Trust between a provider and a patient is not instantaneous. Several factors may contribute to or inhibit the creation of a trusting relationship. Length of time with a physician, ethnicity/race and gender concordance, and a physician's cultural sensitivity all play important roles in bolstering or diminishing trust.

A qualitative study regarding complaints about physicians indicated that patients are sensitive to both verbal and nonverbal elements of care. The most commonly identified category was disrespect (36%), followed by disagreement about expectations of care (23%), inadequate information (20%), distrust (18%), perceived unavailability (15%), interdisciplinary miscommunication (4%), and misinformation (4%).[12] Patients' trust in their physician may also be related to having a choice of physicians, having a longer relationship with their physician, and trusting their managed care organization. Most patients are unaware of how their physicians are reimbursed for care, but many are concerned that some of these payment methods might discourage medical use.[13]

Caring and comfort, technical competency, and communication are the physician behaviors most strongly associated with patient trust.[14] Yet other factors, some immutable (the age and sex of the patient), others modifiable (the training and professional appearance of the physician, positive recommendation by other patients and physicians, and the operation of the physician's office, including staff courtesy, management of messages and laboratory results, and on-call arrangements that ensure accessibility) are important in cementing trust in a relationship.[15]

It is important to recognize that trust must be cultivated. Studies show that patients may switch providers if they perceive their physician to be judgmental or negative. However, do not be offended if they bring in or ask for a second opinion, or question your suggestion by bringing in outside information or data from the Internet or news clippings. It is this active involvement in their personal care that is central to the goal of patient-centeredness. To facilitate this trusting relationship, take steps to listen non-judgmentally, act respectfully, strive to meet patients' expectations, communicate openly and honestly, and be responsive to constructive criticism, such as suggestions collected through patient satisfaction surveys.

### System Changes to Support Patient Health Behaviors

Many providers do not feel that they have been adequately trained to provide counseling on the wide range of health behaviors that patients must learn to embrace in order to prevent or control disease.[16,17] Behavioral counseling for self-management of a chronic condition is less straightforward than prescribing medication and advising patients on its use. Providing counseling on smoking cessation, diet and physical activity, and weight loss may feel foreign to some physicians, and a natural part of care to others. No matter at which point in the continuum of care you see a patient, as a physician it is your responsibility to reinforce healthy behaviors.

In many cases you may have a disease management or wellness program to refer patients to, as well as having other staff to take on key counseling issues (e.g., office staff person, nurse, health educator, NP). Maintaining a good supply of useful reading materials and a list of appropriate websites can facilitate counseling efforts. Again, it is essential to make these counseling efforts patient-centered, personalizing the message and making the recommendation clear (e.g., "Quitting smoking is the most important thing that you can do for your asthma."). Finally, ensure that patients' steps to adopt healthy behaviors are matched to their lifestyle, motivations, and expectations, as well as aligned with a set of realistic goals. This can be accomplished by using collaborative goal-setting strategies. Assessing a patient's conviction (e.g., "How convinced are you that you need to lose weight?") and commitment to making a change can provide important information as to how lofty a goal you both should set. Small achievable goals, with reassessment and readjustment are usually more effective, i.e., "Stop eating chocolate" vs. "limit yourself to one chocolate bar a day." While goal setting appears to have a positive effect, you must be realistic about the long-term success of these strategies, e.g., 95% of those who lose weight will gain it back. [18]

Similar to payment for greater patient satisfaction scores, pay-for-performance initiatives will generally provide greater rewards to physicians who are able to successfully "persuade" their patients to make the types of behavior changes that influence health outcomes measures, such as patients with diabetes starting to exercise, which helps to lower their A1c. Being non-judgmental is essential, as many patients will feel bad if they have not made the recommended changes, and may not share their failures or lapses if they fear disappointing you. Showing your frustration will hamper your relationship with the patient. Using a model of behavior change that incorporates the Transtheoretical Stages of Change Model (TTM), such as the 5 A's, developed and used often for assessing readiness for smoking cessation, will help tailor behavior modification to a patients' readiness to change. [19,20]

## The Importance of Communication

While Chapter 7 delves into specific communication strategies, we would like to stress some key issues that emphasize the importance of thinking through why and how to communicate with patients. Chapters 8 and 12 discuss in further detail risk management strategies and medical malpractice concerns related to relationship and communication barriers between providers and patients.

In relation to utilization and outcomes, patient-centered communication resulted in fewer diagnostic tests, but an increase in length of visit. [21] "A systematic review of randomized clinical trials and analytic studies of physician-patient communication confirmed a positive influence of quality communication on health outcomes." [22]

### Active Listening

Patients often perceive interactions with providers as abrupt and impersonal. Many feel that their provider is not listening to them and is instead focused on reading from or documenting in a chart. Active listening is key to engaging a patient and gleaning important information for care. Often used in psychotherapy, active listening incorporates not only listening to the words, but being aware of non-verbal communication cues and the emotional content. Providers engaged in active listening focus their attention on the patient and, by repeating the patient's concerns without judgment or interpretation, convey that they are listening, undistracted, and understanding what the patient is saying.

An important component of active listening is allowing the patient to speak without interruptions. Phones, beepers, PDAs, and computers have the potential to distract and detract from your active listening efforts. Answering your phone or checking the beeper may not seem offensive to you, but allowing these to interrupt your visit may be perceived by your patients as a lack of respect for their time and issues.

### Health Literacy

In April 2004, The Institute of Medicine (IOM) published a telling report titled *Health Literacy: A Prescription to End Confusion.*[23] This report stressed that "Nearly half of all American adults—90 million people—have difficulty understanding and acting upon health information." The IOM report defines health literacy as "the degree to which individuals have the capacity to obtain, process, and understand basic health information and services needed to make appropriate health decisions." Health literacy requires a greater and varied set of skills including reading, writing, speaking, listening, and understanding numbers. It also relies on cultural and conceptual knowledge, and requires that a patient be able to gather a variety of information, then process and act upon it.

Public and private organizations need to take this issue of health literacy seriously and make programmatic changes to address gaps; it is just as important for physicians to learn how to assess the health literacy of their patients. While it is not feasible to test every patient to determine their health literacy level, there are some ways to ensure that information you share with your patients is understood. It may be useful for physicians to assess the degree to which patients understand and can recall important health information. For example, in a study of conversations between physicians and their patients with diabetes, patients whose physicians asked them about their ability to recall or understand new concepts during visits had better blood sugar control.[24]

### Transitions and Continuity of Care

Chapter 16 goes into greater detail about the actual referral process and issues related to making referrals and appropriate follow-up. However, it is important to recognize how the referral process and the subsequent transitions of care can affect the patient-physician relationship.

Primary care doctors are regarded by many to be care managers for patients. However, older patients, those with chronic conditions, and those needing hospital and other services often see several different doctors in a variety of settings. In many cases, there is no one provider who has complete knowledge of all the care and treatment these patients are receiving. Information required for delivery of the most appropriate, highest quality care may not be conveyed during patient transitions from one type of provider or facility to another. Whether you see the patient as the primary care physician or a specialist, communication across care teams is essential to promote consistent and appropriate care. If you provide care to individuals on an outpatient basis, you may in some cases deal with hospitalists. A hospitalist is a physician who oversees inpatient care. Primary care physicians' satisfaction and acceptance of these relatively new practitioners has been associated with whether the hospitalist program is voluntary or mandatory, and the perceived or real effect of the hospitalists' work on physicians' income.[25] If your tertiary care facility uses hospitalists, it is important to ensure that anyone providing care to your patient has the information needed. Similarly, you should be sure to request information you need from any provider seeing your patient.

Chapter 5 guides you through the development and management of health care teams. Health care teams have been touted as a way of improving quality by providing more continuity of care for patients.[1] It is important to recognize that these teams and the resulting continuity have been shown to increase patient satisfaction and improve outcomes of care.[26,27] Beyond office- or hospital-based teams, you may be dealing with teams of providers in health plan or employer-sponsored disease management programs. While many of the programs can improve your patients' health and health behaviors, it is essential to coordinate with these external programs, just as you would with a hospitalist or a specialist.

### Patient Education

Many patients are taking the initiative to educate themselves. You may find more of your patients, particularly those with chronic conditions, will bring printouts of information they find on the Internet. Be open to discussing these materials with them and prepared to offer additional materials and websites that you know to be accurate and useful.[28] While the Internet has not replaced the provider as the primary source of health information, by some patients' reports, it may have a positive effect on patient-provider relationships by increasing communication and information-sharing.[29]

Patients expect doctors to refer them to useful websites, so it's important for doctors to know which websites are useful; MedlinePlus® is a good source. Patients tend to want to go to reputable websites, so recommending sites like Mayo Clinic and NIH are good bets.[30,31] Otherwise, patients will spend time trying to figure out if the website is reputable or not, rather than focusing on the content.

### Use of Technology to Improve Care and Communication

President Bush has called for the widespread adoption of electronic health records (EHRs) by 2014.[32] EHRs are most commonly defined as a centralized collection of individual patient health information from multiple sources, i.e., hospital, physician office, laboratory, radiological imaging, pharmaceuticals, and personal health records. Chapter 6 offers a history and discusses key issues related to acquisitions and the future trends of electronic medical records (EMRs), which are commonly thought of as site-based records, vs. the EHR's more comprehensive content. With the government's push for the U.S. health care system to be paperless by 2014, the practice or organization you enter or establish will most likely have (or be considering) electronic medical or health records. Providers should think of EMRs and other electronic communications and software as tools to promote a patient-centered practice.

Physicians are often resistant to integrate EMR/EHRs and other health technology applications into practice, not only due to acquisition cost, but due to concerns about disruption to work flow and distraction from the patient-provider interaction. As computers become omnipresent in our lives, patients will soon learn to accept the presence of a computer, e-tablet, or PDA in their visits. Research has found that appropriate use of health information technology during an outpatient visit can have a positive effect on the physician-patient interaction and can help to improve overall patient satisfaction with the visit.[33] There are several ways to integrate the use of these technologies without making the patient feel disregarded or ignored. There are several suggestions for best integrating EMR/EHRs into your office visits: [34]

- Use mobile computer monitors
- Learn to type
- Integrate typing around your patients' needs
- Reserve templates for documentation

- Separate some routine data entry and health-care maintenance issues from your patient encounters

- Start with your patients' concerns

- Tell your patients what you are doing, as you're doing it

- Point to the screen. Encourage patients' participation in building their charts

- Look at your patients

Beyond the health care visit, providers are commencing the use of patient portals that allow patients to make appointments, refill prescriptions, receive lab results and reminders, and even interact with the office and provider through email.

Finally, the personal health record (PHR) is still in its infancy in terms of connectivity, but stands to become a powerful tool to ensure quality patient-centered care. You may work with health plans that offer this tool to their members. Though uptake by consumers is still relatively slow, encouraging patients to keep track of their health information and keep you abreast of updates and changes is an important way to ensure decisions are made with all relevant information.

## Measuring and Improving Patient Satisfaction

In recent years, measuring patient satisfaction and patient experiences has become a hot topic of discussion in relation to quality rating and pay for performance programs. Some surveys are administered by health plans, others by hospitals or medical groups. The level of data collected will vary depending on which organization administers the tool. Some information may be useful to individual providers, while other data may not assist a physician in making changes to their practices and procedures. Chapter 3 offers insights into pay for performance systems.

As with the development of a trusting relationship, many elements of care will contribute to a patient's satisfaction with a visit or care episode. Like trust, research has shown that race and ethnicity appear to influence levels of satisfaction. Not only does concordance of race/ethnicity between patient and physician have an effect, but overall ratings of satisfaction appear to be lower in certain racial and ethnic populations, i.e., African Americans, Asian Americans. These differences may stem from trust issues and cultural perceptions of the health care system.[35]

Satisfaction is not driven simply by patient interactions with the physician. It may also be reflective of other environmental issues in relation to making practices patient-centered and culturally sensitive. Do your patients desire longer office hours? Are materials and forms only provided in English? Is your office staff responsive to phone calls? Did it take a long time to get an appointment? Did the patient have to wait for a long time before being seen? Is it difficult to find a parking spot? Answers to these and other questions will influence the satisfaction level of the patient.

There are a variety of tools available to measure patient satisfaction, and more larger-scale assessment tools are under development. Whether you choose a well-known, validated tool to enable you to benchmark and compare your patient satisfaction scores against others, or create a simple direct survey on your own, measuring and utilizing data from patient satisfaction surveys are important components of creating a patient-centered practice. The Patient Satisfaction Questionnaire (PSQ III) and its short form (PSQ-18) were developed by RAND corporation as tools to receive feedback on seven dimensions of ambulatory care; e.g., general satisfaction, technical quality, interpersonal manner, communication, financial aspects, time spent with doctor, and accessibility and convenience.[36] The PSQ measures satisfaction and perceptions of providers and medical care more generally. However, Rubin created a measure that detailed issues like "how long you waited to get an appointment," "convenience of the location of the office," and "getting through to the office by phone." In studies, lower scores on this scale was a predictor of whether a patient might change doctors.[37] These are issues you have more control over than patients' general perceptions about medical care.

## Conclusion

Remember, patient-centered care is not a simple plug-and-play tool. It takes a conscientious effort to craft a staff, practice, hospital ward, and ultimately healthcare system that is sensitive and respectful to patient diversity, encourages collaborative decision making, and promotes healthy behaviors.

## Case Study

Ms. G calls Dr. M's office to make an appointment for a cough and wheezing that is now keeping her up at night. Dr. M's receptionist tells her that she can be seen at 2pm today and Ms. G is surprised and happy to be able to come in right away.

Once she arrives, Ms. G checks in at the desk and is asked to complete a form with any changes to her information, insurance and health status. It also requests the reason for her visit today. Ms. G writes medication for cough.

Within five minutes, Ms. G is brought back to exam room and the medical assistant checks her vitals, including weight, blood pressure, and temperature. When Dr.

M arrives, he notices that she has gained 20 lbs. since her annual visit just three months ago. He notes that her blood pressure is slightly elevated, but she has no temperature. She complains of a cough that kept her up last night and that she would like to have some antibiotics. On exam, he notes that she is well-appearing, has some expiratory wheezing, but is moving air.

Dr. M says that a cough at night is probably indicative of asthma and he would like to send her for pulmonary function tests. In addition, he suggests that she should be more concerned about her weight gain and blood pressure and gives her a pamphlet about losing weight and a list of local weight loss programs.

Ms. G sits quietly, slightly embarrassed, and a bit upset that Dr. M won't give her antibiotics. He hands her a referral slip for a pulmonologist and provides her with a website that she can look at to get more information on asthma. He asks her if she has any other questions, she shakes her head no.

## Study/Discussion Questions

1. What aspects of this scenario demonstrate patient-centeredness?

2. What aspects do not?

3. How would you make changes to provide more patient-centered care to Ms. G?

## Suggested Readings/Websites

Eight Dimensions of Patient-centered Care:

http://nrcpicker.com/Default.aspx?DN=112,22,2,1,Documents

RAND Report Summary: Consumer Use of Information When Making Treatment Decisions
http://www.bcbs.com/coststudies/reports/Rand_Report_Summary.pdf

RAND Health. Patient Satisfaction Questionnaire.
http://www.rand.org/health/surveys_tools/psq/index.html

Davis K, Schoenbaum SC, Audet AM.A 2020 vision of patient-centered primary care. *J Gen Intern Med.* 2005;20:953-957.
http://www.blackwell-synergy.com/doi/abs/10.1111/j.1525-1497.2005.0178.x

Audet AM, Davis K, Schoenbaum SC. Adoption of patient-centered care practices by physicians: results from a national survey. *Arch Intern Med.* 2006;166:754-759.
http://archinte.ama-assn.org/cgi/reprint/166/7/754

## References

1. Institute of Medicine. *Crossing the Quality Chasm: A New Health System for the 21st Century.* Washington. DC: National Academies Press; 2001.

2. Stewart MA. Effective physician-patient communication and health outcomes: a review *Can Med Assoc J.* 1995:152:1423-1433.

3. Committee on Identifying Effective Treatments for Gulf War Veterans' Health Problems, Board on Health Promotion and Disease Prevention, Bernard M. Rosof BM, Hernandez LM, eds. *Gulf War Veterans: Treating Symptoms and Syndromes.* Washington. DC: National Academies Press; 2001.

4. The Office of Minority Health. What Is Cultural Competency? Available at: http://www.omhrc.gov/templates/browse.aspx?lvl=2&lvlID=11 Accessed July 13, 2006.

5. Health Resources and Services Administration Study on Measuring Cultural Competence in Health Care Delivery Settings. Attachment 3: Potential Measures/Indicators of Cultural Competence. Available at: http://www.hrsa.gov/culturalcompetence/measures/attachment3.htm Accessed July 13, 2006.

6. Kravitz RL. Patients' expectations for medical care: an expanded formulation based on review of the literature. *Med Care Res Rev.* 1996;53(1):3-27.

7. Emanuel EJ, Emanuel LL. Four models of the physician–patient relationship. *JAMA.* 1992;267:2221–2226.

8. Charles C, Gafni A, Whelan T. Shared decision-making in the medical encounter: What does it mean? (or it takes at least two to tango). *Soc Sci Med.* 1997;44:681–692.

9. Bugge C, Entwistle VA, Watt IS. The significance for decision-making of information that is not exchanged by patients and health professionals during consultations. *Soc Sci Med.* 2006 Jun 19; [Epub ahead of print].

10. Spranca M. *RAND Report Summary: Consumer Use of Information When Making Treatment Decisions.* Santa Monica, CA: RAND; 2005.

11. Jaber R, Braksmajer A, Trilling J. Group visits for chronic illness care: models, benefits and challenges. *Fam Pract Manag.* 2006;13:37-40.

12. Wofford MM, Wofford JL, Bothra J, Kendrick SB, Smith A, Lichstein PR. Patient complaints about physician behaviors: a qualitative study. *Acad Med.* 2004;79:134-138.

13. Kao AC, Green DC, Davis NA, Koplan JP, Cleary PD. Patients' trust in their physicians: effects of choice, continuity, and payment method. *J Gen Intern Med.* 1998;13(10):681-6.

14. Thom DH; Stanford Trust Study Physicians. Physician behaviors that predict patient trust. *J Fam Pract.* 2001; 500:323-328.

15. Rosser WW, Kasperski J. The benefits of a trusting physician-patient relationship. *J Fam Pract*. 2001;50:329-30.

16. Cantor JC, Baker LC, Hughes RG. Preparedness for practice. Young physicians' views of their professional education. *JAMA*.1993:270:1035-1040.

17. Orleans CT, George LK, Houpt JL, Brodie KH. Health promotion in primary care: a survey of U.S. family practitioners. *Preventive Medicine*. 1985;14:636-647.

18. Wing RR, Phelan S. Long-term weight loss maintenance. *Am J Clin Nutr*. 2005;82(1 Suppl): 222S-225S.

19. Prochaska, JO, DiClemente, CC. Stages and processes of self-change of smoking: Toward an integrative model of change. *J Consult Clin Psychol*; 1983;51:390-395.

20. Whitlock EP, Orleans CT, Pender N, Allan J. Evaluating primary care behavioral counseling interventions: An evidence-based approach. *Am J Prev Med*. 2002;22:267-284.

21. Epstein RM, Franks P, Fiscella K, Shields CG, Meldrum SC, Kravitz RL, Duberstein PR. Measuring patient-centered communication in patient-physician consultations: theoretical and practical issues. *Soc Sci Med*. 2005;611:1516-1528.

22. Teutsch C. Patient-doctor communication. *Med Clin North Am*. 2003;87:1115-45.

23. Committee on Health Literacy Board on Neuroscience and Behavioral Health, Nielsen-Bohlman L, Panzer AM, Kindig DA, eds. *Health Literacy: A Prescription to End Confusion*. Washington, DC: National Academies Press; 2004.

24. Schillinger, D, Piette J. Grumbach K, et al. Closing the loop: physician communication with diabetic patients who have low health literacy. *Arch Intern Med* 2003;163:83-90.

25. Fernandez A, Grumbach K, Goitein L, Vranizan K, Osmond DH, Bindman AB. Friend or foe? How primary care physicians perceive hospitalists. *Arch Intern Med*. 2000;160:2902-2908.

26. Cabana MD, Jee SH. Does continuity of care improve patient outcomes? *J Fam Pract*. 2004;53:974-980.

27. Fan VS, Burman M, McDonell MB, Fihn SD. Continuity of care and other determinants of patient satisfaction with primary care. *J Gen Intern Med*. 2005;20:226-233.

28. Diaz JA, Sciamanna CN, Evangelou E, Stamp MJ, Ferguson T. Brief report: What types of Internet guidance do patients want from their physicians? *J Gen Intern Med*. 2005;20:683-685.

29. Blanch DC, Sciamanna CN, Lawless HK, Diaz JA. Effect of the Internet on the Doctor-patient relationship: a review of the literature. *J Inform Tech Healthcare*. 2005;3:179-201.

30. http://www.mayoclinic.com/

31. http://health.nih.gov/

32. State of the Union Address, 2004. Available at: http://www.whitehouse.gov/news/releases/2004/01/20040120-7.html. Accessed July 14, 2006.

33. Hsu J, Huang J, Fung V, Robertson N, Jimison H, Frankel R. Health information technology and physician-patient interactions: impact of computers on communication during outpatient primary care visits. *J Am Med Inform Assoc*. 2005;12:474-480.

34. Ventres W, Kooienga S, Marlin R. EHRs in the Exam Room: Tips on patient-centered care with a thoughtful approach, you can maintain your focus on the patient. *Fam Prac Mgt*. 2006;13:45-47.

35. Cooper LA, Roter DL, Johnson RL, Ford DE, Steinwachs DM, Powe NR. Patient-centered communication, ratings of care, and concordance of patient and physician race. *Ann Intern Med*. 2003;139:907-915.

36. RAND Health. Patient Satisfaction Questionnaire. Available at: http://www.rand.org/health/surveys_tools/psq/index.html. Accessed July 14, 2006.

37. Rubin HR, Gandek B, Rogers WH, Kosinski M, McHorney CA, Ware JE Jr. Patients' ratings of outpatient visits in different practice settings. Results from the Medical Outcomes Study. *JAMA*. 1993;270:835-840.

# Chapter 5

## *Succeeding as a Member of the Health Care Team*

Christine B. Turley, MD and Jose L. Gonzalez, MD, JD, MSEd

### Executive Summary

In today's complex systems of health care delivery, young physicians' ability to practice quality, cost-effective health care will be challenged not only by rapid increases in medical knowledge and technology that they must master but also by changing patient expectations towards greater participation in their own care. Practicing physicians will be required to understand the varied environments in which they deliver health care and to develop competency in assisting their patients to successfully and efficiently navigate their multiple interactions with the health care system.

To advocate for the health and safety of their patients and achieve the desired outcomes, physicians will need to work collaboratively with a diverse group of health care professionals. Such cooperative interdependence mandates mutual commitment and accountability by all participants to a common goal of patient wellness, a cultural shift quite in contrast to the long-practiced medical training paradigm of physician autonomy and independence.

The successful and effective health care delivery team consists of a small number of providers with complementary health management skills who are committed to quality, safe, and cost-efficient health care with mutual and collective accountability to the desired outcomes. The greatest obstacle to the development and maintenance of such teams lies not in the lack of medical knowledge, technical competency or other medical skills but rather, in the failure of team members to participate in open and reciprocal communication. Physicians, as the principal health care advocates for their patients, must be able and willing to champion the transformation of a group of health care experts into an expert Health Care Team through leadership and cogent, compassionate communication.

**Learning Objectives**

1. Understand the role of the "Health Care Team" in the delivery of medical care in today's complex health care system.

2. Define the skills of team building and team leadership for the development and maintenance of an effective and efficient "Health Care Team."

3. Analyze the importance of interpersonal communications in the delivery of quality health care.

**Keywords**

health care team; systems-based practice; teamwork skills; interpersonal communications; health care delivery; five C's

## Introduction

The health care system in the United States has been evolving over the last 50 years at an ever-increasing pace. The "practice and art" of medicine that once valued the independence of the profession's physician-patient relationship is largely a thing of the past. This basic tenet is now challenged by rapid increases in medical knowledge and technology, changes associated with managed care, and the increasing complexity of health care insurance plans together with decreasing rates of reimbursement. In addition, patients expect not only the best medical knowledge and expertise from their physicians, they also expect their physician to serve as a guide to navigating the complex health care system. To achieve success as a physician, medical learners must dedicate themselves to understanding the inherent interpersonal dynamics and diverse systems involved in delivering health care.

Many individuals approach a career in medicine as a calling. Indeed, the continued ability to attract numerous bright, motivated students to the field singularly attests to this, especially given that much has been written over the past 10 years about the decline in the U.S. health care delivery system.[1,2] The very real demands of day-to-day medical practice can and do contribute to high levels of physician discontent. As many as one-third of physicians report dissatisfaction with their profession and 40% report a decreased ability to advocate for their patients, a malaise that can be attributed to three primary areas of "morbidity": money, time, and control.[3] Financial pressure stems from decreases in payment for services rendered and increasingly arbitrary funding for patient care. As financial resources have shrunk, demands on physicians' time have increased exponentially forcing practitioners to increase patient through-put by scheduling more (and shorter) clinic appointments over a longer workday. Finally, the loss of physician control over clinical decision making and other practice components thought to be at the core of the doctor-patient relationship have been gradually usurped by third parties motivated by economic or financial interests.

## Systems-based Practice of Health Care

In order to mitigate the increasing frustration with these morbidities and re-establish the primacy of the patient's well-being in health care, it is imperative for physicians to take an active role in understanding their practice environment. This paradigm shift is likely to occur only when physicians recognize that every aspect of the health care environment influences and affects the doctor-patient relationship. Given the relative infrequency of business and economic training by physicians, this task may seem daunting. Nonetheless, when broken into its component parts, the process of acquiring competency in systems-based practice becomes more manageable. Achieving an understanding of the integral and complex associations between the practice of medicine and the varied systems of health care delivery, both at the local and national level, must include: [4]

- a personal goal and commitment to effectively advocate for quality and safe patient care;

- a thorough understanding of the complexity associated with the systems of modern health care delivery;

- the ability to assist patients in efficiently navigating the complex health care system;

- a willingness to communicate and effectively partner with other professionals for the benefit of patients; and

- an ability to manage the duality of quality and cost-effectiveness for the benefit of patients.

## The Health Care Team

While each of the above elements of practice includes individual components outside the traditional doctor-patient dyad, to effectively practice medicine in the modern system of health care delivery a physician must be adept at interacting with a diverse team of health care professionals. Recognition of self as a component of the team, either as its leader or as a member in a learning role, is an important concept that must be mastered. Toward this goal, the Institute of Medicine's report, *To Err is Human: Building a Safer Health Care System*, recommended teamwork training as one important approach for improving safe, quality health care for all patients.[1]

A team is a small number of people with complementary skills who are committed to a common purpose, performance goals, and implementation approach for which they hold themselves mutually accountable.[5] Within the context of health care, a health care team (heretofore the "team") is a small number of health care providers with complementary medical, surgical, nursing, pharmacy, case managing, information technology, or systems-based skills, who are committed to the common purpose of providing safe and effective, quality health care with error-free, patient-centered, satisfactory performance outcomes for which they are collectively responsible. Although the concept of collaborative teams, or performance units, is not new to our society, e.g., the aviation industry, it is only recently that the medical profession has begun to accept this performance ethic. In spite of this recent trend, however, most traditional education programs in medicine and nursing still do not include teamwork training within their formal curriculum.[6]

Team care does not equate with group care. The aviation industry has long established that safe and effective cockpit performance requires the teaching and learning of team skills alongside technical skills.[7] Aviation's improved safety record[8] strongly supports that only through a new paradigm of cooperative interdependence within an interdisciplinary team approach will our health care system reach its lofty goals of safe, effective, and cost-efficient quality health care. Team and performance are inseparably connected in the successful achievement of quality and safe health care for which the team is collectively responsible. To succeed, the team requires technical and functional expertise, as well as competency in interpersonal communications, problem-solving, and decision-making skills. Through commitment to effort and team success, health care providers can embark on a process of inquiry and cooperative performance to ensure outcomes in patient care that exceed the capability of any one individual team member.[9] In contrast to a separate collection of individual performances to achieve patient outcome, the collaborative incorporation of the ideas and perspectives of all team members alternatively employs the intellectual resources of all members and converts diversity into an asset for addressing each patient's unique needs.

Effective teamwork in health care requires agreement on Weinger's Five C's: common goals, commitment, competence, communication and coordination.[10] These remind us that an essential component of successful teams is the need for a high level of trust among its members. Only within an atmosphere of tolerance, respect, and allowance will team members be able to challenge each other, to communicate without offense and to work through any differences and conflicts that arise.[11] No less imperative for the pursuit of team health care is a sense of mutual accountability for results among team members.[5] These attributes will serve to transform a group of expert health care providers from different disciplines into an expert team capable of successfully and consistently implementing effective patient care management plans.[12]

Development of a health care team does not in and of itself guarantee effective implementation and outcomes. A significant paradigm shift in medical education and training from one of independent performance to one of cooperative interdependence is needed to achieve the desired results of providing safe, effective, and cost-efficient health care to an increasingly complex patient population. As the principal advocates for patients' health, physicians need to accept responsibility for the integration and coordination of the team's implementation activities. To attain the desired common purpose of safe, quality health care, physicians must develop the requisite leadership skills to influence and direct team performance goals for the benefit of patients. Facility with interpersonal communication and role modeling are two of the most important components of these necessary skills.

## Interpersonal Communication

Misconceptions and various types of failures in communication present prominent obstacles to effective team health care, and likely are the direct result of independent performance training.[10] Communication failures and the resultant lack of teamwork have been cited as major causes of preventable medical errors.[1] Only by improving interpersonal communication skills and the development of a common understanding of how best to communicate important patient information will health care providers be able to deliver quality health care to their patients in an optimum, team-effective manner. Failures in communication can occur not only at the point of initial information transmission, but also at its reception and acknowledgement. At each of these distinct junctures, successful communication may be disrupted by a variety of dysfunctional processes such as the transmission or receipt of wrong information, a lack of message reception, or the misunderstanding of correct information.[10] Additionally, communication failure may result from a failure to acknowledge message reception, to act on the information received, to acknowledge understanding of the information transmitted, or to complete the action requested.[10]

To overcome the many prevalent obstacles to effective communication, it is necessary to understand the cognitive, physical, and emotional limitations of each team member and to possess a keen and clear awareness of the various situations in which physicians practice. Such achievements will also necessitate a mutual tolerance and acceptability of ongoing monitoring and cross-checking across providers, a non-threatening adaptability to ongoing review and modification of patient management plans and, hardest of all, a willingness to participate in open, reciprocal communication in the context of trusting interpersonal relationships among all team members.[6]

An understanding of who and where one is on the team, and where the team resides, bears in-depth consideration. Reflect on the following scenario, and where and how team members are connected to the physician. Consider, too, the changing nature of the team throughout the development of the patients' contacts with the health care system and their shifting needs.

> A 35-year-old patient presents to the Emergency Room with closed head and spine injuries and fractures of both wrists after a fall from a ladder at home.

In this instance, the patient's initial contact with the health care system team might include:

- Emergency Medicine first responders in the field, who are responsible for stabilization and safe transport;

- Emergency Department nurses, technicians and physicians, who continue the initial management and early recognition of the patient's needs;

- The radiology tech, who runs the MRI machine, allowing images of the spine and head for emergent review;

- The Information Services staff, who ensure the functioning of the technology that allows the radiologist attending to review films immediately from home.

- The social worker, who sorts out an appropriate home situation for the patient's young children while their parent seeks emergently care;

- The Emergency Department Billing staff, who manage the insurance notifications so that the insurance does not deny coverage;

- The Hospital Admissions clerical staff member, who allocates the beds in the ICU;

- The nursing manager, who finds an intensive care nurse to work and care for the patient once admitted;

- The respiratory therapy technician, who sees that a ventilator is available and appropriately staffed;

- The Environmental Management staff, who clean the ICU room in a timely manner and limit the risks for nosocomially-acquired infections; and

- The hospital Epidemiology Department for monitoring infections and ensuring that adequate training has occurred to prevent infectious transmission, among many others.

The list of course continues, but the patient counts on each member of the team to function effectively and cohesively to assure him the highest quality and safety of care.

As is evident from the initial care of this patient, the health care systems at work behind the scenes for each patient are exceedingly complex. Each element is important to the whole, and if one considers the above scenario from the perspective of a dysfunction or absence of any one of these elements, the primary outcomes for physicians to work effectively in a health care team, i.e., the patient's health will be significantly diminished. It is thus critical to the patient's health outcomes as well as to the team's effectiveness and efficiency that the patient's primary caregiver, i.e., the physician, possess the skills to coordinate the efforts of each and every team member and to integrate their multiple, varied roles into one cohesive and mutually complementary management plan.

Looking forward in the care of this patient:

> One month following the accident, the patient is ready for hospital discharge and placement in a long-term rehabilitation facility to regain the ability for self-care in light of the long-term effects of spinal cord and head injuries.

At this juncture, the team will be composed of many new members, including:

- Rehabilitation licensed vocational nurses, who provide day-to-day care and support for the patient's residual post-traumatic needs;

- Physical and occupational therapists, who provide care, support, and guidance on the path to recovery;

- The managed care medical director, who authorizes patient placement in a high-quality rehabilitation center as a covered benefit;

- Rehabilitation center billing office staff, who obtain certification as needed when the in-facility stay is extended; and

- The durable medical equipment supplier, who collects the needed documentation for the appropriate home-assistive technology that permits the patient's discharge to proceed in a timely manner.

- These team members are all essential, both individually and collectively, for the patient's high-quality, long-term health care management and optimal overall outcomes. As stated, it is imperative for physicians to understand and ensure that each team member is individually accountable for the high quality and safe care of the patient and that only through effective interpersonal communication and collaboration will patient outcomes be optimized.

Team membership is far from static. As the patient's medical scenario changes, team members will shift accordingly. The examples described above focused on local team members involved in the health and well-being of the individual patient. Although beyond the scope and objectives of this introductory chapter on team health care, different team members may be found in more distant locations when health care delivery is considered from alternate perspectives such as the one described in the following scenario:

> *A 41-year-old man employed by a local small business is diagnosed with advanced colon cancer after a delay in seeking medical care due to a lack of health insurance.*

Although team members in this individual's health care will comprise many of the same health care systems within the local community listed in the initial case, consider for a moment what other more distant and less evident team members may participate in this patient's access to and interactions with the varied systems of health care that he requires. Note that, even though many of the individuals potentially involved in this patient's health care may don business or administrative suits in far away places and engage with the local health team members in different and unique ways, all are still integral and essential members of the team and dictate that physicians be aware of their possible influences on the patient's quality of received care.

## Conclusion

In order to understand and successfully navigate today's U.S. system of health care so as to effectively advocate for patients, it is important for physicians to recognize and be familiar with all of the systems' components. In so doing, it will also be beneficial to reflect on the respective roles of the health care providers and the patient recipients of such care that may exist within the relevant health care delivery system, and how their various interactions will benefit the individual patient. Such reflection will not only allow physicians to maximize their roles as productive and collaborative members of the health care team, but will also open the way for receptive feedback among all team members in an honest and non-threatening manner. Indeed, as described earlier in the chapter, barriers to effective and efficient team functioning are myriad and are based largely in the challenge of effective communication within a large, diverse, and ever-changing group of team members. As fiduciary advocates for our patients, it is thus critical to develop one's interpersonal communication skills alongside medical knowledge, technical proficiency, life-long learning, and professional behaviors so as to improve the quality and safety of health care.

To assist with this task, we close with the following reminders about successful teams:

- Goals are clearly stated and understood.
- Members commit to individual effort and the accomplishment of shared goals.
- Cooperative, complementary performance ensures outcomes that exceed the capability of any one member.
- A keen and clear awareness of the specific practice situation frames all activities.
- Establish and maintain an atmosphere of trust, tolerance, and respect.
- Honest communication, including feedback, is conducted without offense.
- Accept and encourage ongoing monitoring and cross-checking by all members.
- Adapt, in a non-threatening manner, to ongoing review and modification of management plans.
- Challenge and encourage each other to high levels of performance.
- Accountability for patients' outcomes is not delegable.

## Case Study

A 2-month-old, whose family is new to the area, is seen in the local emergency department. The diagnosis is an upper respiratory infection and she is referred for follow-up to your office, as you are on call for patients without a primary care provider (PCP). The family is asked to follow up in one week for a well visit, and to call sooner if she worsens.

## Study/Discussion Questions

1. What elements of the local health care system may engage in this scenario?
2. What is the greatest risk to this patient should she worsen and some aspect of this team fail?

   *You are working in your office two days later when her mom calls your office to say the baby is worse and now has a temperature of 103°. You ask them to come to the clinic immediately.*

3. What members of the team will engage at this time?
4. Where is the greatest likelihood that the team will break down?

*In clinic she is found to be febrile and irritable. As her PCP, you send the patient to the local hospital for admission. She is in the hospital for three days, after which she is discharged to follow-up with you for well care within one week.*

5. How has the composition of the team shifted as the patient's needs have changed?

*In clinic one week later, she is better and you perform her 2-month, well-baby visit while she is there to help the family avoid an additional return visit.*

6. How do this patient's needs for preventative care now affect the composition and activities of the team?

## Suggested Readings/Websites

Kohn LT, Corrigan JM, Donaldson MS, eds. *To Err is Human: Building a Safer Health Care System.* Institute of Medicine. Washington, DC: National Academies Press; 2000.

*Crossing the Quality Chasm: A New Health System for the Twenty-first Century.* Institute of Medicine. Washington, DC: National Academies Press; 2001.

Kassirer JP. Doctor discontent. *N Engl J Med* 1998; 339:1543-1545.

*Teamwork Takes Hold to Improve Patient Safety.* Risk Manager Reporter, Healthcare Risk Control System. Plymouth Meeting, Pennsylvania: ECRI: 2005;24: 1-7.

Jones FG. To Err is Human – The Institute of Medicine Report revisited – How are We Doing? In: Curry W, Linney BJ, eds. *Essentials of Medical Management.* Tampa, FL: American College of Physician Executives, A&A Printing; 2003: 97-109.

Fink LD. *Team Learning: Putting the "sTEAM" into Learning Groups.* http://www.tlcollaborative.org/Docs/Michaelsen-Putting%20sTEAM%20into%20Learning%20Groups.pdf

Hope JM, Lugassy D, Meyer R, et al. Bringing interdisciplinary and multicultural team building to health care education: the downstate team building initiative. *Acad Med.* 2005;80:74-83.

Salas E, Cannon-Bowers JA, Johnston JH. How can you turn a team of experts into an expert team in: Zsambok CE & Klein G, eds. *Naturalistic Decision Making.* Mahwah, NJ: Lawrence Erlbaum Associates, Inc.; 1997.

Patterson K, Grenny J, McMillan R, Switzler A, Covey SR. *Crucial Conversations: Tools for Talking when Stakes are High.* New York, NY: McGraw-Hill; 2002.

Tu HT, Ginsburg PB. Losing Ground: Physician Income, 1995-2003. Center for Studying Health System Change, June 2006. http://www.hschange.com

Kirch W, Schasii C. Misdiagnosis at a university hospital in four medical eras. *Medicine.* 1996;75: 25-40.

Fernandez CV, Gillis-Ring J. Strategies for the prevention of medical errors in pediatrics. *J Pediatr.* 2003;143:155-162.

Patterson K, Grenny J, McMillan R, et al. Crucial conversations: tools for talking when stakes are high. New York, NY: McGraw-Hill; 2002.

## References

1. Kohn LT, Corrigan JM, Donaldson MS, eds. *To Err is Human: Building a Safer Health Care System*. Institute of Medicine. Washington, DC: National Academies Press; 1999.

2. Committee on Quality of Health Care in America. *Crossing the Quality Chasm: A New Health System for the Twenty-first Century*. Institute of Medicine. Washington, DC: National Academies Press; 2001.

3. Kassirer JP. Doctor discontent. *New Engl J Med*. 1998;339:1543-1545.

4. The ACGME Outcomes Project Competencies. Available at: http://www.acgme.org/outcome/comp/compFull.asp. Accessed August 18, 2006.

5. Katzenbach JR, Smith DK. *The Wisdom of Teams*. New York, NY: HarperCollins Publisher; 1999:9-64.

6. ECRI. Teamwork takes hold to improve patient safety. Risk manager reporter, healthcare risk control system. Plymouth Meeting, Pennsylvania: *ECRI*. 2005;24:1-7.

7. Jones FG. To Err is Human – The Institute of Medicine Report revisited – How are We Doing? In: Curry W & Linney BJ, eds. *Essentials of Medical Management*. Tampa, FL: American College of Physician Executives, A&A Printing; 2003: 97-109.

8. Helmreich RL. On error management: lessons from aviation. *BMJ*. 2000;320:781-785.

9. Fink LD. Team Learning: Putting the "sTEAM" into Learning Groups. Available at: http://www.tlcollaborative.org/Docs/Michaelsen-Putting%20sTEAM%20into%20Learning%20Groups.pdf. Accessed August 19, 2006.

10. Weinger MB, Blike GT. Intubation Mishap, Table 3. AHRQ Web M&M. September 2003. Available at: http://www.webmm.ahrq.gov/case.aspx?caseID=29. Accessed August 19, 2006.

11. Hope JM, Lugassy D, Meyer R, et al. Bringing interdisciplinary and multicultural team building to health care education: the downstate team building initiative. *Acad Med*. 2005;80:74-83.

12. Salas E, Cannon-Bowers JA, Johnston JH. How can you turn a team of experts into an expert team. in: Zsambok CE, Klein G, eds. *Naturalistic Decision Making*. Mahwah, NJ: Lawrence Erlbaum Associates, Inc.; 1997.

# Section 2
# Information Management

# Chapter 6

## Ambulatory Information Technology

Albert G. Crawford, PhD, MBA, MSIS

**Executive Summary**

This chapter begins by describing recent trends facilitating the adoption of ambulatory electronic health records (EHRs), including: President George W. Bush's goal, stated in 2004, of universal EHR system use within 10 years; David Brailer's promotion of development of interoperability standards during his tenure in the Office of the National Coordinator for Health Information Technology (ONCHIT); the Centers for Medicare and Medicaid Services' (CMS) Doctor's Office Quality-Information Technology (DOQ-IT) program; and pay for performance (P4P) incentives and other initiatives developed by payors to promote EHR adoption.

Next, the chapter reviews criteria for evaluating ambulatory EHR systems and reviews the current state of the art. Specifically, the chapter describes the predominant system at present in the public sector, the VA Computerized Patient Record System (VistA), and the predominant systems in the private sector, such as GE's Centricity®, Allscripts' TouchWorks™, iMedica's *Patient Relationship Manager*, Epic Systems *EpicCare*®, and others.

The discussion of practical issues in purchasing, implementing, and using ambulatory EHRs includes considerations of system functionality; financing, including performing and interpreting return on investment (ROI) calculations; interoperability issues; and human resources issues, including staff training and organizational culture change.

The chapter concludes with a delineation of likely trends in the future that would support greater use of ambulatory EHRs.

## Learning Objectives

After reading this chapter, the reader should have an understanding of:

1. The recent history of ambulatory EHR systems;

2. Current national policies and private sector initiatives promoting use of ambulatory EHRs;

3. Criteria for evaluating and selecting an EHR system;

4. Predominant ambulatory EHR systems at present, in both the public sector and the private sector;

5. Issues in purchasing, implementing, and using ambulatory EHRs; and

6. Likely future trends promoting use of ambulatory EHRs.

## Keywords

computerized physician order entry (CPOE); electronic health record (EHR); electronic medical record (EMR); health information technology (HIT); interoperability; national health information network (NHIN); pay for performance (P4P); regional health information organization (RHIO)

## Introduction

Electronic health records (EHRs)* have long been promoted as central to the solution of the problems of high cost, inefficiency, and inadequate quality and safety in the U.S. health care system. However, at present, only approximately 24% of physician office practices have adopted ambulatory EHRs.[1] Moreover, adoption of ambulatory EHRs in the United States lags behind adoption rates in many other developed countries, as will be seen below. Nevertheless, we may now be witnessing a turning point in the adoption process, with a constellation of developments combining to promote widespread implementation of ambulatory EHRs.

---

* Electronic health records (EHRs) are distinguished from electronic medical records (EMRs) in that they are more comprehensive, in terms of including information from more providers and aiming for greater continuity over time. While the conceptual distinction is analytically useful, this chapter will generally use the term electronic health records for reasons of simplicity.

## Ambulatory Electronic Health Records: Recent Trends and Cross-Societal Comparisons

Among the recent trends promoting adoption of ambulatory EHRs are decreasing EHR costs (paralleling the general trend in information technology of increasing processing power and decreasing cost); improving return on investment (ROI) calculations; the increasing focus by all parties on quality and safety and, among providers in particular, avoiding malpractice costs; and improved incentives for adoption offered by payors.

### Recent national policies to promote widespread use of ambulatory EHRs

#### *President Bush's Goal of Universal Use within 10 Years*

President Bush gave significant impetus to adoption of EHRs with his 2004 statement of the goal that all Americans should have access to EHRs within 10 years. While studies suggest that this goal will not be attained if current adoption rates and trends continue,[2] the goal is laudable, and its statement has catalyzed numerous serious efforts in the public and private sectors.

#### *Office of the National Coordinator for Health Information Technology's Promotion of Standards*

One of the most significant developments promoting health information technology (HIT) in the Bush presidency to date was the creation of the Office of the National Coordinator for Health Information Technology (ONCHIT) in 2004, and the appointment of David Brailer, MD, PhD, as its first National Coordinator. Given high federal budget deficits, and the Bush administration's preference for private sector initiatives, Brailer's strategy was not to advocate that the federal government provide direct support for physicians to purchase EHRs, but rather for it to encourage the HIT industry to develop standards facilitating interoperability among proprietary EHR systems (and also to facilitate development of Regional Health Information Organizations – RHIOs, i.e., networks connecting patients, providers, and payors throughout a geographical area).

#### *Doctor's Office Quality-Information Technology Program*

Chief among various recent Centers for Medicare and Medicaid Services (CMS) initiatives promoting HIT is its Doctor's Office Quality-Information Technology (DOQ-IT) program, implemented through the national network of regional Quality Improvement Organizations (QIOs). The main goals of the DOQ-IT program are to provide:

- Help in evaluating practice needs and capabilities;

- Education on features, functionality, and options for purchasing EHRs;

- Objective information and assistance with vendor selection;

- Advice on refining processes and office workflow to improve efficiencies and patient care;

- Enhanced knowledge of available technology from an objective and reliable source;

- Understanding of how to achieve optimal use of technology; and

- Access to the latest innovations in health information technology.


### Pay for Performance and Other Initiatives by Payors

Payors in the United States have long been frustrated by the paradox of paying ever-increasing prices for suboptimal quality care. Recently, many payors have developed pay for performance (P4P) initiatives to promote value in health care purchasing. Payors are motivated by the increasingly popular idea that widespread EHR adoption can generate huge cost savings. For example, two recent studies estimate annual cost savings of $81 billion and $77.8 billion, respectively, from national adoption of EHRs.[3,4] P4P systems can promote adoption of ambulatory EHRs in two ways:

1. Directly, as in the case of the Leapfrog Group's statement on safety practices, i.e., "Research shows that if the first three leaps (Computer Physician Order Entry, Intensive Care Unit Physician Staffing and Evidence-Based Hospital Referral) were implemented in all urban hospitals in the United States we could save up to 65,341 lives, prevent as many as 907,600 serious medication errors each year, and save $41.5 billion."[5]

2. Indirectly, by rewarding high quality care, given that a prerequisite for quality, and quality improvement, is an ambulatory EHR that allows quality measurement.


### Recent trends and current levels of adoption

A report published in July 2006 by the Centers for Disease Control and Prevention's National Center for Health Statistics[1] shows that EHR implementation by office-based physicians increased 31% between 2001 and 2005. The survey found that 23.9% of physicians in 2005 used a full or partial EHR system in their office, up from 18.2% in 2001, 17.3% in both 2002 and 2003, and 20.8% in 2004. Results were based on responses from a sample of 3,000 office-based physicians drawn from the master files of the American Medical Association and the American Osteopathic Association. The report also demonstrates how EHR adoption is related to practice size and geography. In 2005, 16% of solo physician practices and 20.2% of practices with two physicians used a full or partial EHR system, while 25.3% of practices with 3-5 physicians, 33.8% of those with 6-10 physicians, and 46.1% of those with 11 or more physicians used full or partial EHR systems. Moreover, 33.4% of physicians in the West and 26.9% in the Midwest were found to use EHRs, compared with 14.4% of those in the Northeast. Finally, 24.8% of metropolitan area physicians use EHRs, compared with 16.9% of those in nonmetropolitan areas.

At the same time, it is important to note that EHR adoption rates vary according to how "adoption" is defined, as demonstrated in a review of 35 surveys on EHR adoption conducted since 1995. The review found that adoption rates vary from 9.3% to 23.9% depending on the definition of "full or partial use." Researchers David Blumenthal and Sara Rosenbaum examined 21 surveys of adoption and rated the quality of the survey instruments used based on their methodology and content. They rated only eight physician surveys and one hospital survey as having high or medium quality, and they concluded that our ability to estimate EHR adoption accurately is limited by lack of available data.[6]

Beyond these national adoption trends, "the United States lags as much as a dozen years behind other industrialized countries in HIT adoption – countries where national governments have played major roles in establishing the rule, and health insurers have paid most of the costs." [7]

## Criteria for Evaluating Ambulatory EHR Systems

### Certification of Ambulatory EHR Systems

In July 2006, 22 commercially available ambulatory EHR systems from 21 vendors met the new criteria for functionality and interoperability developed by the Certification Commission for Healthcare Information Technology (CCHIT), a federally-supported private testing organization.[8] CCHIT designed its voluntary certification program to clarify the confusing HIT market and to promote EHR adoption. Current products meeting the 2006 ambulatory certification criteria can be found at: http://www.cchit.org/certified/products.htm.

### EHR "Buyer's Guide" Criteria and Evaluation of Private Software

A somewhat dated, but excellent and freely available evaluation of ambulatory EHRs was performed in 2003 by Forrester Research for the California Health Care

Foundation (CHCF).[9] The Forrester team analyzed three broad characteristics of ambulatory EHRs:

- "The quality of the current offering, including features, ease of use, support and service, and cost;
- The vendor's strategy, meaning the future plans the company has for its EHR;
- The vendor's market presence, in terms of financial strength, customer base, and partnerships with other firms."

Current offerings, in turn, were evaluated along four dimensions:

- Functionality, reflected in 15 key features, e.g., speed and effectiveness of display of critical information;
- Usability, with six dimensions, e.g., navigation;
- Support, with four aspects, e.g., installation support; and
- Costs, including both financing flexibility and the vendor's approach to modular pricing.

Forrester evaluated ambulatory EHR vendors' strategies in light of both executive vision and product road map.

Forrester also rated five aspects of market presence: installed base, revenues, number of employees, size of sales force, and business partners.

Forrester's evaluation of the eight main ambulatory EHR systems is shown in Table 1 (page 83). It is worth noting that seven of the eight systems evaluated by Forrester (all but Amicore's *Clinical Management*) are now CCHIT-certified.

The web-based Forrester publication is particularly useful because it includes an interactive spreadsheet that allows users to add data for additional vendors' EHR systems and allows them to customize the weightings to reflect their own priorities and preferences.

The Forrester researchers concluded that GE's *Logician*® (now *Centricity*®) led the pack on all three dimensions of its evaluation, with Allscripts' *TouchWorks*™ and iMedica's *PhysicianSuite* close behind. As noted above, readers can download the Forrester group's interactive spreadsheet to perform their own evaluations, revising the Forrester evaluations and weightings, updating existing products' scores as those products evolve, and adding new products as they enter the market. For example, practices can add some or all of the CCHIT-certified products not already included in the Forrester evaluation.

## Table 1. Sorting the Products[9]

| Company Name | Product Name | Current Offering | Strategy | Market Presence |
|---|---|---|---|---|
| Allscripts Healthcare Solutions | *TouchWorks*™ | ** | *** | ** |
| Amicore | *Clinical Management* | ** | ** | * |
| GE Medical Systems Information Technologies (now GE Healthcare) | *Logician®* (now Centricity®) | *** | *** | ** |
| iMedica | *PhysicianSuite* (now *Patient Relationship Manager*) | ** | *** | * |
| Medical Manager Health Systems (now Emdeon Practice Services) | *Intergy*™ | ** | ** | *** |
| Misys Healthcare Systems | *Misys® EMR* | * | * | ** |
| NextGen Healthcare Information Systems | *NextGen® EMR* | ** | * | ** |
| Physician Micro Systems (now Practice Partner) | *Practice Partner®* *Patient Records* | * | * | * |

\* Good    \*\* Better    \*\*\* Best

## Current Leading Ambulatory EHR Systems in the Public Sector

### The VA Computerized Patient Record System (VistA/CPRS)

VistA is a trusted, proven, and economical EHR system. It is an enterprise-wide, fully-integrated, fully functional information system built around an EHR. It is easily customizable and can be configured to fit various types of health care organizations, from clinics and medical practices to nursing homes and large hospitals. VistA has been named one of the best health care information systems in the nation by the Institute of Medicine. Developed by the Department of Veterans Affairs, the VistA health care information system supports thousands of hospitals and clinics serving veterans throughout the United States and abroad. Because VistA is available in the public domain, there are no license fees to use the software. This makes VistA an affordable EHR system for health care organizations, providing them with all of the tools needed to reduce patient errors, lower costs, and improve the quality of care, including CPOE, bar code medication administration, e-prescribing, and clinical guidelines. Various commentators have noted the key role of VistA in the substantial improvements in quality of care provided to veterans over the last decade.

## Issues in Purchasing, Implementing, and Using Ambulatory EHRs

One of the best approaches to the exigencies of evaluating, selecting, buying, and implementing an ambulatory EHR system is the "12-step program" outlined in the Forrester/CHCF "Buyer's Guide."[9] The 12 steps are as follows:

1.  List high-priority needs.

2.  List the EMR product features most likely to meet those needs.

3.  Factor in future requirements.

4.  Write up a simple request for proposal (RFP).

5.  Make the commitment to having doctors enter data.

6.  Choose either keyboard and mouse or stylus and touch-screen.

7.  Test-drive each system using common scenarios prepared beforehand.

8.  Obtain three physician references from each vendor.

9.  Score competing candidates.

10. Settle on a purchase plan.

11. Nail down commitments on initial implementation and technical support.

12. Take advantage of a buyer's market.

### System Functionality

As noted above, an excellent discussion of functionality is available in the Forrester/CHCF "Buyer's Guide." The Forrester team identified 15 dimensions of functionality (Table 2, page 85).

## Table 2. EMR Functions and Features[9]

| Functionality | How quickly and effectively can the doctor: |
|---|---|
| View | View the patient's problem list, med list, test results, and other information critical to the clinical purposes of the visit? |
| Document | Document the visit and the clinical decision-making process? |
| Identify | Identify clinical issues by means of alerts and reminders? |
| Decide | Decide clinical issues with the support of knowledge references and databases? |
| Prescribe | Authorize and manage prescription refills within the system? Access formulary information in electronic form for new scripts? Consult drug utilization review (DUR) databases integrated into the system? ePrescribe – route new scripts to pharmacies electronically without reliance on faxing? |
| Order | Order labs, images, and other non-medications? |
| Communicate | Communicate electronically with colleagues? Exchange secure email with patients? Structure patient communications in a clinically relevant way that facilitates physician decision making? |
| Code | Match ICD and CPT codes to the details of the patient encounter, integrate an E&M coding tool, and also integrate the SNOMED controlled clinical vocabulary? |
| Comply | Comply with rules and regulations on privacy, consent, et cetera? |
| Aggregate | Aggregate individual data into longitudinal records for easy viewing and graphing? |
| Manage | Manage the individual patient's chronic diseases and conditions? |
| Standardize | Standardize disease management goals for subgroups of chronic disease sufferers within the practice? |
| Query | Query the system's database to produce both individual and group reports on clinical issues – care, quality, outcomes, and associated costs? |
| Conduct | Conduct research, registry, and clinical trial-related efforts? |
| Incorporate | Incorporate information originating with the patient and, as a separate matter, with medical or patient devices? |

### Return on Investment (ROI) Calculations

Return on investment (ROI) calculations require calculation of the ratio of annual net benefits to the sum of amortized initial installation costs and annual operating costs. Clearly, the ROI ratio must be positive; in fact, it must be superior to other alternatives, e.g., investment in new diagnostic technology, practice redesign, or advanced staff training.

Specifically, ROI calculations require identification and measurement, or prediction, of all substantial costs and benefits. A partial list of potential costs and benefits follows:

**Costs:**

- Hardware
- Software licenses and maintenance fees, over time
- Staff training
- Data "backfilling" to convert from paper to electronic records during the initial implementation phase

**Benefits:**

- Reduced labor costs, e.g., elimination of medical records staff position(s)
- Improved productivity/efficiency, e.g., fewer missing charts, reduced chart retrieval time
- Enhanced quality and related pay-for-performance bonuses
- Improved patient satisfaction and lower patient turnover

Clearly, calculating each of these costs and benefits can be problematic, especially when considering the more subjective factors and those related to outcomes rather than processes.

### Financing

Sources of financing include limited federal funds; limited funds from several regional public-private consortia; limited funds from payors, e.g., Blue Cross Blue Shield plans and other health plans; and self-financing. The main federal source is the DOQ-IT program, with some additional grant support by the Agency for Healthcare Research and Quality (AHRQ). Chief among regional consortia is the CHCF. Blue plans figure prominently in several regional consortia, and several individual Blue plans offer grants or incentives.

Still, unless there is new federal legislation, or practices are qualified to seek demonstration or other funding from AHRQ or a similar state or regional program, practices must acquire commercial financing or self-finance their EHR implementations. Given typical installation costs of $20,000 to $30,000 or more per physician, this is a daunting challenge.

### Interoperability Issues

The major thrust of the ONCHIT has been to encourage the HIT industry to develop standards facilitating interoperability of proprietary EHR systems. The process has not yet had much of an impact on improving interoperability. However, the mid-2006 CCHIT certification of 22 EHR systems should have an effect, especially if interoperability requirements become more rigorous in the future. In any event, physician practices must be careful to evaluate the interoperability of candidate EHR systems, particularly in combination with the key systems they already use, i.e., for billing, order entry, result reporting, etc.

### Worker Productivity and Other Human Resources Issues

The impact of EHR implementation on the productivity of professional and clerical staff is complex and difficult to predict. Some research indicates the potential for reducing labor costs, e.g., allowing reductions in clerical staff costs of $13,000 per physician per year.[10] On the other hand, other studies indicate the opposite effect on physician productivity, i.e., a 17% increase in physician documentation time with an EHR and a 98% increase with CPOE.[11] A recent article by Jaan Sidorov seeks to deflate expectations of EHRs, concluding that "The EHR often leads to higher billings and declines in provider productivity with no change in provider-to-patient ratios. Error reduction is inconsistent and has yet to be linked to savings or malpractice premiums."[12] Even those with more optimistic expectations must be sensitive to the complexities of workflow changes, staff training requirements, "backfilling" to convert from a paper-based system to an EHR system, and coping with inevitable defects and other issues requiring technical support.

## Conclusion

This chapter has reviewed recent developments, and the state of the art, in ambulatory information technology, specifically EHR systems.

Trends to date facilitating adoption of ambulatory EHRs include support by President Bush's administration and, specifically, the work of the ONCHIT; the initiatives of CMS, chiefly the DOQ-IT program; and P4P initiatives by payors that explicitly reward EHR adoption or encourage its use by rewarding quality measurement and improvement.

Key criteria for evaluating ambulatory EHR systems include product quality, vendor strategy, and vendor market presence. Each of these criteria has multiple dimensions and indicators. The VA's VistA/CPRS is the dominant EHR system in the public sector. There are numerous strong competitors in the private sector, including GE's *Centricity®*, Allscripts' *TouchWorks™*, iMedica's *Patient Relationship Manager*, and Epic Systems *EpicCare®*. The initial round of certification of ambulatory EHRs in mid-2006 by the public-private CCHIT was a key milestone; practices should only consider adopting EHR systems that have achieved high scores on the CCHIT certification criteria.

Once an EHR system has been selected, there will be numerous challenges in implementing and using it. Critical factors to consider are financial issues (performing and interpreting return on investment (ROI) calculations and obtaining financing), issues regarding functionality and interoperability with other information systems, and human resources issues (including staff training, managing culture change, and obtaining "buy-in" by prospective users).

It is highly likely that a number of trends will facilitate, and may ultimately require, adoption of ambulatory EHR systems, i.e., simultaneous demands for greater efficiency and improved quality and safety. As these trends continue and even accelerate, we may soon reach a "tipping point" and a quantum leap in adoption, where using an EHR system will be a requirement of practice. In any event, it is hoped that physicians beginning their careers in practice will benefit from this chapter and the resources on which it draws.

## Case Study
### The Hudson Valley's Taconic Health Information Network and Community

It is quite a challenge to create an EHR system for a 3,000-physician IPA with mostly small, dispersed practices. But Taconic IPA, Inc., headquartered in Fishkill, NY, has met that challenge. In late 2001, the IPA established a plan to implement a health information exchange (HIE) model among physicians, hospitals, laboratories, and insurers. Currently, about 600 of the IPA's physicians, in two of the eight counties it covers, participate in the data exchange, called Taconic Health Information Network and Community (THINC). THINC allows physicians to manage health care data electronically via a clinical messaging system, a key feature of any EHR. Physicians use a secure password to log in to a main portal from either laptop computers or personal digital assistants to retrieve lab reports, x-rays, and other clinical data. As the HIE model evolves, more physicians have been added, along with the additional functions of e-prescribing and EHR access.

With a three-year, $1.5 million grant from the AHRQ, Taconic staff are moving the project to the next level. The grant focuses on two priorities: 1) hiring an independent clinical investigator to study the HIE's impact on health care quality, and 2) expanding the program by helping more of the IPA's primary care physicians offset the costs of participating in the electronic network.

The impact study is assessing outcomes among three groups, each comprising approximately 100 physicians: a control group still using paper-based medical records, an e-prescribing group, and a group using fully-integrated EHRs. The grant also helps Taconic IPA's physicians surmount the cost barrier of joining the network by providing technical assistance during implementation. While start-up costs for EHRs are typically $30,000 per physician, Taconic IPA physicians pay approximately $500 per month to use the system.

The program also allows primary care physicians to qualify for some pay for performance incentive programs offered by insurers and employers to providers who use EHRs. A primary care physician can receive as much as $400 per month in such incentives.

## Study/Discussion Questions

1. Is it feasible to generalize from the practice in this case study to other practices? If not, why not? What differences preclude generalization?

2. How would you perform an ROI analysis for this practice or your own practice? What factors would you need to include, on both the cost side and the benefit side?

3. How can an ambulatory EHR system like THINC improve a practice? Specifically, how can it improve quality of care and safety?

## Suggested readings/websites

"Electronic Medical Records: A Buyer's Guide for Small Physician Practices": http://www.chcf.org/documents/ihealth/ForresterEMRBuyersGuideRevise.pdf; Download the interactive Excel spreadsheet tool at http://www.chcf.org/topics/view.cfm?itemID=21520.

Extensive vendor profiles: www.EMRConsultant.com:

Reviews "best of breed" products: www.Telemedicalrecord.com:

Information on more than 70 products, including a report with a matrix of features by vendor, brief vendor descriptions, a discussion forum, and links to vendor web sites: www.elmr-electronic-medical-records-emr.com/

"Family Practice Management Vendor Survey": www.aafp.org/fpm/20010100/45elec.html: Information on 28 vendor products, including rankings of products; a vendor characteristics matrix; and a matrix of features by vendor (unfortunately, the data have not been updated since January, 2001).

"Advance 2004 EHR Systems Review":
www.Health-care-it.advanceweb.com/Common/editorial/editorial.aspx?CTIID=1593;
Published by Advance for Health Information Executives; vendor profiles and a matrix based on criteria developed by the Institute of Medicine (IOM); published annually.

AAFP Center for Health Information Technology: www.centerforhit.org:
Requires membership in the American Academy of Family Physicians:
Contains physician EHR product reviews and other tools.

ACP Practice Management Center: http://www.acponline.org/pmc/index.html:
Requires membership in the American College of Physicians and completion of a brief online evaluation; provides free summary evaluations of office software products (including EHRs).

## References

1. Burt CW, Hing E, Woodwell D. Electronic medical record use by office-based physicians: United States, 2005. *NCHS Health and Stats.* Available at: http://www.cdc.gov/nchs/products/pubs/pubd/hestats/electronic/electronic.htm. Accessed July 31, 2006.

2. Ford EW, Menachemi N, Phillips MT. Predicting the adoption of electronic health records by physicians: When will health care be paperless? *J Am Med Inform Assoc.* 2006;13:106-112.

3. Hillestad R, Bigelow J, Bower A, et al. Can electronic medical record systems transform health care: Potential health benefits, savings, and costs. *Health Affairs.* 2005;24:1103-1117.

4. Walker J, Pan E, Johnston D, Adler-Milstein J, Bates DW, Middleton B. The value of health care information exchange and interoperability. *Health Affairs.* 2005;Suppl Web Exclusives:W5-10-W5-18.

5. Birkmeyer JD, Dimick JB. Potential benefits of the new Leapfrog standards: effect of process and outcomes measures. *Surgery.* 2004;135:569-575.

6. Blumenthal D, Rosenbaum S. EHR adoption rates vary by definition. American Health Information Community EHR Workgroup. 2006.

7. Anderson GF, Frogner BK, Johns RA, Reinhardt UE. Health care spending and use of information technology in OECD countries. *Health Affairs.* 2006;25:819-831.

8. Certification Commission for Healthcare Information Technology. CCHIT certified products by product. Available at: http://www.cchit.org/certified/2006/CCHIT+Certified+Products+by+Product.htm. Accessed August 2, 2006.

9.  Forrester Research. *Electronic medical records: A buyer's guide for small physician practices.* California Health Care Foundation; 2003.

10. Miller RH, West C, Brown TM, Sim I, Ganchoff C. The value of electronic health records in solo or small group practices. *Health Affairs.* 2005;24:1127-1137.

11. Poissant L, Pereira J, Tamblyn R, Kawasumi Y. The impact of electronic health records on time efficiency of physicians and nurses: A systematic review. *J Am Med Inform Assoc.* 2005;12:505-516.

12. Sidorov J. It ain't necessarily so: The electronic health record and the unlikely prospect of reducing health care costs. *Health Affairs.* 2006;25:1079-1084.

# Chapter 7

## Communication: The Key to Good Medicine

Nancy B. Finn

### Executive Summary

Communication is transmission of a thought from one individual to another. A complex activity, involving verbal and non-verbal content, which can be oral, written, or computer-mediated, communication is the linchpin around which the work of a physician revolves. Communication inherently involves words, gestures, and facial expressions. These words and expressions can be easily misunderstood because people's perception of the world is influenced by their home environment, genealogy and ancestry, schooling, regional and parental influences, personality and experiences. A 21$^{st}$ century physician does not have the luxury of communications that go awry, are misunderstood or poorly executed. Doctors must use every resource available to deploy communication that is cost-effective, efficient, and, most importantly, clear and persuasive.

In this chapter, physicians will learn how to brand themselves and integrate into the communities where they practice. They will learn how to use evolving communication and information technology to improve efficiency and effectiveness. They will understand how to make each communication encounter with a patient meaningful. They will read tips and suggestions on how to leverage their knowledge and skills to help their patients become more self-sufficient and able to manage their own health care. They will learn practical guidelines for improving their communication behaviors.

### Learning Objectives

1. To learn how to establish a new medical practice in the community with an appropriate outreach program that includes networking, mailings, collateral, and a website.

2. To understand how to structure the first visit with a patient to establish a trusting, ongoing relationship.

3. To investigate various methods to follow up with patients using the telephone, email, and patient portal consultations.

4. To insure that all communication with patients are conducted in an environment of confidentiality and privacy.

5. To determine how to handle communications in a crisis.

6. To explore the reasons why written and oral communication skills are important and discuss methods to develop and improve them.

## Keywords

adherence; asynchronous communication; brand identity; communication; electronic health record; email; e-newsletter; encrypted; listening; Medline Plus®; patient portal; telephone tag

## Introduction

There is a new health care consumer in America. One who is smarter, better informed, busier, and less *"patient"* than the patients of previous generations. The ubiquitous nature of the Internet; the flood of health care reports in the mass media, particularly television; and the ease with which everyone uses email, feed the appetites of consumers. These new information resources are not bound by time or geography, or dependent solely upon a physician's advice.

Health care professionals have always believed that they put their patients first. For generations, doctoring was a one-way relationship that consumers accepted as totally appropriate, because they were convinced that their doctors were trained to make the right decisions.   Patients felt that they had neither the knowledge nor the will to challenge those decisions. However, today's health care consumers demand that a visit to the doctor include full two-way discussions about health care options and treatment plans.   They expect their physicians to communicate with them as equals, and to be as savvy about communication and information as other business associates. They extend respect to their physicians and want that respect returned. They also expect prompt responses to calls, emails, and queries; minimal waiting times for appointments; and appropriate, courteous treatment at a visit. This chapter offers tips and suggestions on how to make all of that happen without infringing upon the physician's ability to deliver high quality care with limited resources.

## Creating your Brand Identity

It might seem strange to think of a medical practice needing a brand identity. We link the concept of a brand identity with the myriad products that the media constantly push in front of us. However, when establishing a new medical practice it is also important to create a brand identity in order to construct the right messages and impressions that you want to convey to potential patients. For an individual physician, creating a brand identity means establishing a certain persona, conveying specific impressions, and creating the appropriate messages that will capture mindshare in the community where you want to have a presence. To get your message out, you should devise ways to grab and keep the attention of your intended audience.

There are media strategies that can help you establish your brand, whether you are joining an existing practice or establishing a new practice. These include a website, an e-newsletter, general mailings, local advertising, listings in important directories, and membership in community organizations. As you introduce yourself to the community you should project a brand identity that says you are competent, credible, caring, and compassionate.

## Launching a Website

As a 21st century medical practitioner, you must be computer- and web-savvy. Most of your patients already use the web to communicate in their business and personal lives and expect the same level of technological expertise from their health care providers. Early on you should consider establishing a website where patients and prospective patients can go to find information about you and your practice, including: hours of operation, hospital affiliations, educational background, and those unique qualities related to your approach and your practice of medicine, i.e., what differentiates you. Include a video clip to introduce yourself. As your practice grows, you may wish to transform your website into a secure patient portal (more on this topic later), offering your patients a tool to schedule appointments, request referrals, find links to credible information on health issues, and maintain their own personal health records.

A website is not only a way to create your brand identity; it also provides a platform for maintaining ongoing communication with your patients about the issues that affect them. It is a way to encourage better adherence in the use of medications; a way to help your patients understand how to sift through their own information overload and cull out credible information resources; and a way to help your patients manage their medical conditions.

## Writing an E-newsletter

As your website evolves, you might want to include an e-newsletter and offer patients the option to subscribe to the newsletter via email. With all of the information available to you as a physician, you can easily publish a bimonthly e-newsletter that focuses on a specific topic of current interest in the health field. The e-newsletter generates worthwhile content for your website and provides an ongoing vehicle for communication with patients. This is a great way to keep in touch and establish a reputation for caring, while offering valuable advice on issues that may affect many people in your community. The content of the e-newsletter can easily be culled from medical bulletins issued by various government agencies, such as the Centers for Disease Control and Prevention (CDC) and the U.S. Department of Health and Human Services (DHHS). Other articles can consist of synopses of material from the myriad journals and magazines that cross your desk, and health websites that you access. With a little effort and ingenuity you can write your own material using these and other resources.

## Announcing Yourself with a Mailing

Among the first things you should do when you open a practice is send out a postcard mailing introducing yourself to the community. Invite prospective patients to contact you for an appointment, or call with questions or issues. Include your website address, which then allows you to push people to the site where they will find value-added information that will not fit on a small postcard.

## Advertising

Tasteful, professional black-and-white advertisements in the local newspaper are another effective communication vehicle. The advertisements should include your name, credentials, office location, phone, fax, website address, and a simple greeting. Committing to six insertions over a period of three months should be sufficient to provide the visibility you need.

## Joining Organizations/Networks

If you are opening a new practice, particularly in a small community, you will want to join the local chamber of commerce, Rotary club, and other organizations that will acquaint you with local leaders, issues, and health problems specific to the community. You may not have time to participate actively in these organizations as your practice grows, but joining is an essential part of a communication strategy.

## Getting Yourself Listed

To further promote your practice, submit your name to online lists and published directories of physicians. You can usually identify those lists by doing an online search for doctors by zip code. Review the directories and lists that appear and choose those that will give you the most exposure and credibility.

Some of the online directories to review:

Medline Plus® Directories: http://www.nlm.nih.gov/medlineplus/directories.html

Doctor Directory: www.doctorpage.com

Web MD Physician Directory: http://doctor.webmd.com/physician_finder/

Health Pages: www.healthpages.com

## Communicating with Patients

Today's patients are consumers who come to a physician with preconceived expectations about the services that they will receive. These empowered consumers are more sophisticated, with vast information resources from which to draw upon to make judgments, comparisons and choices about your services and their own medical care.

Ralph Waldo Emerson, 19th century writer and philosopher, stated in one of his essays, "It is a luxury to be understood." As a doctor, you do not have that luxury. Your communications with your patients must be absolutely clear. They must also be sensitive to the expectations, interests, needs, and values of your patients. Because your patients' needs are not only informational, but emotional and psychological, what you say can be viewed with suspicion and antagonism. In 21st century medicine, physicians must see their patients as people and not as cases. Listening skills are critical. Listening with an open mind and empathetic concern is the difference between a good doctor and a great doctor.

## The Patient Visit

When a patient walks into your office, you want to create an experience that is warm, welcoming, reassuring, and satisfying. The first impression that a patient will have of you is conveyed by the ambience of your office, so make sure that it is neat, bright, warm, and inviting. Have a variety of reading material to keep people occupied while they wait. Make certain that your staff is trained in patient-centered communications, and that they understand and speak coherent English and other languages, where applicable. It is crucial that they are polite and courteous.

Nothing sets a negative tone more than an abrupt, cold reception by the office staff, or an interaction with someone who cannot speak fluently in the patient's native language.

## The Informational Brochure

An informative brochure strategically placed in your office is one communication vehicle that indicates to patients that you have thought a lot about what you are trying to say to them. The brochure should address general health issues and pro-mote your practice. The messages must be clear, crisp, understandable, simple, and complete. If you have a diverse patient population, you might want to have brochures translated into their native language. The look and feel (design and colors) should relay what you want the reader to think and feel about your practice and services – bright, cheery, and caring. Have enough copies available so patients can take one home for themselves, their family, and friends.

There are many websites that offer advice on creation of brochures for medical practices. A local graphic artist can help you put together a low-cost, simple, informative, tri-fold, four-color brochure. It can be printed at a local copy shop to keep the cost down.

## Health History Forms

In most doctors' offices, patients are asked to fill out a health history form as soon as they check in. Be sure these forms are at an appropriate reading and compre-hension level for your populations.. Research indicates that more than 90 million people in the United States have difficulty filling out the forms in doctor's offices.[1] Best practices dictate that you should mail or email patient history forms to your patients and have them filled out and emailed, faxed, or mailed back in advance of their visit. You should review the completed form before the patient's appointment so the time you spend together is devoted to addressing specific problems and answering questions. If you have a patient portal these details can be handled online, in advance of the visit. The result of this advance information is a better patient experience.

If you insist on having the patient complete or update their medical history at the time of the visit, then build a few minutes into your schedule to read that informa-tion before seeing the patient. No matter how tight your schedule, you should come to the patient visit completely informed and ready to discuss the prevailing issues. From the patient point of view, being asked to respond to the same question multi-ple times creates the impression of wasted time and effort.

### The Face-to-Face Encounter

Lack of communication can often result in a dissonance between a doctor's and the patient's perception of their relationship. To the doctor, illness is a disease process that can be measured and understood through tests and clinical observations. To the patient, illness is a disrupted life. While doctors must keep up with the latest practices in medicine, it is imperative for them to address the humanistic side of medicine as well, understanding the patient's feelings. The doctor views a problem as a "find it and fix it" situation. A patient wants to be heard, understood, and viewed as an individual with a unique situation rather than just *another case.* Listening is the key to successful patient-provider relations. Listening means devoting full attention to the patient, hearing what the patient has to say and paying close attention to the way it is said, including non-verbal cues, such as voice inflections and facial expressions. Appropriate responses include kind, caring expressions of understanding, and repeating what you have heard so the patient knows you understand.

### Guidelines for proper communication at an office visit:

- Read the patient's chart before seeing the individual.
- Greet the patient with a warm handshake and a smile.
- Establish the reason for the visit with a warm, caring tone.
- Outline the agenda for the visit — tell the patient exactly what to expect.
- Make a personal connection by referencing something important to the patient that they have listed in their history or is relevant to their lives.
- Elicit information from the patient about their health problems – not only the physical/physiological factors but also the psychosocial/emotional factors.
- Discuss treatment options and explain their rationales.
- Discuss how the health problem(s) affect the individual's lifestyle and family.
- Encourage patients to open up and discuss their feelings by asking questions. Give them your undivided attention so they know you really care.
- Check your posture and body language to be sure that you appear receptive: sitting down and making eye contact are critical.
- Work on establishing trust so the patient will take your advice and follow it.
- Develop a system to communicate test results to your patients and let them know the details of the system.

- Respect patients for their knowledge of their illness and their problems.
- Provide patients with resources so they can learn more about their illness.
- Work together as partners to manage chronic or acute conditions.
- Clarify any misunderstandings or confusion before you end the visit.
- Review next steps for both the patient and the physician.

During the visit, focus your complete attention on the patient, ignoring phone calls and email, and making a concerted effort not to look at a clock or a watch. Although you have to take notes while the patient is talking in order to have an accurate medical record, you must balance that need with the essential requirement of focusing your attention on the patient. That comes with practice and a truly empathetic attitude. A shoulder shrug, lack of eye contact, a hand gesture – the nonverbal behavior of the physician – will influence not only the patient's satisfaction with the clinical visit but the patient's compliance with the doctor's instructions.

Research and literature reviews find that that over half the people who use medications do not use them correctly.[2] Since 1982, the National Council on Patient Information and Education (NCPIE) has focused on raising awareness about the role of the physician in engaging proper communication to promote safe, appropriate use of medicines.[3] It is imperative that you communicate the importance of adherence and make sure that your patients understand the consequences if they do not follow the regimen.

## Follow-up Communications

After the patient has left your office, you cannot assume that is the end of your need to communicate until the next visit, six months or a year away. You must have a plan for staying in touch with patients on a regular basis and following up with their questions and inquiries. There are a variety of strategies, though some approaches may work better for you than others.

## Telephone Communications

The traditional method that doctors have used when patients contact them with a question or a problem between visits is to call back on the telephone. However, telephone tag is a very unsatisfactory way to engage in patient-centered communications. It is irritating to patients and time-consuming for doctors. Too often the connection is never made and patient's questions go unanswered. That situation can lead to serious complications down the road. Instruct your patients to page you in an emergency, and provide them with the pager number. Advise your patients on how to distinguish between a genuine emergency and a less urgent medical need. Provide some guidelines that apply directly to the individual patient. Telephone tag is one reason why so many patients end up going to a hospital emergency room unnecessarily.

The prevalence of cellular telephones may alleviate some of the problems with telephone tag. Most likely you, and many of your patients, carry a cell phone, which reduces the need to sit and wait at home for a return call. However, many physicians are reluctant to give out their cell phone number to patients – and for good reason: there is no one to filter these calls. Physicians need to carefully manage their time and retain some degree of personal privacy; though helpful at times, the use of cell phones may not be ideal for all physicians.

## Snail Mail vs. Email and Patient Portals

Another traditional way doctors communicate with patients, especially to report on test results is to send a letter — often weeks and sometimes months after the tests were done. This mode of communication is often slow, and can cause much anguish to patients who want to know their results quickly. Depending on your patient load, mailing may also be labor intensive, particulary for smaller offices with limited staff and time to undertake all the paperwork required of them. Much more rapid communication is now available via email and patient portals.

### Email

Modern physicians need to use modern tools of communication – email and online options. Conventional email is used by almost everyone to communicate with business associates, family, and friends. Because it is inexpensive or free, and available "24-7," email is a direct, albeit asynchronous, means of contact between patients and doctors. It enables quick and efficient follow-up without the constraints of time pressure or the irritation of telephone tag. By its very nature, email encourages concise messages, permits quick response, and facilitates a dialogue, essential in good doctor-patient communication. Email is particularly effective in treating patients with chronic conditions such as diabetes, hypertension, and congestive heart failure. Using email, these patients can send daily or weekly updates of test results, enabling the physician to easily monitor their condition and make necessary changes in their medication or diet. Email allows patients to send graphical images so that wounds, rashes, and other external injuries can be viewed and resolved often without the need for an office visit. All of this results in better quality medicine for the patient.

### The Privacy Pitfall

You are probably well aware of the Health Insurance Portability and Accountability Act (HIPAA) and its privacy requirements (for detailed information see Chapter 9). One downside of using email for patient communications is that privacy could be compromised. Because email messages are generally transmitted over the global computer network and are not usually encrypted (coded so others cannot read them), people other than the intended recipient can accidentally receive and read them. This happens most often when messages carry the wrong address. However, when employees send an email through the company server those emails can also be intercepted and read. When dealing with health issues, most patients are sensitive to the confidentiality of their discussions with their physician. Although the bulk of messages that a patient might send have a low level of sensitivity, there is a risk that a patient's information could land in the wrong hands, just as a postcard sent in the mail could land in the wrong hands. The solution is for the physician and the patient to agree on the parameters of what should be contained in an email message, what situations require a call to the doctor's page line, and what requires secure communications. Institute an email policy in your office and distribute written guidelines in your office and through your website. These guidelines may include the following:

- Do not use email for emergencies and other time-sensitive issues.

- Do not use email for sensitive information because you cannot assume that email is confidential.

- Do not use email for situations where you need a quick response because the physician response could be delayed.

- Be concise in all email communications.

- Patients should always include their name and medical record number in the subject line.

- Patients need to keep copies of email they receive from a physician.

- The doctor should also keep a copy of the email in the medical record.

- It should be understood that email messages might be shared with members of the doctor's staff where necessary or efficient.

### Patient Portals

An alternative to conventional email is the use of a patient portal. A patient portal is a secure website where you and your patients can have personal discussions and send and receive email messages, using password protection and encryption.

Though patient portal designs vary, these software programs can offer patients the opportunity to view their medical chart (if in an electronic form), including their laboratory test results.

Portal software enables your patients to request referrals and prescription renewals, which can be directed to the proper source without the doctor becoming involved unless needed. By using the portal as a communication vehicle to address non-critical issues, you will be able to devote more time to those patients who need the personal encounter. The patient portal changes the context of the face-to-face visit, and enables you to deliver care that results in an enhanced patient-provider relationship.

For patients with chronic diseases such as diabetes, heart disease, asthma, or depression, a patient portal offers a place to upload personal data, and the ability track their disease on a daily basis. All patients should be encouraged to use the portal to maintain a personal health record, which contains their medical history, all of their conditions, medications, allergies, names of their specialists, past surgeries, and test results. Many portals integrate with electronic health records to provide a complete patient record in one location, accessible to both doctor and patient. This will reduce the chance of medical error and provide a consolidated approach to patient care.

Delivering patient care using this asynchronous communication over the Internet means that doctors and their patients have a means to communicate with each other at all times. By using a portal and establishing the appropriate process among your office staff, you are able to triage many of the electronic communications for better patient interaction.

## Collaborating with Colleagues, Suppliers, and Other Providers

In a successful medical practice your communication does not end with the patient. You have to communicate with colleagues, suppliers, and other providers on patient matters and possibly on public health issues. One of the most effective and efficient ways of communicating with all of these partners is to use online technology, ideally starting with the electronic health record. Keeping an up-to-date, accurate, electronic record that can be encrypted and sent via secure email saves time, money, and aggravation. If you refer a patient to a colleague, you need to communicate all relevant information about the patient's history and current condition. You should request that you receive back a comprehensive record of the treatment provided to that patient. While sharing patient information for the delivery of care does not require patient consent, at their first visit to your office, each patient should receive and sign a HIPAA authorization regarding use of their personal health information (See chapter 9 for more information.).

Using electronic technology also enables you to send a group message to patients on a matter of public health that might affect them. A new discovery, a warning, and a reminder about flu shots can be easily posted online to every patient you see. You must make a concerted effort to collect patients' email addresses, and urge them to update their information when it changes. Those initiatives must come from the physician.

## Conclusion

The 21ˢᵗ century is a new era where medical expertise and skill are no longer enough. Communication and the use of information technology are essential for providing the best medical care available. Physicians must hone their listening and communication skills to have satisfying interaction with patients. Email and the Internet enable doctors not only to engage in messaging with patients and colleagues but also to be a part of the exciting communication opportunities that continue to open new vistas for health care providers. Electronic health records are becoming an integral part of health delivery systems, and will enable doctors and patients to experience better, safer, higher quality health care. All of this technology, when used with the skill and deliberation that you apply in your day to day patient care, will insure that you succeed as a doctor and your patients are given every opportunity for good health.

## Case Study/Communication Practicum

### I. Patient–Physician Communication

Review the two scenarios below and determine what communication elements are incorrectly handled.

#### Scenario One

*Jim is a 73-year-old man with diabetes, high blood pressure, and questionable kidney function. He calls his primary care physician because he has had a persistent cough for about a week. The doctor's assistant schedules him for a visit two days later. At the visit, the doctor examines Jim and diagnoses a bronchial infection. He checks Jim's paper chart where he looks over Jim's medications and reviews his notes about drug allergies. He writes out a prescription for an antibiotic, which Jim carries to his pharmacy where he is informed that his health plan will not cover this particular drug. While Jim waits, they call the doctor, whom they cannot reach. They advise Jim to return the next day. Meanwhile, they keep trying to call the doctor.*

*Jim goes back the next day, but the doctor still has not responded. He goes home and waits for the pharmacy to notify him that they have filled a prescription for an alternative medication. Two days later the prescription is filled. Jim takes his first dose of the medication and spends the entire night vomiting. He calls the doctor in the morning and the doctor prescribes a different antibiotic which makes him very sleepy. He stops that medication and two days later is admitted to the hospital with pneumonia.*

### Scenario Two

*Jim, a 73-year-old man with diabetes, high blood pressure, and questionable kidney function, sends his doctor an email about a persistent cough. The doctor replies, asking Jim to come in to be checked, and within a couple of hours Jim is at the doctor's office. After examining Jim and confirming the presence of a bronchial infection, the doctor logs into his computer and accesses the medication database. The computer returns with a list of three antibiotics to treat the infection, one of which is flagged as unacceptable to Jim's health plan. The computer searches the other two medications to see if any of them will cause an interaction with Jim's diabetes drugs. The doctor chooses the only available option compatible with Jim's medications. He electronically transmits the prescription to Jim's local pharmacy which also prints a concise set of instructions for Jim to use in administering the drug, and a warning on potential side effects. While Jim is at the doctor's office, they bring up his electronic medical record, and go over any other problems. Jim recovers from the infection without any adverse events.*

Nothing in either of these scenarios indicates that the doctor did anything wrong, or did not follow standard procedure. However, the outcome was not the same. What led to a better situation for Jim?

1. Email got Jim's message to the doctor faster and more efficiently with the result that he was seen sooner, medicated sooner and healed faster.

2. Email also sent the prescription directly to the pharmacy to be filled. Jim did not have to physically go to the pharmacy until the medication was ready for him.

3. Use of an electronic medical record enabled the doctor to review all of the medications Jim was on and check for drug-to-drug interactions so there would not be any errors.

4. The e-prescribing system provided Jim with a comprehensive set of instructions about how to take the antibiotic medication with the other medications he currently uses.

5. Jim's visit with the doctor was a better experience. The doctor did not have to spend a portion of the visit searching through the paper chart for information on Jim's medications. As a result, he was able to give Jim more quality time discussing his problems.

6. A good outcome for Jim depended upon fast, efficient communication and administering of medication. In the first scenario, the medication was not given for several days and Jim stopped taking it because he suffered side effects. Thus he landed in the hospital even sicker than he had been when he saw the doctor.

## II. Communication Best Practices

The 21ˢᵗ century physician is constantly barraged with the need to communicate with insurance companies, with Medicare and other government agencies, with attorneys, with colleagues and especially with patients. Most research shows that patient complaints typically have little to do with quality of care but are focused on better service – shorter wait in the office, a friendly staff, and a caring, compassionate physician who knows how to communicate. Your skills as a communicator directly affect your success as a health care professional.

The following suggestions for good communication practices should increase the efficiency of your practice and avoid disconnect between what you are trying to convey and what others will come away with. Because you have a short time – generally 15 minutes – to spend with each patient, you want to make each of those minutes count.

### Clarity

With all of the communications you are asked to generate each day – patient letters, medical forms, emails – it is essential that all your messages are clear. To check a document for clarity, ask these questions:

- Are equal points given equal emphasis?

- Do you have proper transition between thoughts?

- Are you using medical terminology that an average non-medical person will understand?

- Do you tend to repeat the same thing over and over?

### Concise

Are you using as few words as possible to get your total thought across? Rule of thumb in written English is no more than 15 words in a sentence – and 75% of those words should consist of one syllable.

### Complete

Have you included everything that you need to communicate? Are all of the relevant ideas, data, and observations in the document?

### Tone

Is your tone natural, courteous, and positive vs. stilted, abrupt, hurried, and negative? Do people infer from your tone that you are willing to listen with undivided attention?

### Voice

Are your communications sent from the patient viewpoint?

### Format

Appearances count. Communications must be easy to read, positioned correctly on the page and set up in a format that delivers a positive impression.

### Presentation Skills

- Look friendly, smile.
- Make eye contact; don't look at your notes or a clock on the wall.
- Open with a question that captures attention.
- Present a quick overview of what you are going to talk about.
- Introduce yourself by relaying an anecdote or sharing a story.
- Invite questions.
- Explain clearly.
- Be persuasive – talk about benefits and results.
- Speak in short phrases.
- Gesture naturally – keep your hands relaxed at your sides and use them for emphasis where needed.
- Always speak truthfully and admit when you do not know an answer, but offer to do research and get an answer.

## Suggested Readings/ Websites

### Books (can be viewed at www.amazon.com)

Barnard S, Hughes KT, St. James D, and Health Care Communication Group. *Writing, Speaking and Communication Skills for Health Professionals*. New Haven, CT: Yale University Press; 2001.

Goodman N, Edwards MB, Black A. *Medical Writing A Prescription for Clarity*, 3rd ed. Cambridge, UK: Cambridge University Press; 2006.

Herzlinger R. *Market Driven Health Care: Who Wins, Who Loses in the Transformation of America's Largest Service Industry*. New York, NY: Perseus Books; 1997.

Hughes, Mark, *Buzz Marketing: Get People to Talk About Your Stuff*. New York, NY: Penguin Group; 2005.

Marram Van Servellan G. *Communication Skills for the Health Care Professional*. Gaithersburg, MD: Aspen Publishers Inc.; 1997.

Peters P. *The Ultimate Marketing Toolkit: Ads that Attract, Customer Brochures that Create Buzz, Websites that Wow*. Avon, MA: Adams Media Corporation, F&W Publications Company; 2006.

### Websites

Provides a 12-step marketing guide for a professional practice: www.cypressmedia.net

Outlines the seven sins that professional services groups commit when marketing online: www.marketingprofs.com

Search engine to find the best medical websites: www.google.com.top/health/medicine

Centers for Disease Control and Prevention website with the most current information on public health issues, disease control, and information on specific diseases. Good resource for an e-health newsletter: www.cdc.gov

Internet Healthcare Coalition — an independent, non-industry, website that focuses on information to educate health care professionals on the uses of the Internet for health care related issues: www.ihcc.com

Website sponsored by the National Heart Lung and Blood Institute with definitive reliable, current information on these conditions: www.nhlbi.nhi.gov

Sponsored by the National Cancer Institute — good reference for physicians to recommend to cancer patients: www.nci.gov

Sponsored by the National Library of Medicine and the National Institute of Health — includes general health care topics and other relevant data. Good resources for an e-health newsletter and link for patients to look up drug information or other health related issues: www.medlineplus.gov

National Council on Patient Information and Education: www.talkaboutrx.org/med_compliance.jsp

## References

1. Committee on Health Literacy Board on Neuroscience and Behavioral Health. Nielsen-Bohlman L, Panzer AM, Kindig DA, eds. *Health Literacy: A Prescription to End Confusion*. Washington, DC: National Academies Press; 2004.

2. Haynes RB, Yao X, Degani A, Kripalani S, Garg A, McDonald HP. Interventions for helping patients to follow prescriptions for medications. *Cochrane Database Syst Rev.* 2005 Oct 19;(4): CD000011.

3. National Council on Patient Information and Education. Available at: http://www.talkaboutrx.org/med_compliance.jsp. Accessed August 18, 2006

# Section 3
# The Practice Environment

# Chapter 8

## Risk Management in Medical Practice Today

Rosemary Gafner, EdD

### Executive Summary

"Risk management" refers to the process of analyzing exposure to risk and determining how to best handle such exposure. In the medical environment, risk management involves review of communication skills, documentation practices, interaction with colleagues, and systems analysis, to ensure that physicians perform their duties in the manner most likely to result in positive outcomes and improved patient safety. Attention to these components reduces the likelihood that a physician may be sued for malpractice. This chapter provides an admittedly brief introduction to key areas of medical risk management:

- Malpractice basics, and what every physician needs to know to protect himself or herself from litigation;

- Communication as a risk management tool;

- Medical office risk factors;

- Informed consent; and

- Medical record documentation.

### Learning Objectives

After reading this chapter, you should be able to:

1. Name the four elements of malpractice.

2. Discuss the risk management implications of communication with colleagues and with patients.

3. Identify common areas of risk in the medical office setting.

4. Document patient care in a defensible manner.

**Keywords**

communication; documentation; liability; malpractice; medical records; negligence; risk management

## Introduction

"Risk management" is one approach to reducing the frequency and severity of malpractice suits. The practice of risk management involves identifying problem practice patterns or behaviors (those which affect the commencement or pursuit of a claim), then eliminating or controlling them to reduce the likelihood that a malpractice claim will be filed. Medical record charting, patient scheduling, prescription writing, and communicating with patients are only a few of the common activities that may affect the likelihood or course of litigation.

## The Basic Elements of Malpractice

Although some patients may perceive that malpractice has occurred when there is a poor or unexpected outcome, physicians know that's not true. A bad outcome, in and of itself, does not warrant a claim of malpractice. In fact, a physician's act, error or omission need not warrant a claim of malpractice, as long as the act, error or omission was reasonable under the circumstances.

For our purposes, medical malpractice may be defined as any deviation from the accepted medical standard of care that causes injury to a patient.[1] To prove that malpractice took place, the plaintiff should be able to prove, by a preponderance of the credible evidence, four elements: duty, breach of duty, causation, and damages. If any one of these four is not proven, there should be no judgment of medical malpractice; the defense must negate only one element in order to prevail.

### Duty

Physicians do not have a legal duty to treat anyone who walks into the office. In order for a legal duty to exist, there must be a physician-patient relationship. This relationship is usually established when the patient retains the doctor, but in some instances the relationship can be established by a third party, including a partner or a colleague with whom you consult. And, increasingly in the era of managed care, a physician–patient relationship can be established by an HMO or network to which you belong.

**Consults and referrals.** To avoid inhibiting the free exchange of knowledge between physicians, the courts have generally held that informal consultations do not create a physician–patient relationship.[2] When approached by a colleague for your opinion regarding a patient, you can reduce your own liability without alienating your colleagues by making sure that all parties clearly understand whether you're giving gratuitous advice or assuming an active role in patient care. If the latter, a duty is established. If the former, emphasize that you are responding in general terms only, and ask your colleague to request a formal consultation if he or she wants more specific information.

### Breach of Duty (Negligence)

Once duty has been established, a plaintiff must demonstrate that the physician failed to render the required *standard of care*, traditionally defined as that level of care a reasonably prudent physician would provide under similar circumstances.[3] Failure to do so results in the breach of duty, which constitutes negligence.

Who establishes the standard of care? In court, expert witnesses for each side will give their opinions regarding the standard of care. Standards set by specialty societies also are being promulgated as the "standard of care." And more and more, practice parameters (also known as practice guidelines, practice policies, and clinical pathways) are used as evidence of the standard of care. It's important to remember that such guidelines are designed to assist—not govern—your clinical decision making.

Where do parameters come from? They are developed by specialty societies, the federal and state governments, academic medical centers, hospitals, and other sources. They usually have their source in the medical literature and hospital studies, which then are adapted to local practice. Evidence-based medicine also provides material that may be incorporated into practice parameters.

### Causation

Next, it must be proven that the breach of duty was the cause of the patient's injury – in other words, that the physician's failure to adhere to the standard of care caused a situation or event that resulted in harm to the patient.

The jury can find that a physician failed to conform to the standard of care, yet decide that this failure was not the cause of injury. In *Neal v. Welker*, the patient fell and sought treatment at a hospital emergency room. The defendant physician failed to discover a skull fracture and, after prescribing aspirin, sent the patient home to bed. The patient suffered severe brain damage and eventually died. The defense prevailed, however, despite the defendant's negligence, by showing that proper treatment (i.e., timely diagnosis and treatment of the skull fracture) would have made no difference in outcome.[4]

### Damages

The final element that the plaintiff must prove is damages, which is the amount of money a court or jury awards as compensation for a tort or breach of contract. There are different types of damages. *Monetary or economic* damages include money that the plaintiff must spend in order to rectify or manage the injury allegedly caused by the physician. Included would be the cost of items, which are readily quantifiable: repeated surgeries, round-the-clock nursing care, institutionalization, the cost of household help, special equipment or clothing, etc. Monetary damages also include money lost due to the plaintiff's inability to work. *Non-economic* damages include compensation for the plaintiff and/or the plaintiff's family for alleged pain and suffering or mental anguish. Other types of non-economic damage are alleged loss of consortium and interference with the ability to enjoy life. *Punitive or exemplary* damages are money sought for the purpose of punishing the defendant for an intentional tort or gross negligence, or for the purpose of deterring others from taking a similar approach to patient management.

## Communication as a Risk Management Tool

Much of the above material focused on the technical nature of the physician-patient relationship, or duty. However, the interpersonal side of the relationship is also a factor in risk management. Physician-patient relationships play an enormous part in the patient's decision to sue. Some studies suggest that as many as 63% of suits are based on communication issues: failure to keep the family informed; the patient's desire for revenge; or the perception that the physician or other members of the health care team were avoiding the family.[5]

"Poor relationships with patients" and "poor communication" play a surprisingly large role in a patient's decision to sue. Of course, patients don't sue exclusively because their doctors don't communicate well, but if things go wrong during the course of treatment, or if there is an unexpected outcome, poor relationships make it much more inviting for the patient to file suit. In fact, it has been stated that "the critical variable in the filing of a malpractice claim is neither clinical error nor iatrogenic injury: it is the patient or the patient's family."[6] A noted plaintiff's attorney agrees, saying that many patients turn to lawyers when they feel they can't get information, or believe the doctor is avoiding them or giving them the runaround. "The family wants answers," says Jim Perdue. He tells doctors that the best way to avoid being involved in a lawsuit is to maintain good patient rapport.[7]

Among common patient complaints related to communication are the following:

**"He interrupts me too often."** In fact, some studies have shown that the average length of time a doctor allows a patient to speak before interrupting is only *18 seconds*.[8] Why is it so common for physicians to interrupt? Most physicians are taught to keep patient interviews on track and, if they perceive that the patient is starting to ramble, they interrupt to bring the conversation back on course. However, it is important to remember that patients, like most of us, are brought up to believe that it is not polite to interrupt, and they may well perceive the physician's interruption as rude, even if it is clinically necessary.

**"She doesn't answer my questions."** This is one of the most frequent factors cited in a patient's decision to file a suit. When the patient or family member has a question that isn't answered to their satisfaction, or if they feel ignored, they become anxious, then angry, and may think that the physician is ignoring them because there is something to hide. In such cases they may seek answers in the medical record, which often leads to outside evaluation by attorneys and hired experts—evaluation that can lead to litigation if the medical record suggests that care was questionable.

**"She doesn't spend enough time with me."** A sick patient is an anxious, nervous human being who longs for reassurance, or at least acknowledgment from the physician that efforts are being made to make things better. However, if the physician seems to give the patient only a cursory visit, or doesn't spend "enough" time, the patient may resent that. Although the doctor may be able to do everything that's needed during that time, the patient probably will feel shortchanged—especially if he is presented with a bill that doesn't adequately reflect the *perceived value* of the amount of time spent with the doctor.

**"The doctor doesn't <u>listen</u> to me."** This complaint underlies most other grievances. If the patient's question is ignored or answered flippantly, or if the patient wants to hear about what's happening to him but the doctor doesn't stay long enough, the underlying perception may be that the physician is a poor listener.

A point to remember: many patients may complain to your staff instead of you. They may not want to bother you with what they think is a personal perception; or they fear that you will become angry if they bring up something negative.

## Countering Complaints

The above are common patient complaints that can produce relationship problems if allowed to progress. In addition to posing risks, they can also affect the patient's *perception* of the quality of care. Here are some tips to counter them and some pitfalls to avoid.

**Show that you're listening.** Of the four traditional communication skills, we spend most of our time listening and the least amount of time reading and writing. However, the time spent learning how to do each is reversed. In school, we're taught reading and writing from the first grade up, but listening is seldom a part of our formal education. Why? Possibly because there's a tendency to equate "listening" with "hearing," but the two are very different. Listening takes effort, and there are definite factors which get in the way of effective listening. For example:

**Thinking about what you will say next.** This type of dysfunctional communication is called a duologue. When one person speaks it is very common for the listener to hear the first part of what is said, and then start to formulate his response while the speaker is still talking. As a result, the listener doesn't really hear the last part of what is said and may miss a critical part of the conversation.

**Keying in on facts and details while ignoring the broader message.** In medicine you must gather as much information as you can, but it is easy to let facts get in the way of understanding the patient's overall message. This is a learned habit: our educational system encourages paying attention to facts and details by testing us on them as we go through school. As a result, when a patient says, "I first noticed these symptoms about two weeks ago; it was right after I got back from vacation," the physician may zero in on the fact ("two weeks ago") and overlook the part about the vacation. Doing so may make a difference if the vacation site or events may have played a part in the patient's symptoms.

**Faking attention.** With increased emphasis on good patient relations as both a practice management and risk management technique, most doctors today know the power of listening. Unfortunately, knowing what to do and actually doing it are often quite different. While the patient is talking, many doctors may be guilty of reading the chart, making notes, or even thinking about what to say next. However, since they know they *should* be listening instead of doing these other things they may well "fake" attention, thus running the risk of missing an important piece of information or of alienating an astute patient.

**Try active listening as both a diagnostic and quality improvement tool.** Active listening is a technique that encourages the patient to talk and gives you valuable information you won't get by asking straight "yes" or "no" questions. Most listening is passive: the speaker talks and the listener just sits there. Active listening takes things up a notch. The active listener takes part in the conversation, by periodically summarizing what the speaker says, searching for content, and not judging. Here's how it works:

**Ask the patient an open-ended question,** one that can't be answered "yes" or "no" and requires the patient to think before responding. When she responds, use nonverbal cues that show you are paying attention: nod, frown, raise an eyebrow, or demonstrate other "attending" behaviors. When the patient is through, paraphrase what she said by feeding it back to her, using your own words to summarize the meaning.

**When you are actively listening, watch out for traps.** It's easy to get caught up in what the patient is saying, or to judge or evaluate what she is saying, or to let your mind wander. Doing so will sabotage your active listening efforts and you will probably appear insincere to your patient. Active listening is appropriate for counseling situations, but you may not want to use it during yes/no interactions, such as taking a history.

**Spend quality time.** As noted above, a major patient complaint is that the physician doesn't spend enough time with the patient. This complaint is rooted in perception, such as the perception that the patient doesn't get enough time and attention from the physician to justify the bill. One way to maximize the quality of time with patients is to *sit down.* Pull up a chair within easy conversational distance, and look at the patient while you're asking questions and getting answers. Do this either before or after the physical examination, and the impact of your behavior will go a long way toward improving relationships.

## The Impact of Health Literacy

Another factor that can affect your communication with patients is their level of health literacy—the ability to access, comprehend, and utilize health care information. Patients with low health literacy are at increased risk of poor outcomes because they are less likely to make use of health care knowledge at every stage in which it could help them. Because they are less aware of the risk factors for a disease, they are more likely to expose themselves to it. Literacy is more than just the ability to decode written words—it's also the ability to comprehend them well enough to understand the information presented, and act on it. Using this definition, the 1993 National Adult Literacy Survey estimated that between 40 million and 44 million American adults could not read a medication label or simple written instructions.[9] An additional 50 million were found to be only marginally literate. This means that over 90 million American adults, or 37% of the population, lack functional reading skills.

What can a busy physician do to counter risks of patients' low health literacy? Some tips:

**Always perform an oral review** with the patient of any forms that he or she filled out, and verify the information given. If a patient doesn't understand a question, he's unlikely to give an accurate answer.

**With your staff, ensure that the patient knows the answers** to three key questions at the end of every visit: "What is my main problem?", "what do I need to do?", and "why is it important for me to do this?" If the patient knows the answers to those questions, he's much more likely to comply with your treatment and become involved in his care.

**Use "teach back" to verify understanding.** After you explain a topic to the patient, have him feed back to you, in his own words, the essence of his understanding. That way you can correct any misunderstandings.

**Choose simple words,** like "sickness" instead of "ailment," or "work together" instead of "collaborate."

For more information on communicating with patients with low health literacy, see the references at the end of this chapter.

## Medical Office Risk Factors

Most physician-patient interactions take place not in the hospital, but in the medical office. That's why you need to pay attention to risks associated with appointments and scheduling, the patient history, the general office environment, and telephone communication.

### Appointments and Scheduling

When patients have to endure long waits, they perceive that you really don't care about them, you're indifferent to their needs, and you don't need them. No one likes feeling that way and, if something goes wrong, the patient may well be predisposed to seek out reasons to "get back" at the doctor. There are risk management implications as well. For example, if there is an adverse outcome, one of the first questions asked will be, "Was the patient able to see the doctor in a timely manner?" Your appointment book or software will be a valuable aid in your defense, as long as records are maintained properly.

Missed or canceled appointments should be followed up as appropriate. Some no-shows are critical: those where a patient may suffer if treatment is delayed, or those where you must monitor medication or treatment. In these cases, always phone the patient to try to get her back in. If you can't reach the patient by phone, or if the patient refuses to come in, send a certified letter to show that you did make the effort to reschedule. Some no-shows are less important for follow-up: a new patient who skips the first appointment, for example. It's a good idea to call those patients and, if they were referred by another doctor, to notify him or her as well. Document these contacts in the medical record as well as in the appointment log.

Keep appointment logs well past the statute of limitations. If you treat only adults, keeping the logs for five years should suffice. If you treat children, keep the logs until the patient reaches his or her twentieth birthday. Keep the logs in addition to documenting no-shows or cancellations in the medical record. Note: These suggestions are for appointment logs. Medical records should be kept indefinitely.

### Taking the Patient's History

One of the most important opportunities for physician-patient interaction comes during the initial history. During this appointment you can elicit important medical clues that will enable you to plan treatment for the patient. It also provides an opportunity for the patient to evaluate the doctor as a person, based on the quality of human interaction and compassion displayed.

The history is important in medical risk management as well. Studies by the Physician Insurers Association of America (PIAA) have shown that a major problem in cases where the physician missed a diagnosis of cancer was a "serious deficiency" in doctors taking histories from their patients. For example, in 15% of cases of missed lung cancer diagnoses, the doctor did not determine if the patient had ever smoked or worked in environments where he or she might be exposed to toxic agents.[10] In 37% of breast cancer cases, a family history was not taken.[11]

Review any written history questionnaires with the patient to make sure the information is accurate. Patients who are sick or in pain can't be relied on to even read the questions carefully, let alone provide thoughtful answers. Many patients will simply respond with a "no" to all prior diseases without reading the list and some patients, as discussed early, may not even be able to read or understand the questions. Review the responses verbally with the patient to make sure that you really do have a useful medical history.

Hear the patient out while taking the history and don't interrupt. Physicians are often overworked, overbooked, and scrambling to stay on schedule. This can leave them anxious to get to the point of a patient visit. A previously-cited study found that physicians, on average, interrupted patients only 18 seconds into the explanation of the reason for the visit.[8] This is significant because patients typically have a list of several complaints or observations they would like to discuss, yet rarely get beyond the first or second before being interrupted.

Encourage the patient to bring written lists of symptoms, complaints, and questions. Patients who have a lot going on may sometimes forget important details that could be critical to your diagnosis. Written lists not only avoid this problem, but help you quickly sort through the symptoms and determine which are related and which are most important.

End the visit with an open-ended question along the lines of "Is there anything else?" or "Have we covered everything you came here for?" This demonstrates to the patient that you're genuinely concerned about providing quality care.

### Telephone Communication

The telephone has been called "one of the great instruments of malpractice." Why? One of the most important reasons is lack of documentation. Document all phone communication with patients. If you take or make a call while you are in the office, it is most convenient to pull the chart and document the call immediately. If you are away from your office, use a pocket notepad to write down the nature of the call and what action you took. Alternatively, use a pocket dictation device and have the tape transcribed when you get back to the office. Allow no exceptions: all staff and the doctor should adhere to the same documentation rules.

Other problems arise when the two parties can't make immediate contact. That's when messages are left, and there is potential for miscommunication. Often messages are lost. Sometimes they're received by the wrong person.

Leaving messages on answering devices presents a potential for breach of confidentiality. You don't know who will hear your recorded message. Try to deal with the answering machine problem before it arises. Ask the patient how she wants you to handle messages if you need to phone her. Or, on your patient intake form, have a place where the patient tells you how to handle phone messages. If you must leave a message and don't have instructions from the patient on how to proceed, it's best to leave a call back message only: "This message is for Ellen Powers. Please call Susan at Dr. Connor's office at 932-9980."

Another issue is that of returned phone calls. It's seldom that a patient calls and the matter is handled right away. More frequently, the patient is told that the call will be returned. If that's the case, make sure patients are told when to expect the callback – after 5:00 p.m. or over the lunch hour, for example. Many a patient has become frustrated and angry when told, "The doctor is with a patient and will call you back." Unless told otherwise, the patient will likely think the call will come much more quickly – very likely, in ten minutes or so.

## Informed Consent

Informed consent is a process, not a form or an event, although many physicians and other health care professionals treat it as an event. There are two models of informed consent. The process model involves dialogue and two-way communication resulting in an educational and team-oriented outcome. The event model equates obtaining informed consent with obtaining a signature on a form.

Make informed consent a shared decision. Follow the process model by discussing with the patient the risks and benefits of a proposed treatment or procedure; alternatives to a proposed treatment or procedure; risks and benefits of the alternatives; and risks and benefits of doing nothing.[12] Don't just tell the patient what to expect; ask the patient to feed back to you his or her understanding of what you said. Ask the patient to describe the procedure or tell you what he thinks will happen, for example.

When discussing medical alternatives, do it in language the patient can understand. If the patient doesn't understand English well, speak to him in his own language or get a translator. Even if the patient does understand English, speak to him in jargon-free language. Many times patients are intimidated by their doctors and, if the physician is speaking in clinical terms, the patient may be too shy to admit that he or she doesn't understand.

Document informed consent discussions and patients' decisions, including their informed refusal of treatment, in the office record. Don't rely on the hospital to "get informed consent." All the hospital does is obtain the patient's signature on a form. It's your responsibility as physician to actually discuss the procedure and ensure the patient understands and consents. Document this in your office chart, as a supplement to any forms you may use and those the hospital uses.

Responsibility for the informed consent process rests with you, the physician, and cannot be delegated. However, you may delegate the task of getting forms signed to a nurse or other assistant. This should only be done after you have discussed the procedure, alternatives, and risks with the patient.

If a patient refuses to submit to treatment, document that as informed refusal. Forms are available to facilitate this documentation and the patient should sign and date the form.

## Medical Record Documentation

The medical record serves multiple purposes. First, it's a communication tool. When you document your actions in the chart, you're essentially communicating with subsequent treaters and co-providers about your findings and treatment. Second, the record provides justification for billing and payment decisions. If an insurer finds that a patient's record doesn't justify a claim for payment, the claim may be delayed or denied. Finally, the record is evidence of the care provided, in case the patient wants to file suit against you or a hospital. In that case, if the record shows that care was proper, chances are that no suit will be filed. But if care was not well documented, leaving gaps for a plaintiff's expert to fill in, the case will be much harder to defend, even if the care was appropriate. Medical records are pivotal in determining the course of a malpractice suit, and it's useful to list the characteristics of a defensible record.

### Legibility

Consequences of illegible entries range from inconvenient to deadly. If another practitioner can't read your entry, he or she will have to guess about what you meant. For example, if you intend to write, "Normal exam," but the entry is misread as "No exam," you may be faulted for having failed to conduct an exam when one was warranted.

*"But I can read my writing…why do I have to worry about everyone else?"* First, the medical record is intended as a communication tool. Illegible entries are dangerous because they cannot help others who may treat the patient. And, if something does go wrong and your records are called into question, a hostile expert who attempts to interpret them will always interpret them in a way that reflects poorly on your treatment of the patient.

*"I know my writing is bad, so I dictate. Any problem with that?"* No problem at all—as long as you read the transcription to make sure it says what you intended, then initial and date the document. Don't fall into the trap of using a stamp or automatic entry that says, "Dictated but not read." If the transcriptionist made a mistake, you'd never know it; and would be liable for the error should others rely on it. Always review your notes and initial them.

### Accuracy

The defensible record does not contain entries that are vague, self-serving or subject to misinterpretation. Include only clinically relevant information. Accuracy also requires the use of precise words. Words like "excessive" or "severe" mean different things to different people. Try to avoid entries such as, "Excessive bleeding was noted." To some, that might mean a liter or more of blood; to others, it may mean a few drops. To avoid the possibility of confusion, quantify amounts whenever possible: "Approximately 40 ccs of blood were lost."

### Complete

It's important that your total care of the patient be documented in your office chart. If you order a test, the test results should be in the chart, initialed and dated to show you reviewed the results. Similarly, if you order a consultation, the consultant's report should be in the chart, also initialed and dated. Include evidence of informed consent and notes regarding patient hospitalizations. This protects you in the event the hospital chart is lost or changed. Remember: omissions provide the opportunity for a plaintiffs' attorney to build his own case about what happened.

### Original

The defensible medical record contains only original, unaltered entries. Any errors should be corrected by drawing a single line through the incorrect entry, then writing the correction above the lined-out entry. The correction should be dated and initialed by the person making the correction. Under no circumstances use correction fluid or ink to obliterate the original text. No matter how well-meaning your intention, obliterations will work against you, suggesting that you intended to "doctor" the record. Always correct errors so the original, incorrect entry is still readable.

## Conclusion

No one who dreams of being a physician wants to consider the darker side of medical practice: the risk of being sued by someone who believes you're delivering poor or even dangerous patient care. However, the real world is such that those risks exist every day. By practicing prudent risk management, including the tips included in this chapter, you'll be better equipped to protect yourself again such allegations – and in the process, better protect your patient.

## Case Study

Marcia Olson* was 22 years old when she first started seeing Dr. James Zeller, an OB/Gyn. She saw him regularly over the next eight years for routine gynecological care, and she was frequently diagnosed as suffering from cervical inflammation.

---

* All are fictional names.

In January 1991, Ms. Olson went to Dr. Zeller's office for her yearly exam. Dr. Zeller was out of the country, and Dr. Zeller's partner, Dr. George Kleimann, examined Marcia and performed a complete physical and Pap smear. The pathology report indicated that the sample revealed inflammation and possible koilocytosis, an abnormal and suspicious finding that requires a follow-up Pap smear within six months. The results of the Pap smear were sent by the pathology lab to Dr. Zeller's office.

In June 1991, Ms. Olson returned to Dr. Zeller's office for a routine exam. She was not notified of the abnormal Pap smear results, nor did she receive a follow-up Pap smear, despite the previous suspicious test results and despite the fact that during this exam, her physician noted that her cervix had an abnormal appearance.

In March 1992, Dr. Zeller again examined Ms. Olson, and performed another Pap test that revealed keratinizing squamous cell carcinoma. On April 13, she underwent a laparotomy, which revealed a 2 cm. iliac node in the left pararectal and paravesical spaces containing metastatic squamous cell carcinoma. Despite chemotherapy and radiation, she died at age 32. She and her husband had no children.

## Study/Discussion Questions

1. How should Drs. Kleimann and Zeller have communicated with each other regarding Marcia Olson's treatment?

2. What information should either or both physicians have conveyed to Ms. Olson so that she could assume an acceptable level of responsibility for her care?

3. What office procedures may have contributed to this poor outcome?

4. What duty do consultants have to communicate with referring physicians regarding unexpected test results?

## Suggested Readings/Websites

### Printed Materials

Yedidia MJ, Gillespie CC, Kachur E, et al. Effect of communications training on medical student performance. JAMA. 2003;290:1157-1165.

Kohn L, Corrigan J, Donaldson M, eds. *To Err Is Human. Building a Safer Health System.* Institute of Medicine. Washington, DC: National Academies Press; 2000.

Epstein RM. Communication between primary care physicians and consultants. *Arch Fam Med*. 1995;4:403-409.

Helmreich RL, Schaefer HG. *Team performance in the operating room*. In: Bogner MS, ed. *Human Error in Medicine*. Hillsdale, NJ: Lawrence Erlbaum Assoc; 1994:179-196.

Leape LL. Error in medicine. JAMA. 1994;272:1851-1857.

Herz DA, Looman JE, Lewis SK. Informed consent: is it a myth? *Neurosurgery*. 1992;30:453-458.

**Internet and web sites:**

Medical Risk Management, Inc.: http://www.medrisk.com.

Yale-New Haven Hospital Issues in Risk Management:
http://info.med.yale.edu/caim/risk/contents.html

Agency for Healthcare Research and Quality. Making Health Care Safer: A Critical Analysis of Patient Safety Practices: http://www.ahcpr.gov/clinic/ptsafety/

Partnership for Patient Safety: http://www.p4ps.org/

# References

1. Louisiana Medical Mutual Insurance Company. *Malpractice: Don't Be a Target*. Metairie, LA: LAMMICO; 2000.

2. *Ranier vs. Grossman*, 31 Cal App. 3rd 539, Ct. of App. 2nd Dist., April 11, 1973.

3. Harney DM. *Medical Malpractice*. Charlottesville, VA: The Michie Company; 2001, 506.

4. *Neal v. Welker*, 426 S.W.2nd 476 (Ky. App. 1968).

5. Hickson GB, Clayton EW, Githens PB, Sloan FA. Factors that prompted families to file medical malpractice claims following perinatal injuries. JAMA. 1992;267:1359-1363.

6. Orlikoff JE, Vanagunas, AM. *Malpractice Prevention and Liability Control for Hospitals*. Chicago, IL: American Hospital Publishing; 1988, 113.

7. Perdue J. *Touched by an angel*. *The Perdue Law Firm*. Available at: http://www.perduelaw.com/sub/?contentid=o9sQeQ76fBkzWpRh66whv4dZ. Accessed August 10, 2006.

8. Beckman HB, Frankel RM. The effect of physician behavior on the collection of data. *Ann Intern Med*. 1994;101:692-696.

9. Kirsch IS, Jungeblut A, Jenkins L, Andrew Kolstad A. *Adult Literacy in America: A First Look at the National Adult Literacy Survey*. Washington, DC: U.S. Department of Education; 1993.

10. Physician Insurers Association of America. Lung Cancer Study. Lawrenceville, NJ: Physician Insurers Association of America; 2005.

11. Physician Insurers Association of America. *Breast Cancer Study.* Lawrenceville, NJ: Physician Insurers Association of America; 2002.

12. Lidz CW, Appelbaum PA, Meisel A. Two models of implementing informed consent. *Archives Int Med.* 1988; 148:1385-1389.

# Chapter 9

## Health Care and the Law

Sarah Freymann Fontenot, JD

### Executive Summary

This chapter provides an introduction to Health Law, a very broad topic, in a concise format. Although it is not an exhaustive resource, and does not constitute legal advice, it is meant to provide the reader with a list of issues for further research and consideration. More than anything, it is intended to help new physicians to become *informed* consumers of legal services.

After an explanation of the breadth of Health Law, guidance is provided for how appropriate legal consultation can be obtained, with an explanation of the difference kinds of legal disputes that might involve a physician.

The discussion of specific legal issues begins with patient legal rights, focusing first on informed consent. This section includes the required elements of informed consent, documentation of consent, the role of parents and other patient representatives, incompetency, consent in emergency care, and how to best obtain interpretation when obtaining consent. The second focus on patient rights is privacy rights created by the Privacy Rule of the Health Insurance Portability and Accountability Act [HIPAA]. The four privacy rights of all patients are explained, as are actions physicians must take to be HIPAA compliant. Penalties for failure to comply are explained, and directions are provided for how to obtain free, accurate HIPAA guidance.

The chapter includes a discussion of the common elements of tort reform initiatives.

Corporate and regulatory issues affecting physicians are reviewed briefly, with specific examples of each, an explanation of potential liabilities in corporate and regulatory arena, and guidance on how to seek legal advice in these areas.

Finally, this chapter gives a brief nod to a very important area of health law:

medical ethics. The chapter concludes with a plea for appropriate physician lobbying and leadership in future legal interventions that could negatively impact patient care and the physician/patient relationship.

## Learning Objectives

1. Understand patients' rights under the HIPAA Privacy Rule.

2. Recognize the common elements of tort reform.

3. Consider corporate and regulatory issues related to a medical practice.

4. Learn where to get answers to health law questions.

## Keywords

antitrust; bar-designated specialty; civil penalties; corporate issues; criminal penalties; fraud and abuse; Health Insurance Portability and Accountability Act (HIPAA); HIPAA Privacy Rule; incompetency; informed consent; medical ethics; mental health care record; parental rights; patient rights under HIPAA; physician advocacy; protected health information; regulatory issues; tort reform

## Introduction

### The Scope of Health Law

Health law is a very broad topic. The field extends from patient rights to lawsuits involving claims of negligence; from compliance with multiple state and federal regulations to a physician's response to a request to end a patient's life.

Issues involving "health law" could land you in court and needing a lawyer's assistance. If you are in a civil court, you are being sued by another private party for an alleged harm. Medical malpractice is certainly the biggest concern, but civil suits could also include claims brought against you by a disgruntled ex-employee, contract disputes with a managed care company, or issues involving hazardous conditions on your property.

If you lose in civil court, you face financial damages, and maybe even punitive damages. You could also face a court order or injunction, requiring you to re-hire an employee or repair a dangerous parking lot. Civil claims are what you are insured for, through your own personal liability insurance against malpractice claims and other insurance policies addressing your role as an employer and as a property owner.

You could also find yourself in a criminal court, where your concern, understandably, is the potential of serving jail time and/or paying large fines. What could subject you to criminal charges? Claims of patient abuse can rise to a criminal level; most wrongful deaths are resolved on the civil side but criminal claims against physicians for murder are not impossible (think physician-assisted suicide).

Violations of the federal and state laws may have both civil and criminal components. Stark is only civil in nature, but fraud and abuse, kickbacks and even Health Insurance Portability and Accountability Act (HIPAA) have both civil and criminal penalties attached for violators.[1]

While all of these topics are discussed, this chapter is not meant to be an exhaustive reference, nor does it constitute legal advice. The purposes of this chapter are to leave you with an appreciation for the breadth of health law, and a respect for the significant implications of health law for medicine. Most of all, this chapter is meant to educate you on why you might need legal advice throughout your career, and how to find a lawyer suitable for the issue at hand.

### Finding a Lawyer

Few, if any, "Health Lawyers" practice in all aspects of the field. When seeking legal advice, you need to find a lawyer with expertise in the appropriate area of the law. If your state has made "Health Law" a bar-designated specialty, that would be an obvious place to start. However, you will still need to inquire as to the particular emphasis and expertise of any attorney you locate. Ask around. Your specialty society or colleagues who have faced similar legal issues may have a recommendation. If you are still in residency, or if you practice close to your residency institution, lawyers who work for your *alma mater* may have a referral for you.

It is wise for physicians seeking assistance to contact the American Health Lawyers Association (www.ahla.org), which has a finder's service. Even though a lawyer may be a member of AHLA, it does not mean he or she has particular expertise in the area you need; however, it will narrow your search. When you find an attorney, interview him or her about experience, track record, and additional training. You should be able to get an estimate on fees. Ask for references, and call those references. Be a smart consumer of legal services.

## Patient Rights

Patients have many rights, including the right to be treated politely, promptly, and in a non-discriminatory manner. The reverse of the duty to practice the standard of care (see below) implies the patient has the right to be treated according to the standard of care. As discussed elsewhere in this text, the patient has a right to be treated in a safe environment with appropriately maintained equipment and by well-trained and supervised staff.

In the midst of all these rights, however, two areas deserve special attention: the patient's right to consent to care, and their privacy rights under the HIPAA Privacy Rule.[2]

### The Right to Consent to Treatment

American medicine operates within the context of "informed consent." The U.S. Supreme Court, as well as each individual state court system, has recognized the right of competent adults to consent to their own care. Consent also extends to the right to *refuse* recommended care, even if that care is necessary to save the patient's life.

This right is limited to "competent adults." There are times in any state when a minor can consent to their own care, such as in cases of suspected abuse. In the absence of any state-sanctioned exception, however, the minor's parents are given both the legal *duty* to provide adequate medical care and the *right* to consent to that care. Both parents maintain that right, unless their parental rights have been limited (often the case in divorce) or terminated (as in abuse cases) by the state. Resolution of these conflicts will rely on the court's rulings and are the sole province of the state law where you practice. (For more information regarding these rights, responsibilities, and exceptions available in your state, please consult a local authority, such as your state medical association.)

People who are not competent, such as an elderly patient with dementia or a young adult with mental retardation, require a guardian or state-recognized representative to act on their behalf. People who are in a persistent vegetative state or otherwise unable to consent for themselves will also need an appointed representative, unless they executed a document such as a Living Will when they were competent and that document is in keeping with relevant state law.

It is possible that a parent or a guardian may act in a manner deemed negligent or potentially hazardous to their child or charge; again, state law will dictate the appropriate intervention of state agencies, law enforcement officials and, ultimately, the state courts. If you believe your recommended care is being inappropriately refused by your patient's legal representative, you need to contact proper state authorities.

Regardless of age or competency, an exception to informed consent must always be made in an emergency. If the patient is at risk of loss of life or bodily function, care must be initiated, even if the person cannot speak for themselves or is not legally competent to do so. Simultaneous, aggressive attempts must be made (and documented) to contact a parent, legal guardian, or next of kin, but that should not delay necessary emergency treatment.

Having set aside all of the exceptions, following is a discussion of what constitutes "informed consent."

First of all, the patient needs to understand what is being said. There are legal mandates for providing interpreters under the Civil Rights Act,[3] U.S. Department of Health and Human Services (DHHS) Rules, the Americans with Disabilities Act (ADA),[4] and state law. Clearly "consent" requires understanding and, in many circumstances, will require an interpreter.

A family member or friend of the patient should not serve as the interpreter for purposes of consent. These people may be very helpful in obtaining a patient's history, in explaining post-operative instructions, and assisting you to understand a patient's concerns. However, the moment of consent is a legal moment. Proceeding with non-emergency treatment without consent can be the basis of a lawsuit against you. Evidence of what was said in obtaining consent can be critical. For this reason, interpreters for the consent process should be impartial third parties.

If consent is being obtained in the hospital, the hospital will likely have interpreters available. Local colleges or churches may also offer interpreter services. When the language needed outstrips local capabilities, you may rely on the interpreters available through the phone companies. Regardless of the method you use to obtain consent, the first question should be "Please ask her if she consents to obtaining translation in this manner." Document in your chart "Consent obtained via AT&T interpreter" or whatever would be appropriate to the situation.

The next item to consider is what information a patient needs in order to give informed consent. The rule of thumb is "anything a reasonable person would want to know." At a minimum, this should include:

1) What the suggested treatment entails;

2) Why the treatment is suggested;

3) The expected benefit(s) and risk(s) of the suggested treatment;

4) Any alternatives to the suggested treatment, (including doing nothing);

5) What they should expect during and after treatment; and

6) Answers to their questions.

It is also helpful to explain your expertise and experience with the suggested treatment (e.g., the number of times you have performed the recommended procedure). Some states have specific guidance on what information must be transmitted for individual procedures. There are very particular requirements for consent on any experimental procedure. Contact the Investigational Review Board (IRB) at your local hospital for more details.

It is important to allow the patient to ask questions and have them answered. Our culture puts a premium on transparency, and you would be well-served to keep the same level of disclosure you would want from your own physician.

Consent must be clearly documented; all hospitals have forms for this purpose. Those forms, however, are only documentation that consent was obtained, and cannot be construed as "consent." Whoever is providing the treatment is legally responsible for the consent. It is good practice for physicians to obtain their own consent, stored in their own office records, in addition to any form the hospital requires. Hospital forms are by necessity generic; having your own form allows you to create forms specific to the procedures you perform, and allow personalization for each patient. Any state-required elements for a specific procedure must be included in your office form.

Although a proper consent form will not relieve you from a claim of medical malpractice, it may certainly help in your defense against that claim. Many times the claimed harm was not due to negligence, but was a known risk of a procedure. A consent form that clearly demonstrates the patient's choice to proceed, fully-informed of that known risk, will be an asset to your defense.

### Patient Rights under the HIPAA Privacy Rule

The Health Insurance Portability and Accountability Act (HIPAA) was passed in 1996.[1] It covers many issues, such as the portability of insurance from one employer to another, increasing penalties and funding for investigations of fraud and abuse, the protection of patient health information, and achieving the security necessary to accomplish a "paperless" American health care system.

The portion of HIPAA devoted to protecting health care information ("the Privacy Rule") created four new federal patient rights[2]; the Privacy Rule supersedes any state law that sets the standard of privacy below that required under the federal law. Each of the four new federal rights will be discussed separately.

Under the HIPAA Privacy Rule, there are special protections that apply to mental health records. As defined by HIPAA, a "mental health record" is a record created by a "mental health care provider," which includes psychiatrists, psychologists, and licensed counselors.

The determination of what constitutes a mental health care record rests with the type of practice a physician has, not the nature of the patient's care. A physician who is not a psychiatrist may treat mental health conditions, but the records, including prescription records, may be released with the rest of the patient's records under the conventional protections. The records they generate will be released under the "Permissive Disclosure" standard (discussed below). Records that are generated by a mental health care provider, such as a psychiatrist, are afforded the highest possible protections under both state laws and HIPAA:[5]

> *Save for few exceptions, "psychotherapy notes" cannot be disclosed to anyone without the patient's specific authorization. Furthermore, such authorization cannot be compelled for payment, underwriting, or plan enrollment.*

All states have laws that give special protections to the records of mental health care providers. If you are a psychiatrist, you will need to educate yourself on both your state law and the portion of the HIPAA Privacy Rule that pertains specifically to your records. The American Psychiatric Association (APA) website (www.psych.org) is an excellent place to start, as is your state psychiatry organization.

Parents have the right to control the flow of "protected health information" (PHI), and other rights of their children under the HIPAA Privacy Rule. Similarly, once legally recognized, the representative of an incompetent patient can exercise HIPAA privacy rights on their behalf.

### Becoming a HIPAA-Compliant Physician

As you establish your practice, it will be important to ensure that your office is HIPAA-compliant. There are many resources available to assist you, but some of them are misleading or wrong. Following is a brief explanation of how physicians who are not psychiatrists will function in compliance with the HIPAA Privacy Rule.

HIPAA requires a specific form, known as an "Authorization," to be signed by the patient (or legal representative) before PHI is released. While this is the rule, there is a very broad exception, called "Permissive Disclosures," that will apply to most of the information that leaves your office. A permissive disclosure is a release of patient information in any form (on paper, over the phone, via FAX, electronically, or in a face-to-face conversation) by a *non-mental health care provider* that is related to the treatment, payment, or operations of the physician (TPO).

As explained by U.S. Department of Health and Human Services (DHHS) in its Guidance to the HIPAA Privacy Rule released in December 2002,[6] "treatment" includes "the provision, coordination, or management of health care and related services among health care providers…consultation between health care providers regarding a patient, or the referral of a patient from one health care provider to another." The definition of "payment" is similarly broad: "Payment encompasses the various activities of health care providers to obtain payment or be reimbursed for their services and of a health plan to obtain premiums, to fulfill their coverage responsibilities and provide benefits under the plan, and to obtain or provide reimbursement for the provision of health care." "Operations" is defined as "administrative, financial, legal, and quality improvement activities of a covered entity that are necessary to run its business and to support the core functions of treatment and payment." The vast majority of patient information that leaves your office—whether spoken, electronic or written—meets one of these definitions.

In order to be HIPAA-compliant, there are a number of preliminary steps you must take before you make permissive disclosures, such as:

• Designate a "Privacy Officer;"

• Develop or acquire Policies and Procedures consistent with the Privacy Rule;

• Post a "Notice of Privacy Practices" in your office and make a good faith effort to get every patient to acknowledge in writing they have been provided with that copy; and

• Take reasonable measures to protect patient health information from unnecessary disclosure.

Assuming these are in place, and the communication of PHI is in keeping with TPO, communication can occur without any further patient involvement. You do not need a release form, or to have your patient sign a "HIPAA Authorization" form. Be sure to limit any information disclosed to what is minimally necessary to achieve the TPO goal. If patient information must leave your office that does *not* meet the definitions of TPO (or if you are unsure), you must obtain a "HIPAA Authorization" from the patient or their representative.

Please note that under the TPO exception, physicians are not only permitted to share information with other providers, they are expected to do so, as failure to disclose information might become a patient safety issue. "Physicians may release Protected Health Information (PHI) to other providers to "carry out treatment."[7] The one possible exception is when a patient has requested that you not share information with a particular person — for example, their spouse.

It is important not to lose sight of the significance of permissive disclosures in the detail of this answer. To sum it up, you may release information without release authorizations if:

- You are not a mental health care provider;

- You keep track of patients who have made reasonable requests to restrict disclosure of their PHI;

- You set up all the required elements of HIPAA in your office (and meet those requirements); and

- You then exchange information as needed for your TPO functions.

Another portion of the Privacy Rule allows for "Mandatory Disclosures." This section allows you to release patient information as necessary to comply with any other federal or state law or investigation. Similarly, HIPAA allows sharing of patient information with public authorities to deal with public health emergencies, such as a terrorist attack. Examples include complying with State Reporting laws (e.g., communicable disease reporting, reporting suspected abuse), complying with federal law (reporting drug complications to the FDA), complying with governmental investigations (state or federal), complying with law enforcement, or complying with court orders, subpoenas or other requests sanctioned by state law.

**Patient Rights under HIPAA[8]**

*#1: A patient has the right to obtain a copy of his or her medical record.*

Patients have a right under HIPAA to obtain a copy of their medical record under most circumstances.

> [A]n individual has a right of access to inspect and obtain a copy of protected health information about the individual in a designated record set, for as long as the protected health information is maintained in the designated record set[9]."

HIPAA allows a physician to deny a records request, but must notify the patient of the denial in writing.

*Copies may be denied if the physician "believes the access requested is reasonably likely to endanger the life or physical safety of the individual or another person"...with a letter explaining that.[9]*

Other exceptions to the right of a patient to copies of the medical records recognized in HIPAA include:

- Mental health care records

- Notes for legal matters

- Research records (IRB exceptions)

- Information from a third party (not a provider) with promise of confidentiality

- Exceptions with "Right of Review" (a grab bag possibility of getting an exception recognized upon review)

Under HIPAA "your record" includes information received from other physicians/providers, and these should be included in your release. If your record contains letters or records from a mental health care provider, such as a psychiatrist or licensed counselor, you must treat those records differently and release them only under the special precautions required for those records (i.e., with a "HIPAA Authorization").

Many doctors would prefer to create a summary or narrative of their patient's medical record rather than giving them an actual copy of their chart. You should not go to the trouble of preparing one unless you have both the patient's assurances that a summary will be sufficient, and you have agreed upon a price for your efforts. HIPAA requires that any charge for preparing a summary is *pre-approved*. If your patient agrees that a summary will be efficient and agrees to your cost for preparing it (or you are willing to prepare the summary for free), it may make sense to prepare a summary or narrative. Otherwise, give your patient a copy of his or her entire record. (Contact your state medical association for more explanation of when and how you can refuse such requests.)

### #2: A patient has the right to limit the disclosure of the health information.

Many people have been led to believe that they can dictate exactly how and when their PHI is shared or used, but this is not the case. For example, physicians are free to exchange patient information with other providers involved in that patient's care. Obviously this does not extend to gossip or the inappropriate sharing of information, but any information relevant to the patient's care can, and should, be shared. No patient permission is required.

Patients do not have an unlimited right to restrict their PHI under HIPAA. They also do not have the right to demand that information be kept out of their record, even if that information is highly confidential, such as HIV status.

The right granted to all patients under HIPAA is to have reasonable requests to limit the disclosure of their PHI accommodated. You should, therefore, follow those reasonable requests ("please do not talk directly to my spouse"). It is important that your office track and comply with these types of request in order to protect that patient's right. However, it is not "reasonable" to restrict information from other physicians involved in the patient's care, and you are under no obligation to agree to a patient's request to limit information to other providers.

### #3: A patient has the right to amend their medical record.

The most common misunderstanding about a patient's "Right to Amend" their medical record is that the public (and most physicians) have been led to believe that this right gives a patient the right to change what the physician and staff have put in their record.

The "Right to Amend" gives a patient the right to *add* to his or her record. These additions (amendments) could clarify a patient's perspective of their health, add information they think is relevant to their medical record, or even argue against what the physician wrote in their record or express general dissatisfaction with their care. The amendments should be clearly labeled. If you have paper records, they should be on a separate page; in an electronic record, the beginning and the end of the amendment should be clearly marked.

Amendments become part of the patient's permanent medical record. As such, they must be maintained with the record for the length of time required, included with the record any time it is sent out, and added to the copy of your medical record that might already be in another location, if the amendment is relevant to the purpose of that copy (e.g., if the amendment pertains to a billing issue, it would be appropriate to share it with your billing service).

There are some records the patient cannot amend under "Denial with No Right to Review," usually because the patient has no right to access these records in the first place, including psychiatric records, records maintained in anticipation of legal action, records that can not be changed because of Clinical Laboratory Improvement Amendments (CLIA)[10] and, for the most part, records relating to a research study.

Other requests to amend fall under "Denial with Right to Review," which means that the patient can challenge your decision to deny a patient's amendment. Any time you deny a request to amend, you must state that in writing to the patient. The review process contains a series of appeal rights and administrative procedures which could extend the debate. Because the time required to fight an amendment request can be a distraction from patient care, and because the denial sets up a complaint to the government, a good rule of thumb would be to allow the patient to make amendments (additions) to their chart unless you feel the denial is important enough to warrant the time involved.

### #4: A patient has the right to obtain an accounting of disclosures of health care information.

The language in HIPAA creating this right is as follows:

> *An individual has a right to receive an accounting of disclosures of protected health information made by a covered entity in the six years prior to the date on which the accounting is requested…*[11]

When the Privacy Rule was first released, the prospect of having to account for every disclosure was overwhelming, and resulted in the exception made for any information an office released under the "Permissive Disclosures" exception (TPO). A later modification to the Privacy Rule also removed information released under a HIPAA Authorization from the list of disclosures that had to be included.

Accountings prepared for a patient (upon request) also do not need to include the following:

- information released to the patient
- anything that was an "incidental" disclosure
- information released for national security purposes
- information given to persons involved in the individual's care
- information released to correctional institutions or law enforcement officials
- information released as part of a limited data set (i.e., research)
- information released for disaster relief
- information released for directory compilation
- information released for notification of clergy
- information released with patient present
- information released prior to 4/14/03

There are still, however, some incidences of disclosure of patient information that do need to be included in any requested accounting. These include reports made subject to state or federal laws, such as: disclosures made for public health purposes, including:

- Reportable injuries/deaths under State law (such as suspicious death)
- Child abuse reporting
- Elder abuse reporting
- Communicable diseases
- Cancer/tumor registry
- Blood lead levels
- Childhood immunizations
- Vital statistics
- Fetal deaths/stillbirths
- Medical Examiner/Coroner reports
- Disclosures to funeral homes
- Organ Procurement agencies

Other specific events that should be included are: research that was done on data that did not require the patient's authorization/permission (i.e., under an IRB waiver), (possibly) peer review reports and security breaches under HIPAA.

Offices can either account for all of these disclosures on all patients or create an accounting on a patient after the request has been made. If they choose to wait to create these accountings on an "as needed" basis, they must be confident that they can accurately create an accounting for the patient based on the information that is available in the patient's record.

### Penalties Under HIPAA

The penalty for most violations (i.e., the unintended mistakes made in the course of delivering quality patient care or running an efficient office) under HIPAA is a fine (civil monetary penalty) of $100 per incident. You can be fined for as many as 250 identical violations a year, which could result in a fine of $25,000.

There are criminal penalties under HIPAA, but these do not apply to innocent mistakes. Criminal penalties apply when you intentionally violate a patient's privacy for malicious or fraudulent reasons or for your *own personal financial gain*:

Criminal Penalties under HIPAA:

- Up to $50,000 and one year in prison for knowingly and improperly obtaining or disclosing PHI (or using a unique health identifier)

- Up to $100,000 and 5 years if the offense is committed under false pretenses

- Up to $250,000 and 10 years in prison for obtaining or disclosing PHI with the intention to sell it or use it for malicious purposes

A violation of a patient's privacy might result in a suit by that patient in state court. Inappropriate, careless, or malicious revelation of information as confidential as health care information is punishable under state civil law.

### Obtaining Accurate HIPAA Information

Many physicians, especially those just entering practice, have been preyed on by unscrupulous "HIPAA consultants" with false information. Far more have been led into unnecessary HIPAA precautions by well-intentioned resources that have been misinformed.

The best place to get HIPAA information is from the government itself. The DHHS, to its credit, has been answering "Frequently Asked Questions" (FAQs) since early in the Privacy Rule creation process, and posting the questions and answers on the web. This is, without a doubt, the most definitive information you can obtain about HIPAA. It is *free*, accessible, and undeniably accurate. It is a good practice for all physician offices (presumably the Privacy Officer) to consult the government's resource frequently. Go to http://www.hhs.gov/ocr/hipaa and click on "Your Frequently Asked Questions on Privacy." You can also search the FAQs data-bank by key word or phrase, and submit your own question if it has not already been addressed.

Medical malpractice is discussed very capably in Chapter 12 of this reference, as well as in Chapter 8, addressing Risk Management.

## Tort Reform

Tort reform is of primary importance to most physicians, as many are convinced that the traditional medical malpractice litigation system has been surpassed by the complexities of modern medicine, and that the current system has led to a litigation crisis in our country. Multiple states are experiencing an impact in the availability of care as physicians retire prematurely, choose to stop performing high-risk procedures, or move to another state with more favorable laws in place. (More on this topic can be obtained through the American Medical Association, which tracks "States in Crisis.")[12]

For years there have been calls for federal tort reform; a federal law would improve the climate for physicians and other providers, uniformly and simultaneously. Many proposed tort reform laws have been introduced in the U.S. Congress; all have to date been unsuccessful. In the absence of federal legislation, all tort reform efforts must be fought and won on a state-by-state basis. You can obtain more information on the status of tort reform from your state medical association; all tort reform proposals are largely modeled after the California Tort Reform law, The Medical Injury Compensation Reform Act of 1975 (MICRA).[13]

## Common Elements of Tort Reform

### Cap on Economic Damages

Only a small minority of proposals involve limiting economic damages; most tort reform initiatives allow economic damages to be determined by the court as proved by the plaintiff. In contrast, non-economic damages (such as pain and suffering, disfigurement, and mental anguish) can significantly compound the amount of a jury verdict. Capping these damages (usually at $250,000) is a fundamental element of most tort reform proposals.

### The Collateral Source Rule

The "Collateral Source Rule" is the traditional rule that requires a jury to make a judgment on damages without other relevant information:

> If an injured person receives compensation…from a source wholly independent of the [defendant/s], the payment should not be deducted from the damages which he would otherwise collect…[14]

Advocates of tort reform argue that this rule also inflates jury verdicts. It is believed that waiving this rule in medical malpractice claims allows the jury to make a fairer assessment of a defendant's liability. For example, without the collateral source rule, a jury might be told about relevant insurance payments, state assistance, and other claims against other defendants that will all assist the plaintiff in obtaining care and living expenses.

### Revision of the Statute of Limitations

As discussed above, a state's statute of limitations could allow a claim against a physician decades after any claimed act of negligence. Tort reform proposals usually include a deviation from the traditional rule, especially as it applies to minors. Many want to limit the length of time physicians can be exposed to liability, especially those who treat children or are involved in obstetric deliveries.

### Limiting Attorney Fees

Under these proposals, in lieu of a straight contingency fee (usually limited to a certain percentage of recovery under state laws), plaintiff lawyers would be paid on a decreasing scale as the size of the recovery grows. It is thought that the financial benefits in multi-million dollar claims disproportionately favor attorneys.

### Other Components of Tort Reform Initiatives

There are many other components frequently included in tort reform proposals, such as replacing "joint and several" liability with a "fair share" rule, limiting punitive damages, and allowing for periodic payment of damages over time, to name a few.

A full discussion of all the various possible initiatives exceed the scope of this resource, but physicians are encouraged to consult texts on the topic, as well as state and national physician advocacy groups for more information.

### Establishing an Entirely Different System

The elements just discussed, although valuable, all attempt to modify the current medical malpractice litigation system in our country. Many argue, however, that the system does not need to be altered; it needs to be replaced. Proposals include possibly establishing a separate court system that deals exclusively with medical malpractice, or replacing the court with a panel of physicians. Interested readers should contact state and federal physician organizations for more information about these proposals.

### Corporate and Regulatory Issues in Health Law

A large portion of health law is devoted to corporate and regulatory issues. Corporate issues include the planning and organization of a joint venture between physicians, such as a free-standing surgery center; issues involving contracts with managed care, and how to negotiate managed care contracts without violating antitrust laws; establishing corporations; managing a practice; leasing the building where the practice operates; hiring, maintaining, training, and firing employees; and relationships between hospitals and physicians.

Regulatory issues involve dealing with the myriad laws, rules, regulations and licensing requirements that impact practice management. This is the "alphabet soup" of health law: Emergency Medical Treatment and Active Labor Act (EMTA-LA), HIPAA, CLIA, and regulations on health and safety, such as Occupational Safety and Health Administration (OSHA).[1,10,15,16] Regulatory health law also involves laws regarding how and how much physicians get paid. Fraud and abuse legislation, penalties for offering or accepting kickbacks, and prohibitions against physician self-referral fall under Physician Self-Referral Law, also known as Stark.[17] State and municipal laws may also apply.

### Corporate Issues: Questions to Ponder

Corporate issues emerge before you ever open your doors to patients. Are you a corporation? Are you practicing alone or with other physicians? If practicing with others, are you truly "partners" or have you established a corporate identity collectively? Hiring your employees, establishing the business practices of your office and meeting state requirements for employee safety, the use and storage of potentially hazardous materials, and the storage and distribution of pharmaceutical samples must all be planned with an eye to both state and federal laws.

In establishing your medical record system, you want records that are complete, relevant, and will assist you in the event you are sued. Do your records reflect the competency of your care? How do you fire a patient? How do you protect yourself from a claim of "abandonment?"

Most physicians need managed care contracts in order to keep their practice full; the contract is what brings the patients into your waiting room. What rights do you have under that contract? Many states have legislated reforms that control against the most egregious managed care abuses of the past, but you certainly cannot assume that a contract is all right because "everyone else signed it." Speaking of which, if you have been talking to your colleagues, but they are not physicians who are in your practice (e.g., same tax ID number, provider number, etc.), you better not have talked about what fees they are getting under the contract "everybody signed;" if you did, you have violated antitrust laws.

You set up a billing system and signed contracts with a few managed care companies, but what rights do they have over your records? Can a payor obtain copies of a patient's record from before she was insured, that is, can the managed care plan go "fishing" in your patient's prior medical history? What should you do when a managed care company unilaterally changes your fee? What if they don't pay you at all?

Do you understand your obligations under the Hospital Medical Staff Bylaws? Will you serve on the Hospital Peer Review committee, and if so, what procedures must you follow to avoid allegations of antitrust violations? How are you going to respond if you feel you are being squeezed out by your colleagues? What recourse do you have if there is an unfavorable peer review decision against you?

When moving to an underserved area, it is possible that you can legally accept incentives to establish your practice in that area, but what can you accept, and what value is permitted? Do you yourself qualify as a physician who can accept incentives, and how do you know if your desired location is truly "underserved"?

When you retire, can you sell your charts? Can you guarantee your patients will follow the purchaser after the sale? What if they want their chart? What is good will and how should it be valued? Do you keep your license after retirement? Should you maintain your insurance?

### Regulatory Issues: Questions to Ponder

Emergency Medical Treatment and Active Labor Act (EMTALA)[15] is a federal law that dictates when and how patients can be transferred in emergency situations. Do you understand what "stable" means in your field of practice? What are your EMTALA obligations if you are on call? What are your obligations if the patient was referred to your office for follow-up?

What precautions should you establish to prevent fraudulent or abusive billing? Will you have regular audits of your charts? If so, will they be internal or external? Will they be prospective or retrospective? Do you already have policies and procedures in place regarding all aspects of your practice, and do they also address billing issues? Do you have an avenue for employees to notify you anonymously of possible billing violations?

What can you accept from drug company representatives? Is the nice dinner for you and your spouse during a CME presentation legal? How about the cruise the drug company treated you to last spring?

If you are referring to a particular hospital, home health agency, or skilled nursing facility, is that because you are getting anything of value in return? If you have an ownership interest in the MRI center or laboratory, has that been fully disclosed? What if your spouse has the ownership interest?

Will you be involved in a joint venture with your local hospital? What referral patterns will you establish, and where will you establish your hospital privileges? Are the two connected to any ownership interest or gifts in return (kickbacks)?

Are you establishing a paperless office, or is it at least partially-electronic? If so, then you need to understand the requirements of the HIPAA Security rule.

Do you have employees? There are precautions you must take, notices you must post, and employee rights you must protect. Have you taken into consideration all the aspects of the Equal Employment Opportunity Commission (EEOC), OSHA and the ADA.[4, 16, 18]

Do you have a laboratory in your office? There are federal and state laws that apply. Are there controlled drugs on the premises? How about flammable liquids, such as acetone? Do your halls and doorways meet your local fire code? Are your fire alarms and extinguishers compliant?

### Corporate and Regulatory Issues: Get Help

In the last two sections many questions were posed without the accompanying answers, for two reasons. First, it is important to understand that the practice of medicine is inextricably entwined with state and federal laws and regulations, and will be throughout your career. It will be important to stay informed and obtain assistance from people you can trust.

A suitably trained and supported office manager can help with most of these issues, but many physicians will have offices too small to afford the expense of a full-time management position. Even with an outstanding manager, physicians will continuously need advice on how to operate a practice within the confines of relevant laws.

Where can you obtain good practice management advice? The second, and most important, reason questions were listed without answers, is that the entire area of corporate and regulatory health law is an area physicians should not enter alone. You need appropriate legal advice to navigate through these issues. As explained in the beginning of this chapter, "appropriate" means a lawyer with expertise in the area in which you are seeking help.

There is no doubt that physicians are able to master these legal issues, but is it a good use of time to spend your evenings working through a contracting textbook? Common sense tells us that a physician will not be as effective as a lawyer practicing in this field. The laws change too swiftly, the interpretation of contracts is too nuanced, and compliance with state and federal laws is too detailed for a casual student.

It is not necessary to have a lawyer on retainer. Many corporate and regulatory issues can be answered through seminars or services from state medical associations and specialty societies. The AMA offers a wealth of information to members. Support your office manager and/or staff in attending professional training programs through PAHCOM (the Professional Association of Healthcare Office Management, www.pahcom.com) or MGMA (Medical Group Management Association, www.mgma.org). There are consultants available, particularly in the areas of establishing a practice and practice management issues. Ideally you will find a consultant through your local or state medical association, your specialty society, or recommendations from your colleagues. Always check references and credentials; know who you are hiring.

Finally, it is a good idea to have an established relationship with a lawyer who is well versed in corporate and regulatory issues. Maybe it is the lawyer that established your corporation; perhaps he reviewed your employment contract before you joined the multi-physician practice where you now work. You certainly don't need him on retainer, but it will be useful to know whom to call as new corporate and regulatory issues arise.

### Possible Penalties in Corporate and Regulatory Issues

There are many possible repercussions for failure to comply with corporate and regulatory issues; basically these fall into two general areas: private civil action and claims brought against you by a government in either civil or criminal court.

Private civil actions would include all the possible ways to get sued by another private party (e.g., an ex-employee suing for wrongful termination, a landlord suing for violation of the lease, or a managed care company bringing an action for violation of the provider contract). Medical malpractice suits are included in this private civil claims category. Generally speaking, physicians can be sued in state court by another private party for any claim involving treatment, their role as an employer, or their obligations under a contract. If you lose, these claims may result in financial damages and/or a court order to stop doing something or compelling you to take a specific action. These cases will not result in jail or criminal liability.

If you violate a state or federal regulation, you will be answering to an agency or department of the government. Do you have discriminatory hiring practices? You might find yourself dealing with the EEOC. Did you violate the HIPAA Privacy Rule? The Office of Civil Rights at DHHS will want to know. Fraudulent billing? The Office of Inspector General, the Attorney General, and even the FBI might be paying you a visit.

You could be charged with violating both a state and a federal statute, as they often mirror each other. The two government agencies might coordinate their efforts against you, or you might face two separate investigations. Similarly, you could find yourself involved in both a private and a government action over the same activity. For example, an improper denial of hospital privileges to a possible competitor, if those privileges were denied in order to prevent local competition, could bring both federal and state criminal claims as well as a private suit by the physician who was kept out of your community (if successful, he or she is entitled to treble damages).

Sometimes violation of a federal law will result in a fine only, such as the Stark Law or civil penalties under HIPAA. Financial penalties are also frequently the outcome of successful actions by state governments against their physicians.

There are some activities that can send you to jail, such as fraudulent billing practices or participating in a kickback scheme for the referral of Medicare patients. Sometimes the government will threaten you with jail, but will allow you to enter a settlement agreement that will include a monetary fine, high enough to be punitive, and might also allow the court jurisdiction over your practice for a period of time. You could be ordered to disband your IPA (Independent Physician Association), your practice, or your ownership interest in a facility or other entity.

Your activities could preclude you from participating in any government payment program (Medicare, Medicaid, State Children Health Insurance Programs), which is known as "Exclusion." Physicians who have had a number of claims for billing improprieties could find themselves excluded for five years, or even permanently, but even a one-year exclusion will put most physicians out of business.

Last, but certainly not least, any action against you could result in a loss of your reputation and even your business. Reports to the National Practitioner Data Bank must be revealed any time a physician is credentialed. Activity in your office by law enforcement can embarrass you and your staff, and frighten your patients. Colleagues may be wary of continuing to refer to you if you are under investigation for questionable practices. At the end of the day, your reputation with the lay public may dictate whether you might have to close your practice.

The point in painting this bleak picture is not to dissuade you from practicing medicine, but to dissuade you from taking a *laissez faire* approach. You need to be informed, surround yourself with competent people, and always be watchful for forces that would have you compromise your integrity.

## Medical Ethics

By the very nature of health care, physicians are involved in a number of ethical issues. One cannot adequately introduce health law without at least a brief acknowledgement of this important aspect of the field.

Physicians encounter ethical issues on a daily basis. When dealing with a pregnant teenager, what are your responsibilities beyond what the law demands? What are your personal political leanings, and should that matter? How about the elderly man with end-stage cancer who requests a lethal dose of medication? How should you respond? How can you respond? Do you terminate the life supports of a person in a permanent vegetative state with a legal Living Will, or are you cowed by the strident family members who insist on care at all costs? Do you notify authorities that your partner has a substance abuse problem? When your psychiatrist colleague admits to sexual relations with his female patients?

Medicine is an ethical profession. The ethics of medicine are broader than, and in many ways more important than, the law of medicine. This is not to suggest that you follow your ethics in conflict with the law, but your ethics might dictate controls well beyond what is mandated by law.

It is a strong personal belief that physicians must stay actively involved in the ethics of the medical profession. These issues are ripe for political intervention, but it is almost impossible to legislate ethics. It is preferable for physicians to make professional decisions on a patient-by-patient basis than to have laws arbitrarily passed in the glow of a heated controversial case.

## Future Laws and Physician Advocacy

Legislators can generally be relied upon to pass a new law related to health care at least every two years. As of this writing, we are waiting to see how the Rules and Regulations under the Patient Safety and Quality Improvement Act of 2006 will dictate the implementation of that law. The "paperless" health care system envisioned by many remains a difficult-to-achieve reality. Will the government institute punitive measures to achieve that goal? Is there any chance that the oft-proposed exemptions to antitrust for physicians will result in a more level playing field for managed care contract negotiations? Will Oregon's law allowing physician-assisted suicide be adopted by other states? What will be the future of stem cell research?

It is this author's firm belief that laws that affect patient care should be written with input from physicians, yet physician participation in politics remains low.

Membership in the AMA is not even close to being representative. How many physicians are actually assisting their state medical associations regarding state laws controlling medicine? Specialty associations may also provide opportunities for advocacy. If in reading this chapter you found yourself irritated by a particular law, or desiring another, ask yourself, "Could more physician advocacy have made a difference?" The answer is almost undoubtedly "yes."

Aside from the demands of patient care, physicians are busy people and have other factors in their lives that deserve attention. Many physicians do not feel they have time for activity in a political arena, but please consider at least supporting organizations that represent you and your patients.

## Conclusion

This chapter has covered a very broad topic in a concise format. It is certainly not meant to be all-inclusive or construed as legal advice, but to leave the reader with a list of issues for further research and consideration. More than anything, it has been the intent of this chapter to make you an informed consumer of legal services.

In closing, allow me to conclude with a personal belief that I hold dear in my career teaching physicians about legal issues. Everything explained in this chapter is important. However, ultimately, I hope you will leave the law to the lawyers who work for you. Trust your liability insurance company to represent you well. Hire the best possible employees and support your office manager and staff. Advocate for your profession through participation with your local, state and national physician organizations. But, when all is said and done, nothing is more important than delivering the best possible care to your patients. It is the best for them, the best for you, and ultimately the best for your profession.

## Study/Discussion Questions

1. How does informed consent alter the physician-patient relationship? Does it point to an erosion of faith in physicians, or is it consistent with a cooperative physician-patient relationship?

2. Whose responsibility is it to obtain informed consent? Should that process include information about the physician's own personal experience with a procedure?

3. Are physician fears about criminal liability springing from violations of the HIPAA Privacy Rule realistic?

4. How do the "new" federal privacy rights for all patients change the traditional flow of patient information between physicians carrying for a particular patient?

5. What is the role of physician leadership in legislative matters affecting medicine? How can physicians best participate in advocacy for their patients and for their profession?

## Suggested Readings/Websites

The American Medical Association: www.ama-assn.org

The American Health Lawyers Association: www.ahla.org

"Frequently Asked Questions" about HIPAA: www.hhs.gov/ocr/hipaa

The Professional Association of Healthcare Office Management: www.pahcom.com

Support your office manager and/or staff in attending professional training programs through The Medical Group Management Association: www.mgma.org

## References

1. The Health Insurance Portability and Accountability Act of 1996. Available at: http://www.cms.hhs.gov/HIPAAGenInfo/Downloads/HIPAAlawdetail.pdf. Accessed September 26, 2006.

2. HIPAA Privacy Rule. Available at: http://www.hhs.gov/ocr/hipaa/. Accessed September 26, 2006.

3. Civil Rights Act of 1964. Available at: http://usinfo.state.gov/usa/infousa/laws/majorlaw/civilr19.htm. Accessed September 26, 2006.

4. Americans with Disabilities Acts. Available at: http://www.ada.gov/. Accessed September 26, 2006.

5. The American Psychiatric Association. Psychotherapy Notes Provision of the HIPAA Privacy Rule. March 2002. Available at: http://www.psych.org/edu/other_res/lib_archives/archives/200201.pdf. Accessed September 26, 2006.

6. U.S. DEPARTMENT OF HEALTH AND HUMAN SERVICES. Title 45—Public Welfare PART 164—SECURITY AND PRIVACY. Available at: http://www.access.gpo.gov/nara/cfr/waisidx_02/45cfr164_02.html. Accessed September 26, 2006.

7. U.S. DEPARTMENT OF HEALTH AND HUMAN SERVICES. 45 CFR §164.502. Available at: http://www.access.gpo.gov/nara/cfr/waisidx_02/45cfr164_02.html Accessed September 26, 2006.

8. HIPAA Compliance Program. Patient Rights under HIPAA. Available at: http://www.uthscsa.edu/hipaa/patientrights.html. Accessed September 26, 2006.

9. U.S. DEPARTMENT OF HEALTH AND HUMAN SERVICES. 45 CFR §164.524 Available at: http://www.access.gpo.gov/nara/cfr/waisidx_02/45cfr164_02.html Accessed September 26, 2006.

10. Clinical Laboratory Improvement Act Amendments. Available at: http://www.cms.hhs.gov/clia/. Accessed September 26, 2006.

11. U.S. DEPARTMENT OF HEALTH AND HUMAN SERVICES. 45 CFR § 164.528 Available at: http://www.access.gpo.gov/nara/cfr/waisidx_02/45cfr164_02.html Accessed September 26, 2006.

12. American Medical Association. Medical liability crisis map. Available at: http://www.ama-assn.org/ama/noindex/category/11871.html. Accessed September 26, 2006.

13. Californians Allied for Patient Protection. About MIRCA. Available at: http://www.micra.org/AboutMICRA.htm. Accessed September 26, 2006.

14. Black HC. *Black's Law Dictionary*, 5th Ed. Eagan, MN: West Publishing Co.; 1983, 137.

15. Emergency Medical Treatment and Active Labor Act (EMTALA). Available at: http://www.emtala.com/. Accessed September 26, 2006.

16. Occupational Safety and Health Administration. Available at: http://www.osha.gov/. Accessed September 26, 2006.

17. Self-Referral Law. Available at: http://www.cms.hhs.gov/PhysicianSelfReferral/. Accessed September 26, 2006.

18. U.S. Equal Employment Opportunity Commission. Available at: http://www.eeoc.gov/. Accessed September 26, 2006.

# Chapter 10

## Practicing Medicine in a Managed Care Environment

Ralph O. Bischof, MD, MBA, FAAFP

### Executive Summary

This chapter provides an in-depth look at the practice of medicine in the context of managed care. The goal is to provide the reader with a better understanding of how to effectively practice in the managed care environment.

The chapter begins with a look at the term "managed care" and the different meanings and uses of the term. Next, there is a discussion regarding the way managed care has changed over time and how it will continue to evolve. A large portion of the chapter examines the importance of the business aspects of practice, coding, and reimbursement and reviews approaches to mastering these aspects of medical practice. There is also a discussion of how best to interact with managed care organizations and effectively appeal claim denials.

In addition to the practical aspects of practice management, the chapter takes a broader look at the driving forces behind changes in health care insurance and the health care system as a whole. There is a review of specific health care insurance changes that are on the horizon, such as consumer-directed health care, transparency, tiered networks and benefits, and pay for performance. Suggestions for how to become a more active participant in these changes in the health care system are also discussed.

### Learning Objectives

1. Understand the different meanings of the term "managed care."

2. Review the tools and concepts to successfully practice medicine in a managed care environment.

3. Understand the accelerated pace of change in the health care system and its effects on the evolution of the managed care environment.

4. Demonstrate the ability to appeal denials effectively.

## Keywords

appeals; consumer-directed health care; health care system; health maintenance organization (HMO); health plan; health reimbursement accounts (HRAs); health savings accounts (HSAs); indemnity insurance; insurance; managed care; managed care organization (MCO); managed care plans; medical coding; medical necessity; payment policies; point of service (POS); preferred provider organization (PPO); practice management; reimbursement policies; tiered benefit structure; tiered networks; transparency

## Introduction

The early 21ˢᵗ century is an exciting time to practice medicine. There has never been a greater need for the effective practice of medicine, and the whole health care system is undergoing rapid change. The American health care system seems to be on the verge of monumental changes. The successful medical practitioner will not only need to anticipate these changes, but also be aware of the drivers of those changes and be able to adapt the practice to those changes.

Managed care has been a key change agent in the health care system since the late 1970s. The Health Maintenance Organization (HMO) Act of 1973 set into play a series of changes that will continue well into this century. The original HMOs were the precursors of what eventually became known as managed care. But over the subsequent decades, the term "managed care" has evolved and taken on different meanings. This chapter examines those meanings, and how managed care influences the practice of medicine.

This chapter will focus on providing a general overview and discussion of practical considerations. Other chapters in this book address a number of specific managed care-related topics in greater depth.

## Managed Care – What is it?

To most health care practitioners, the term "managed care" usually refers to the insurance companies that offer managed care plans, also known as managed care organizations (MCOs). Administration of these plans was relatively simple in the 1970s and 1980s when there were two very distinct types of health care insurance companies: traditional indemnity insurance companies and HMOs. HMOs offered a different type of coverage than traditional insurance companies. These HMO plans were "managed," and shared certain distinctive characteristics. In this context, being managed meant that they were more actively involved in the delivery of the health care than traditional indemnity insurance plans. Traditional insurance companies focused on the payment of medical service claims and the insurance aspects of the business, but did relatively little in terms of quality, network issues, and the delivery of health care. Some of the classic features that distinguished managed care plans from traditional insurance plans are listed in Figure 1, below. However, as time has passed, traditional insurance companies and MCOs have cross-fertilized, and most health insurance companies today offer a broad spectrum of products with combinations of features.

**Figure 1.  Classic Distinguishing Features of Managed Care Plans**

Provider Networks

Fee Schedules

Payment in Advance for Health Care Services

Financial Risk

Shared Risk Through Provider Payment Capitation

Quality Improvement Initiatives and Mechanisms

Precertification Requirements

Referrals

"Gatekeepers"

Concurrent Utilization Review

Discharge Planning

Disease Management

Case Management

Today, health plans are usually grouped into two major types, "HMO" (managed) and "PPO" (Preferred Provider Organizations, based on the traditional model). But interestingly, today's traditional plans are not the same as those of the 1970s. Today's traditional plans have adapted some elements of managed care, e.g., quality improvement programs, patient management tools, precertification requirements, and case management. In many situations today, the classification of a health plan as an HMO or PPO type plan is based more on how the plan is filed with state regulators than the plan's specific characteristics.

Managed care as a broad concept is a different perspective of the traditional term. At its simplest, it is the integration of the delivery and financing of health care. With such a broad definition, it is easy to understand how the term often functions as a proxy for the health care system in discussions about the health care system and the challenges that the health care system faces.

The use of the term managed care is actually decreasing today, particularly in the context of insurance companies. Some have even declared managed care dead, but as Mark Twain might have commented, rumors of its death are greatly exaggerated. The tools and concepts of managed care have become an integral part of the American health care system. Discharge planning, case management, disease management, cost containment, quality improvement, and population health are now components of many institutions in the health care system.

Since there are so many aspects of managed care incorporated into these organizations and plans, what are they to be called if not MCOs and managed care plans? The "insurance company" moniker is again gaining favor, although some dislike that term because today's insurance companies are very different from those of 30 years ago. "Third-party payor" is another term that is used, but it is very generic. The term that appears to be gaining favor is "health plan." This relatively new term reflects the new hybrid organization that has evolved over the last 30 years or so. In this chapter, the terms managed care, health plan, plan, health care insurance, and insurance will be used interchangeably in describing both plans and organizations.

## Alphabet Soup: What is that Acronym?

A decade ago, understanding managed care required a detailed knowledge of the different categories of managed care plans, each known by a unique acronym. At one point, the number of new acronyms seemed to multiply exponentially, creating a haze of acronym confusion across the health care landscape. However, this has changed as health plans have evolved to meet ever-increasing employer and consumer demands. One helpful remnant of that era is the concept of the basic plan categories, and how they vary in terms of the degree to which they are "managed" (see Figure 2, page 159). The different categories of plans can be arranged so they represent a continuum of the degree to which they are managed, from the most to the least managed. However, in actual practice today, the safest approach is to view each plan as a unique combination of features rather than one of a certain category of plans that all share the same characteristics.

The acronyms for the three very basic plan types are worth understanding, as they are still frequently used today. The Health Maintenance Organization (HMO) is

**Figure 2. The Continuum of "Management" in Health Plan Categories**

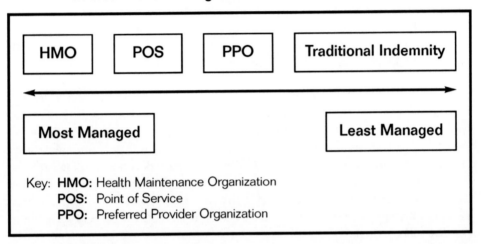

the original managed care plan of the modern era, and is the most tightly controlled of the managed care plans. Consequently, HMOs typically use most, if not all, of the classic features of MCOs listed in Figure 1. HMOs typically cover services in full (although that is changing in today's environment), but provide no benefits for services outside the plan's network of providers. Point of Service (POS) plans couple a tightly managed plan, similar to an HMO, with a lower benefit for services that are obtained outside of the established provider network. The level of benefits for a service under a POS plan is determined at the point of service, depending on the network status of the provider. The Preferred Provider Organization (PPO) was originally not considered a managed care plan, but rather a variant of traditional health insurance. The central tenet of a PPO is a network of providers with a negotiated fee schedule. PPO members receive a higher benefit for using providers in the network, and a lower benefit for services received outside the network. Although the main feature of a PPO is the network, many PPOs today offer several of the classic features of managed care plans, such as case management, disease management, concurrent review, quality improvement initiatives, and precertification. While the acronyms have remained the same, today's health plans often are hybrids with features crossing the traditional boundaries of the original HMO, POS, and PPO plans.

## Manage the Business Aspects of the Practice

One of the most fundamental elements of a successful practice is recognizing that a medical practice is a business. No matter how altruistic the goals of an organization are, it cannot exist without funding and proper financial management.

If the thought of managing a business is not appealing, you can delegate these duties to a skilled office manager or other staff member. In order to have time to practice medicine, you will need to delegate many administrative responsibilities, even if you are interested in the business aspects of the practice. Outsourcing some business functions to a practice management company is also an option or, if the whole concept is too unappealing, one can always become a salaried employee.

The spectrum of involvement in the business aspects of a practice varies from getting a Master of Business Administration (MBA) degree to learning just a few key basics. In the last decade, interest in these business aspects has grown, and over 50 medical schools now offer dual MD/MBA degree programs. There are many other options that don't require obtaining a business degree. Become familiar with the variety of practice management resources that are available to you locally and nationally: websites, local colleges, specialty societies, practice management journals, a proficient office manager, etc. All these resources can be very valuable in practice management.

## Learn the Basics of Coding and Reimbursement

Medical coding is the common language that a practice uses to track the services that it performs and to generate its income. Knowledge of the basics of coding is essential for understanding reimbursement and to be in compliance with standard coding convention and government regulations. Physicians should learn the fundamentals of coding, at least in their own specialty, or ensure that the practice either has an employee knowledgeable in coding or hires an expert vendor. In any case, the ultimate responsibility and accountability for a practice's appropriate coding lies with the physicians.

Learning coding is very much like learning a foreign language: there are new words (codes), as well as rules, conventions, and nuances in how to use them. Different dialects are reflected in the variations in coding for different specialties and in different coding systems. The Health Insurance Portability and Accountability Act (HIPAA) has helped to greatly simplify medical coding by requiring providers and insurers to use standardized coding sets.

It can be relatively easy to learn coding by becoming familiar with and using the many available coding resources. The American Academy of Professional Coders and its local chapters offer courses, seminars, and certification. Professional coders, office staff, practice management organizations, consultants, specialty societies, managed care organizations, books, and coding publications are other valuable resources.

On a practical level, there are two basic and relatively simple steps for a physician to take regarding coding and related reimbursement. First, obtain a copy of the professional edition of the American Medical Association's (AMA) *Current Procedural Terminology* (CPT) manual. Read the introduction to the manual, the introduction to each section, and the sections dealing with your specialty and your most frequent services. There is a wealth of important coding information in these brief introductions. Second, become very familiar with the coding for your ten most frequent services/procedures, as well as the reimbursement policies of the three largest insurance companies in your practice for those services. These simple steps will provide a foundation for understanding coding, and maybe even whet the appetite for a more in-depth understanding.

## Understand Your Health Plans

One of the keys to a successful practice is your knowledge of your patients' health plans, and how to resolve day-to-day issues that may arise. To keep things running smoothly, get acquainted with a key contact at each plan who can help identify the appropriate resources. Figure 3, below, lists seven important things to know about each health plan. And in a pinch, the back of the member's insurance card generally contains key plan information and contact resources.

## Figure 3. Seven Key Things to Know About a Managed Care Organization (MCO)

1. The single (preferably) point of contact for any issues you may have.

2. Your area medical director(s) and how to contact them.

3. Your network representative(s) and how to contact them.

4. The details of your contract with the MCO.

5. Keep a copy of the provider administration manual.

6. The MCOs website address and location of reference tools.

7. How to file a claim and an appeal.

## Appeal Denials Efficiently

Understanding how to appeal a denial can save an incredible amount of time and frustration. Knowing the ground rules of the appeal process is important, and the health plan should provide you with a copy of the appeal procedure. Most health plans have two appeal processes — one for members and one for providers. (Some health plans may not offer appeal processes for providers unless there is a state mandate to do so.) The member appeal process is more regulated, and generally more involved, than the provider appeal process since state and federal legislation focus on the rights of members. Other parties, including physicians, typically can act on behalf of the member provided that the appropriate release and authorization are obtained from the member.

Some important factors must be considered to make the most of the appeal process. The first and most important action is to take advantage of the appeal process that is offered and file the appeal. If an appeal is not filed, there is no chance of the denial being overturned. Second, remember that the health plan bases its decisions upon the documentation you submit in the form of medical records and narrative summaries. If there is no detailed documentation of the service, it is unlikely to be reimbursed, no matter how medically necessary it was, and even if a plan has a specific benefit for the service. If there are unusual or atypical circumstances about the patient or the clinical situation, be sure to include that information in the appeal. Exceptions to guidelines or policies may be considered in some situations if there is documentation of unusual or extenuating case-specific circumstances.

There are several important considerations that must be taken into account when filing an appeal. If it is not clear why the claim was denied, ask for an explanation of the exact denial reason. You can then focus your appeal on that reason. Don't make the common mistake of assuming that every denial is based on a determination of medical necessity. Otherwise, your efforts may be wasted and you will needlessly use up all of the levels of appeal that are offered. Also, maximize the return on your efforts by appealing those cases where there is the greatest chance of reversing the initial decision. It may be more fruitful, for example, to appeal a medical necessity denial where there were unusual clinical circumstances rather than a situation where there is a black and white contractual exclusion.

If your initial appeal is unsuccessful, take advantage of all avenues of recourse offered. There may be multiple appeal levels, different appeal tracks for members and practitioners, state-sponsored external reviews, health plan-sponsored external reviews, or reviews with the plan sponsor (employer). Additional reviews are seen by some as unnecessary barriers, but they increase your chances for a successful outcome. These are opportunities not only for additional reviews, but sometimes also for a different reviewer (who may view the situation differently), independent reviewers, and to supply any additionally identified missing information. Figure 4, below, summarizes the key steps to successful appeals.

## Figure 4. Five Key Steps to Successful Appeals

1. Ask for an explanation of the exact denial reason.

2. Focus your appeal on that exact denial reason.

3. Don't assume every denial is based on medical necessity.

4. Appeal selectively where you have the greatest chance of affecting the outcome.

5. Document any case-specific circumstances that may affect the outcome.

## Prepare for Consumer-Directed Health Care

Consumer-directed health care is the newest wave in insurance and is receiving a lot of interest from employers. This trend is born from the parallel movements towards consumerism and transparency in today's society. Consumers have become savvy about their health care, particularly with the explosion of health care-related information available on the Internet. The information age has created a new breed of consumers who have researched their interests, are tuned in to the latest developments in their field of interest, and are demanding a new level of service.

A new age of transparency has begun among insurers. This benefits not only their members, but also their providers. Many detailed policies that previously were difficult to understand or obtain are now being made available on easy-to-access websites. The types of information available include not only the standard insurance information, but also clinical policies, reimbursement policies, payment policies, provider reimbursement schedules, and provider quality ratings. This transparency has obvious benefits for the practitioner who needs to get a service approved or a claim paid, but it also gives patients the tools and information they need to better understand and direct their own health care.

Health Savings Accounts (HSAs) and Health Reimbursement Accounts (HRAs) are two new products that have been at the forefront of the move toward consumer-directed health care. These products typically are offered with a high deductible health plan and tools to help make informed health care decisions. There are specific federal mandates governing how these plans operate. One key element is that any funds remaining in these special accounts at the end of a calendar year may be carried forward to future years. These accounts generally also provide tax benefits for the member and employer. The funds from HSAs may also be made available to the member under certain conditions when coverage under a plan is terminated. As a result, the member has a financial incentive to be more informed about health care decisions and spending. Employers are increasingly in favor of these initiatives that encourage employees to be more directly involved in their health care.

As a practicing physician you need to be aware of consumerism and consumer-directed health care, and the potential impacts on your practice (see Figure 5, below). Be prepared for patients to ask specific questions about quality measures or about fees, and even begin to negotiate fees. Be prepared for your fee schedules and quality measures to be made available to the public. Your awareness of these coming changes will help you to anticipate patients' questions and issues, and begin to formulate responses and strategies. Think about what quality measures matter most in your particular practice niche and how to measure them. While quality measurement has received much attention and debate in recent years, its use and dissemination have been limited to specific measures and provider types. Still, quality measurement will soon be more widespread and pervasive, affecting all aspects of the health care system.

## Figure 5.  Impacts of Consumer-Directed Health Care on Physicians

1. Fee schedules will be widely published.

2. Quality measures will be widely published.

3. Patients will ask about your fee schedules and quality measures.

4. Patients will begin to negotiate fees.

5. Enhanced electronic tools to provide benefit and reimbursement information.

The structure of health plan benefits may become more complex as consumer-directed health care gains momentum. The special savings and reimbursement accounts unique to these plans will add another layer of complexity to the standard layers of deductibles, flexible spending accounts, co-insurance, out-of-pocket maximums, and benefit caps. The good news is that insurers are working to make these plan designs simpler for both members and providers by making electronic tools available to quickly answer benefit and reimbursement questions.

In summary, consumer-directed health care is the newest wave in health care insurance. It reflects the larger trend of consumerism, which will impact all sectors of our economy, not only health care. As with other new trends, there is greater opportunity for those who anticipate and plan for the changes.

## Expect Ongoing Change

Change is the one constant in both managed care and health care in general. The nature of the health care insurance industry has been one of rapid change over the last half century, and the pace of change seems to constantly accelerate. Change often happens when there is a large degree of dissatisfaction with the status quo. When the dissatisfaction is great, there may be a "tipping point" that triggers a sudden, dramatic, and pervasive change. Many feel that health care is nearing such a point. The high level of medical costs in this country and the rapid year-to-year increase in those costs serve as ongoing catalysts for change, and the situation is not likely to stabilize anytime soon.

Modifications in the health care system and health care insurance industry in response to employers' needs and other forces will also drive change in managed care plans, procedures, contracts, and policies. Some of the key changes on the horizon involve tiered networks and pay for performance. Although both have been around for some time, their influence and implementation have not been widespread. With greater pressures toward improvements in quality and reductions in cost, these will likely become more widely used in the health care system.

Tiered networks involve a graduated level of benefits available to the patient, based on the tier ranking of the provider. The preferred tier—usually including those providers with the best quality records—provides the highest level of benefits, while the lowest tier provides the lowest level of benefits. Tiered benefit levels have been used more commonly for prescription drug benefits. Their use is expanding to other types of health plan benefits as well. The use of tiers helps to steer patients to the highest quality and most efficient providers, yet allows members to participate in the decision making, and have a choice of options beyond the traditional all-or-nothing benefit structure. Figure 6, page 166, shows an example of a tiered benefit structure.

## Figure 6. Example of a Tiered Benefit Structure with Four Tiers

| Tier | Status | Member's Benefit |
|------|--------|------------------|
| 1 | Most preferred | 90% |
| 2 | 2nd most preferred | 70% |
| 3 | 3rd most preferred | 50% |
| 4 | Least preferred | 30% |

Pay for performance is currently a hot topic. In the past, most pay for performance initiatives have been implemented for select geographic regions and providers; the new generation of pay for performance programs will be more widespread. The government, employers, and others have given strong support to this initiative. Physicians in practice need to think about what measures make the most sense in their specialty and participate actively in the discussions. This topic is addressed in detail in Chapters 3 and 21.

Other notable changes in health care plans are also occurring. Disease management is receiving increased attention as a means to help identify where intervention efforts may have the largest impact. Wellness interventions continue to grow to aid in the prevention of disease. There is an expansion of the more recent drug interventions to optimize a patient's pharmacotherapy and also avert potential adverse drug interactions and reactions. In order for these efforts to be most effective, information must be shared among different systems; this is most easily accomplished where electronic medical records are in use. The general public is increasingly expecting these important interventions to occur; the ongoing challenge for the health care system is to bring all records into electronic format and improve the capability of disparate electronic systems to communicate with each other.

## Understanding the Driving Forces Behind Managed Care

In order to fully comprehend the issues surrounding managed care and its evolution in today's health care landscape, it is essential to have a working knowledge of the forces driving change in the health care system. To a large degree, managed care is driven by a combination of the rising cost of health care and the employer-based health insurance system in the United States. Health care inflation has consistently outpaced the rate of general inflation, thereby creating pervasive financial challenges. Employers have been the largest purchaser of health insurance in the commercial (non-government) insurance market since World War II. Managed care has a long-standing association with employer-based health care coverage. The earliest roots of managed care date back to the 19th century, when large employers purchased pre-paid health care for their employees. Employers have a stake in the health care of their employees for a variety of important reasons, including avoiding occupational injuries, promoting general health and productivity, providing a level of benefits that allow them to attract and retain the most skilled employees, and more recently, controlling the dramatically increasing costs of health insurance. Managed care is the vehicle that provides employers the primary tools to accomplish these goals. Change in managed care typically results from an underlying need among employers.

One way to anticipate changes in the insurance or managed care industry is to pay attention to the large employers in the United States. Often, the issues being faced by large employers will be reflected in their needs from the insurance industry. As employer profits shrink, for example, the pressure to cut costs affects the benefits that the employer offers, and managed care plans adapt their offerings. One of the simplest ways to watch for these employer changes and trends is to keep up with business news. Watching a daily business newscast, reading business headlines, or reading a newspaper such as the *Wall Street Journal* are all good ways to help a busy physician keep up-to-date and thinking about future trends in health plans.

With the high level of concern over the rising costs of health care, dramatic change is possible. Universal coverage, a single-payer system, and individual insurance markets similar to auto and homeowner's insurance are just some of the possibilities being discussed.

Amidst all this change, however, there is one constant: the physician-patient relationship. Many things may change dramatically about the health care system, but the one common denominator that will always remain is the physician-patient relationship and the unique role it plays in the delivery of health care. Building strong physician-patient relationships will always be as important as anticipating and adjusting to changes in the health care system.

## Be an Active Participant

In the midst of a rapidly changing environment, one of the most important things a physician can do is to be an active participant. Medicine is a demanding profession, and it is easy to become fully-absorbed in the clinical aspects. However, feedback from physicians is vital to shaping the future of the health care system. Being an active participant also provides a unique satisfaction that comes from knowing you are helping shape the future of health care.

There are many ways to actively participate and provide feedback to decision makers. Be vocal about issues with which you agree and disagree. Seek out committee positions in your group, your hospital, your community, your local, state, and national medical societies. Figure 7, below, lists some examples of ways to become a more active participant in the health care system.

**Figure 7. Ways to be a More Active Participant in the Health Care System**

1. Join a hospital committee.

2. Volunteer some clinical time at a community health clinic or service.

3. Be available to speak to local community groups.

4. Run for an elected position in a local, state, or national medical or specialty society.

5. Ask your local health plans about committees and other ways to participate.

6. Become a part time medical director at a local health plan.

7. Become a specialty reviewer for an independent review organization.

## Conclusion

Practicing medicine in the 21ˢᵗ century will bring unique challenges. Managed care will continue to be an influential part of the health care landscape, although it will be more integrated into the health care system as a whole, rather than simply a type of health care insurance. This chapter has provided an oversight of some of the key elements of managed care in the future practice of medicine. Those who understand these elements and their key driving forces will be well positioned to succeed in the practice of 21ˢᵗ century medicine.

## Case Study

At the office staff meeting for your ophthalmology practice, your office manager reports that one of the area insurance companies apparently has a new policy that denies corneal topography. Historically, the policy for this service has been that it is conditionally eligible for certain indications, and you confirm the current policy by checking the clinical policy section on the insurance company's website. Your office manager insists that there has been a change and shows you a stack of 20 claims that have been denied. You ask that she contact the insurance company for more specific details.

After reviewing the denied claims with the insurance company, your office manager reports the following;

- two claims had typographical errors in the patient identification number, and the claim system did not recognize the numbers.

- two claims were submitted for patients who were insured with a different insurance company.

- three claims were denied as duplicate claim submissions, but had already been reimbursed on a prior submission.

- two claims were for an entirely different service that the insurance company considers to be experimental/investigational.

- four claims were for corneal topography, but were submitted with diagnosis codes that are not among the indications considered reimbursable by the insurance company's clinical policy.

- three claims were denied because the patients' insurance coverage had terminated prior to the date of service.

- four claims were denied as duplicate claim submissions for claims that had previously been denied for one of the other above reasons.

After correction of the claims with the correct identification numbers, insurance policies, and diagnosis codes, all of the claims for corneal topography were eventually reimbursed. What had originally appeared to the office staff to be a change in a clinical policy by the insurance company turned out on further investigation in this case to be a collection of miscellaneous other issues.

## Study/Discussion Questions

1. How will managed care impact my practice in the future?

2. What are some of the different uses and meanings of the term "managed care"?

3. How can my practice operate most effectively in a managed care environment?

4. What are the tools and techniques that my practice can use to interact most effectively with managed care organizations?

5. What are the drivers of change in the health care system?

6. How can my practice anticipate and best adapt to the rapid changes in the health care system?

7. What are some specific changes on the horizon for health care insurance, and how will they impact my practice?

8. How can I be an active participant in the changing health care system?

## Suggested Readings/Websites

| | |
|---|---|
| Aetna Inc. | www.aetna.com |
| American Academy of Family Physicians | www.aafp.org |
| American Academy of Professional Coders | www.aapc.com |
| America's Health Insurance Plans | www.ahip.org |
| American Medical Association | www.ama-assn.org |
| CIGNA | www.cigna.com |
| Center for Studying Health System Change | www.hschange.org |
| National Committee for Quality Assurance | www.ncqa.org |
| The Commonwealth Fund | www.cmwf.org |

*Family Practice Management*

*The Journal of Medical Practice Management*

Bischof, RO, Nash, DB. Managed care: Past, present, and future. Medical Clinics of North America, 1996; 80: 225-244.

# Chapter 11

## What Every Doctor Needs to Know About Medicare and Medicaid

Joshua J. Gagne, PharmD and Vittorio Maio, PharmD, MS, MSPH

### Executive Summary

Almost half of all Americans receive publicly-funded health insurance, with the majority of these individuals receiving it through programs sponsored by the Centers for Medicare and Medicaid Services (CMS). Navigating all of the components of the CMS programs can be challenging for patients and providers alike. CMS administers Medicare to provide hospital and medical insurance to elderly persons and individuals with certain disabilities via three major components – Parts A, B, and D. The Medicare Prescription Drug Improvement and Modernization Act of 2003 (MMA) represents the most drastic change to the Medicare program since its inception, with the addition of prescription drug coverage for beneficiaries. CMS also offers Medicaid to provide medical assistance for individuals and families with low incomes, and the State Children's Health Program (SCHIP) as the newest coverage tool for children and families. Medicare is a federally-sponsored program, whereas Medicaid is jointly-administered by the federal and state governments. Some individuals qualify for both programs. Each program offers different benefit structures, payment mechanisms, and models of reimbursement. Increasing costs, compounded by federal and state budget constraints, are challenging the ability of these programs to provide health care services for millions of individuals in the most vulnerable segments of the U.S. population. A fundamental understanding of these programs will help physicians in their quest to deliver high quality care to patients.

### Learning Objectives

1. To describe the purposes of Medicare, Medicaid, and State Children's Health Insurance Program (SCHIP).

2. To define patient eligibility criteria and covered benefits of these programs.

3. To explain how Medicare and Medicaid are financed and how providers are reimbursed by these programs.

4. To discuss the futures of these programs.

## Keywords

Centers for Medicare and Medicaid Services (CMS); government health care financing; Medicaid; Medicare; State Children's Health Insurance Plan (SCHIP)

## Introduction/History

Most developed countries have national health insurance programs that cover the vast majority of their citizens. The United States is the most notable exception. The first efforts to establish some form of government health insurance in the United States were initiated at the state level between 1915 and 1920, but to no avail. In the 1930s, interest in government health insurance resurfaced at the federal level, but nothing came to fruition beyond limited provisions in the Social Security Act that supported state activities related to public health and health care services for mothers and children.

From then on, most people desired some form of health insurance to guard against unpredictable and potentially catastrophic medical costs and, eventually, private insurance prevailed for the majority of the U.S. population. In 1950, Congress agreed to provide access to medical care for needy persons who were receiving public assistance, permitting, for the first time, federal participation in the financing of state payments made directly to health care providers. Congress also agreed that older individuals, like those with low incomes, required improved access to medical care.

After lengthy national debate, Congress passed legislation in 1965 establishing the Medicare and Medicaid programs as Title XVIII and Title XIX, respectively, of the Social Security Act. Medicare was established to address the specific medical care needs of the elderly, and Medicaid to mend the inadequacy of welfare medical care under public assistance. Responsibility for administering these two programs was entrusted to the Department of Health, Education, and Welfare, the precursor to the current U.S. Department of Health and Human Services (DHHS). Until 1977, the Social Security Administration (SSA) managed the Medicare program, and the Social and Rehabilitation Service (SRS) managed the Medicaid program. The duties were then transferred from SSA and SRS to the newly formed Health Care Financing Administration (HCFA), renamed in 2001 to the Centers for Medicare and Medicaid Services (CMS) as it is still known today.[1-4]

## CMS

Housed within the U.S. Department of Health and Human Services, the Centers for Medicare and Medicaid Services (CMS) are charged with assuring health care security for beneficiaries of the Medicare, Medicaid, and SCHIP programs. Essentially, CMS assures that these government-sponsored health insurance programs are properly run by its contractors and state agencies. In addition, CMS establishes policies for paying health care providers, conducts research on the effectiveness of various methods of health care management, treatment, and financing, and assesses the quality of care facilities and services and takes enforcement actions as appropriate. In 2004, public insurance accounted for nearly half of all health care spending, with the CMS-run programs constituting a considerable proportion of this spending (Figure, below).

**Figure. Sources of National Health Care Expenditures, 2004**

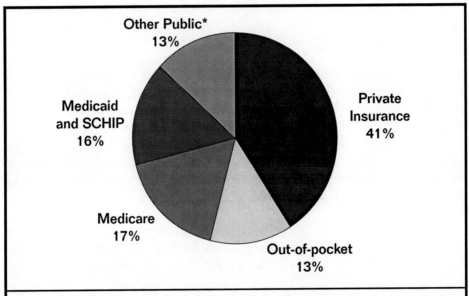

\* Other public includes programs such as workers' compensation, public health activity, Department of Defense, Department of Veterans Affairs, Indian Health Services, State and local hospital subsidies, and school health.
Source: Centers for Medicare & Medicaid Services, Office of the Actuary, National Health Statistics Group

## Medicare

### Overview

Established as a federal government program under Title XVIII of the Social Security Act of 1965, Medicare provides hospital and medical expense insurance to elderly persons and individuals with certain disabilities, as well as all people with end-stage renal disease. Originally, Medicare consisted of two parts, which still exist – A and B. Part A covers most inpatient care in hospitals, critical access hospitals, and skilled nursing facilities, but not custodial or long-term care services. Individuals pay into Medicare Part A throughout their working lives, and generally become eligible to receive benefits at age 65. Part B covers some physician and outpatient services that are not covered by Part A, including physical and occupational therapy, and some home health care. Unlike Part A, patients who opt for Part B coverage must pay a monthly premium in order to receive benefits. Recently, CMS introduced Medicare prescription drug coverage, also known as Medicare Part D, as part of the Medicare Prescription Drug Improvement and Modernization Act of 2003 (MMA). Beneficiaries of Medicare Part A are eligible to enroll in Part D as long as they are willing to participate in the payment structure. The MMA represents the most significant change to the Medicare program since its inception. While the MMA contains language pertaining to many facets of the Medicare program, such as chronic care improvement and medication therapy management, the most notable change is the addition of prescription drug coverage.

### Population Covered/Eligibility

As of 2005, Medicare provided health insurance for nearly 42 million Americans – 35.4 million elderly individuals and 6.3 million non-elderly individuals with permanent disabilities. The median age of Medicare beneficiaries is 73 years, and many have multiple chronic conditions. More than half of beneficiaries have two or more chronic conditions and more than a quarter of beneficiaries report their health as fair or poor. More than 2 million beneficiaries reside in long-term care facilities. One-quarter of all Medicare beneficiaries have problems with mental functioning or cognitive impairments.[3]

Although beneficiaries are eligible for Medicare despite income status, most Medicare beneficiaries rely on Social Security for the bulk of their income, and almost 40% of beneficiaries have incomes 200% below the established federal poverty level.[3]

### Component Structure and Benefits

Medicare provides coverage for basic health services such as inpatient hospital care (Part A), ambulatory care including physician and preventive services (Part B), and outpatient prescription medications (Part D). The program provides limited long-term care benefits, but does not cover eyeglasses, hearing aids, or dental care. Medicare-covered benefits are generally subject to deductibles and cost-sharing requirements.

### Part A

Often referred to as Hospital Insurance, Part A covers services such as inpatient hospital, skilled nursing facilities, hospice care, and some home health care (Table 1, page 176). It is funded mainly by a payroll tax on employers and workers. Part A is generally provided automatically, and free of premiums, to persons age 65 or over who are eligible for Social Security or Railroad Retirement benefits, whether or not they have claimed these monthly cash benefits. Even though most people do not have to pay for Part A if they paid Medicare taxes while working, patient deductibles and co-insurance apply.

### Part B

Medicare Part B, also known as Supplementary Medical Insurance, extends Medicare coverage to physician professional services in various settings, outpatient hospital care, ambulance services, medical supplies and equipment, diagnostic tests, physical and occupational therapists, and some home health care (Table 2, page 177). Although voluntary, most individuals participating in Part A also enroll in Part B, which requires premiums and co-payments.

### Part C

Medicare Part C, formerly and more commonly known as the Medicare+Choice program, was recently renamed the Medicare Advantage program as a result of the MMA. The new Medicare Advantage program expands beneficiaries' options for participation in private-sector health care plans, which include HMO plans; point-of-service plans, in which beneficiaries may choose providers upon approval of their primary care physicians; and preferred provider organization plans (PPOs), in which beneficiaries may choose from a network of providers based on their specific needs.

### Part D

Medicare Part D, also known as the Medicare Prescription Drug Benefit, was added to the Medicare program as part of the MMA beginning January 1, 2006 (Table 3, page 178). This program provides, for the first time, prescription drug coverage for Medicare beneficiaries. Medicare beneficiaries may enroll in either a stand-alone prescription drug plan (PDP) or an integrated Medicare Advantage Plan or other Medicare Health Plans offering Part D coverage. The benefit offers coverage for most medications and biological agents approved by the U.S. Food and Drug Administration. Organizations providing the prescription drug coverage must offer formularies that conform to the model guidelines set forth by the U.S. Pharmacopeia. The model guidelines consist of drug categories and therapeutic

## Table 1.  Summary of Medicare Part A as of 2006

| Eligibility |
| --- |
| • Beginning at age 65, individuals (and their spouses) who are eligible for Social Security are automatically enrolled in Medicare regardless of retirement status |
| • Individuals who have been receiving Social Security disability benefits for at least 24 months, and government employees with Medicare-only coverage who have been disabled for at least 29 months |
| • Insured workers with end-stage renal disease |

| Financing |
| --- |
| Financed by the Social Security system |
| • Employers and employees pay a tax rate of 1.45% of salaries and wages, respectively |
| • Self-employed individuals pay a tax rate of 2.90% of earnings |

**Services Covered**

| Service | Benefit | Patient payment |
| --- | --- | --- |
| *Hospital care* Includes a semi-private room, meals, general nursing, intensive care, inpatient prescription medications, lab tests, X-rays, inpatient mental care, inpatient rehabilitation, long-term care (if needed), and other hospital services and supplies | For each benefit period[a]: Days 1-60 Days 61-90 Days 91-150 Beyond 150 days | $952 deductible $238/day $476/day All costs |
| *Skilled nursing facility care* Under certain conditions for a limited time, includes services similar to those for inpatients but also includes rehabilitation care | Days 1-20 Days 21-100 Beyond 100 days | None $119/day All costs |
| *Home health care* Has to be approved by the Medicare program and includes skilled nursing care and certain medical supplies | 100 visits following hospitalization or skilled nursing facility stay | None |
| *Hospice care* Has to be certified by a doctor and provides services for terminally ill individuals with life expectancies of 6 months or less, including pain relief, supportive medical and social services, physical therapy, and nursing services | | None for most services |

[a] A benefit period begins when the beneficiary enters a hospital and ends 60 days after discharge from the hospital or from a skilled nursing facility. There is no limit to the number of benefit periods covered; however, some limitations in the number of consecutive hospital days covered during a benefit period may apply.

Source: a) CMS. Brief Summaries of Medicare & Medicaid. Available at:
http://www.cms.hhs.gov/MedicareProgramRatesStats/02_SummaryMedicareMedicaid.asp;
b) CMS. Your Medicare Benefits. Available at: http://www.medicare.gov/Publications/Pubs/pdf/10116.pdf

## Table 2. Summary of Medicare Part B as of 2006

| Eligibility |
|---|
| • Individuals who are eligible for Part A and who decide to enroll in Part B paying a premium of $88.50 per month |

| Financing |
|---|
| Financed by general federal revenues and beneficiary monthly premiums |

**Services Covered**

| Service | Benefit | Patient payment |
|---|---|---|
| *Outpatient services* Includes emergency room services or outpatient clinics, physicians' and surgeons' services; home health care; diagnostic tests; physical, occupational, and speech therapy; mental health care, and; durable medical equipment for home use (e.g., wheelchairs, oxygen, walkers) | Services must be deemed medically necessary | Subject to an annual deductible of $124 and coinsurance (usually 20% of the approved charges) |
| *Preventive care* Includes certain screening tests, such as colorectal and prostate cancer, mammograms, Pap smears, glaucoma, influenza, hepatitis B, and pneumococcal vaccinations | | Included in medical expenses |

Source: a) CMS. Brief Summaries of Medicare & Medicaid. Available at: http://www.cms.hhs.gov/MedicareProgramRatesStats/02_SummaryMedicareMedicaid.asp; b) CMS. Your Medicare Benefits. Available at: http://www.medicare.gov/Publications/Pubs/pdf/10116.pdf

classes that Medicare prescription drug plans must include on their formularies. The formulary must include at least two drugs in each category and class, as well as meet certain other standards. Despite inclusion on the formulary, certain drugs may be subject to prior authorization by the prescribing physician.[5,6]

### Spending

In fiscal year 2004, Medicare benefit payments totaled $295 billion, accounting for almost one-fifth of the $1.4 trillion in U.S. personal health care expenditures, and as much as 12% of the entire federal budget. Inpatient hospital services account for 39% of Medicare benefits spending, but spending proportions are shifting with the addition of the Part D prescription drug benefit. By 2010, prescription drugs are projected to account for more than 20% of total Medicare benefit spending. On a per capita basis, Medicare spending has grown at a rate slightly lower than that in

## Table 3.  Summary of Medicare Part D as of 2006

| Eligibility |
| --- |
| • Individuals eligible for Part A or enrolled in Part B paying a monthly premium |
| • Low-income beneficiaries may benefit from premium and cost-sharing subsidies |
| • Individuals may enroll in either a stand-alone prescription drug plan (PDP) or an integrated Medicare Advantage Plan or other Medicare Health Plans offering Part D coverage |

| Financing |
| --- |
| Financed by general federal and state revenues and beneficiary monthly premiums |

**Services Covered**

| Services | Benefit | Patient payment |
| --- | --- | --- |
| *Outpatient prescription medications* Includes most FDA-approved medications and biological agents. The US Pharmacopeia has created formulary model guidelines— a list of drug categories and therapeutic classes that Medicare prescription drug plans may use as they design their formularies. The formulary must include at least two drugs in each category and class, as well as meet certain other standards. Specific drugs may be subject to prior authorization programs. | Annual total drug costs: Up to $250 $251-$2,250 $2,251-$5,100 Above $5,100 | All costs 25% of costs All costs 5% of costs |

Source: a) CMS. Brief Summaries of Medicare & Medicaid. Available at: http://www.cms.hhs.gov/MedicareProgramRatesStats/02_SummaryMedicareMedicaid.asp;
b) CMS. Your Medicare Benefits. Available at: http://www.medicare.gov/Publications/Pubs/pdf/10116.pdf

the private insurance sector.  Private insurance spending grew at an annual rate of 10.1% between 1970 and 2003, while Medicare grew at a rate of about 9.0% per year.[3,7,8]

Medicare spending averaged just more than $6,000 per covered life in 2002, but is highly concentrated among a small proportion of beneficiaries.  In 2002, 12% of beneficiaries accounted for approximately 70% of program spending.[3,9]

### Financing/Administration

The various components of Medicare are financed differently through combinations of tax revenues, beneficiary monthly premiums, and other cost-sharing strategies.  For example, Part A is financed primarily through payroll taxes paid by workers and employers.  A tax rate of 1.45% of salaries and wages is paid, respectively, by employers and employees, and a tax rate of 2.9% of earnings is paid by self-employed individuals. Part B is financed by a combination of general tax revenues and beneficiary monthly premiums, which cost $88.50 per month in 2006. Part D is financed by general federal and state revenues and beneficiary monthly premiums. While plans administering the prescription drug benefit are allowed some leeway in determining the specific details of the patient payment structure, each of the plans must adhere to a general structure. For example, patients enrolled in the prescription drug benefit are subject to an annual deductible of $250. Once the deductible is met, patients are required to pay 25% of drug costs up to $2,250 in a year. Subsequently, patients enter what is known as the coverage gap. In this gap, patients are required to pay 100% of annual prescription drug costs between $2,250 and $5,100. Above $5,100, catastrophic coverage sets in, at which point patients pay 5% of drug costs. Each year this payment structure resets, with patients having to pay the deductible at the beginning of each year before Medicare coverage for medications sets in.[3,6,7]

### Models of Payment/Reimbursement for Physicians

Fees are calculated by multiplying the relative value unit (RVU) for a Current Procedural Terminology (CPT) code by a conversion factor. The Medicare physician fee schedule sets Medicare's payment rates for more than 7,000 covered services and procedures. Under Medicare, two physicians can be reimbursed for concurrent care, provided the documentation supports the need and the coding reflects the differences. Physicians who treat Medicare beneficiaries receive 80% of the fee if they are the attending physician and bill Medicare Part B. Providers are required to collect any co-payments from patients.[10]

### Current Issues/Challenges and Future Direction

The biggest challenge facing the Medicare program is that of the aging population. As more and more baby-boomers reach age 65, the Medicare-eligible population continues to grow. This results in a decline in the number of workers contributing to Medicare per Medicare beneficiary. Additionally, an increasing life expectancy is keeping beneficiaries in the Medicare program longer, further compounding the issue.

Another major challenge is the administration and the impact of the prescription drug benefit. Research examining the impact of this benefit is vital, particularly as beneficiaries reach the coverage gap at which point they are forced to pay out-of-pocket for all of their prescription drugs.[11] Another major challenge facing Medicare is continually increasing health care costs, an issue that reverberates throughout the healthcare arena. To tackle increasing expenditures, Medicare is pushing beneficiaries toward managed care organizations and engaging in strategies, such as pay for performance initiatives as set forth by the MMA.[12]

## Medicaid

### Overview

Established as a federal/state government program under Title XIX of the Social Security Act of 1965, Medicaid pays for medical assistance for individuals and families with low incomes (Table 4, page 181). Medicaid is the nation's largest public health insurance program and provides insurance coverage and long-term care services to over 52 million low-income children, families, seniors, and people with disabilities. During periods of economic downturn, Medicaid plays an important safety-net role when enrollment grows as a result of increases in the number of people living in poverty.

Within broad national guidelines established by federal statutes, regulations, and policies, each state establishes its own eligibility standards; determines the type, amount, duration, and scope of services; sets the rate of payment for services; and administers its own program. Medicaid policies for eligibility, services, and payment are complex and vary considerably, even among states of similar size or geographic proximity. Medicaid programs are constantly under intense pressure to control costs because they are typically the second largest programs in most state budgets and their spending generally grows faster than that of other programs.[9,13,14]

### Population Covered/Eligibility

On average, Medicaid covers about one out of every nine Americans. States are required to include certain eligibility groups under their Medicaid plans, including categorically needy, medically needy, and special groups. The categorically needy include children ages 6 to 19 with family income up to 100% of the federal poverty level, and individuals and couples who are living in medical institutions and who have monthly income up to 300% of the SSI income standard, for example. Medically needy includes individuals who exceed the categorically needy income thresholds, but to whom states, under their own eligibility standards, extend Medicaid coverage. If a state offers a program for the medically needy, the program is required to include pregnant women through a 60-day postpartum period, children under age 18, certain newborns for a period of one year, and certain protected blind persons.

### Component Structure and Benefits

A state's Medicaid program must offer certain basic services, including inpatient and outpatient hospital, physician services, and laboratory and x-ray services, as examples. States may also receive federal contribution for offering certain optional

## Table 4.  Summary of Medicaid as of 2006

| Eligibility |
| --- |
| • Individuals and families with low incomes and resources. Each state establishes its own eligibility standards within broad national guidelines set by federal regulations. |
| • The federal government requires that the following groups be eligible for Medicaid coverage: |
| — Low-income families with children meeting specific eligibility requirements |
| — Children under age 6 whose family income is at or below 133% of the federal poverty level |
| — Pregnant women whose family income is below 133% of the federal poverty level |
| — Children under age 19 whose family income is at or below the federal poverty level |
| — Individuals, including elderly, blind, or disabled adults, recipients of cash assistance under the Supplemental Security Income (SSI) program |
| — Low-income children eligible under the State Children's Health Insurance Program (SCHIP) |

| Financing |
| --- |
| The federal government pays between 50% and 83% of total Medicaid costs. The lower the state's per capita income level, the greater the federal contribution. |

**Services Covered**

| Services | Patient payment |
| --- | --- |
| A state's Medicaid program must offer certain basic services including: Inpatient and outpatient hospital, physician, laboratory and x-ray, prenatal, vaccines for children, nursing home, home health care, and other optional services.<br><br>States may also receive federal contribution for offering certain optional services, such as diagnostic services, nursing home care for selected ages, rehabilitation, and home health care for certain impaired individuals. | States may request cost-sharing but not for emergency services. Certain beneficiaries must be exempted from cost-sharing. |

Source: a) CMS. Brief Summaries of Medicare & Medicaid. Available at:
http://www.cms.hhs.gov/MedicareProgramRatesStats/02_SummaryMedicareMedicaid.asp;
b) CMS. Medicaid At-a-Glance. Available at:
http://www.cms.hhs.gov/MedicaidGenInfo/Downloads/MedicaidAtAGlance2005.pdf

services, such as specialized diagnostic testing, nursing home services for selected ages, rehabilitation, and home health care for individuals with certain impairments.

## Spending

Medicaid spending in fiscal years 2003 and 2004 grew faster than other state programs; however, it also grew slower than private health insurance. In 2004, total Medicaid expenditures were expected to exceed $300 billion. In response to pressures to contain costs in Medicaid, every state has adopted budget-driven Medicaid cost containment policies and initiatives, including reductions in eligibility, benefits, and provider payments. Specific strategies have included provider payment rate changes, pharmacy utilization and cost control initiatives, benefit changes, and co-payment requirements. While these measures may have been successful in reducing spending, they have also placed additional burdens on Medicaid beneficiaries and the providers who serve them.[9,13,14]

## Financing/Administration

The federal government pays between 50% and 83% of total Medicaid costs. The lower the state's per capita income level, the more the state receives in federal contribution. In fiscal year 2005, the average federal contribution was approximately 57% (excluding federal contribution through the SCHIP program); the highest federal contribution was 77% in Mississippi.[2,15]

Except for emergency services and family planning services, cost sharing may be imposed by states at their own discretion. However, specific beneficiaries, including pregnant women, children under age 18, and certain hospital or nursing patients, must be excluded from cost sharing.

## Models of Payment/Reimbursement for Physicians

Medicaid operates as a vendor payment program. States may pay health care providers directly on a fee-for-service basis, or through prepayment arrangements such as health maintenance organizations (HMOs). Rates for physician reimbursement vary and are published by each state.[16]

## Current Issues/Challenges and Future Direction

As Medicaid costs continue to grow, states are faced with the increasingly difficult challenge of accounting for these expenses in the face of budget shortfalls. In addition, state budgets and Medicaid programs will continue to face a host of new challenges. Specifically, Medicaid will be pressured by increasing poverty and eroding employer-sponsored health insurance. Because of this, states will look for additional strategies to contain costs, and may resort to limiting eligibility or eliminating various covered services.

## Dual Eligibles

More than 7 million low-income elderly and individuals with disabilities are eligible for both Medicare and Medicaid. For these individuals, Medicare continues to pay for basic health services, but Medicaid pays for the Medicare premiums and cost sharing and also covers critical benefits, such as long-term care, that Medicare does not cover. Previously, prescription medications for these beneficiaries were covered under Medicaid; however, with the enactment of the MMA, coverage for drugs has shifted to Medicare Part D.

## SCHIP

The State Children's Health Insurance Program (SCHIP) was established by Congress through the Balanced Budget Act of 1997 as a federal-state partnership to extend health coverage to uninsured children in low-income families. Thereafter, states acted quickly to implement their programs, with children in some states first gaining SCHIP coverage as early as January 1998. Within broad federal guidelines, each state determines the design of its program, eligibility groups, benefit packages, payment levels for coverage, and administrative and operating procedures. By federal law, a child who is eligible for Medicaid, or who has any employer-sponsored health insurance coverage, is not eligible to enroll in SCHIP. SCHIP provides a capped amount of funds to states on a matching basis for federal fiscal years (FY) 1998 through 2007.[1,17]

## Conclusion

Federal and state health insurance programs, including Medicare, Medicaid, and SCHIP, pay for health services for many of America's vulnerable populations, such as the elderly and those with low incomes. A large proportion of the U.S. population, however, remains without any source of coverage. Understanding the basic structures, covered benefits, payment methods, and systems of finance will help providers better serve the individuals covered by these programs. Changes and challenges to the Medicare and Medicaid programs, such as those imposed by the MMA and by state budgetary shortfalls, continue to shape these programs more than 40 years after their creation.

## Case Study

### Medicaid in Pennsylvania

The Pennsylvania Medical Assistance (MA) program purchases health care services for Pennsylvania's most needy and vulnerable citizens, including the elderly and disabled people, and low-income individuals. The Department of Public Welfare's Office of Medical Assistance Program (OMAP) is responsible for administering the joint state/federal program. OMAP is responsible for defining eligibility criteria for program recipients in accordance with federal government regulations. Other OMAP responsibilities include monitoring fraud and abuse activities, and evaluating the quality of care provided to beneficiaries. OMAP runs four major programs: managed care services purchased on a prepaid capitation basis; long-term care; inpatient care; and outpatient services purchased on a fee-for-service or cost-reimbursement basis.

There has been a steady increase in MA enrollment since 2000. In fiscal year 2004-2005, the MA program provided services for approximately 1.8 million residents in Pennsylvania. Children and families represented about 60% of the total number of recipients, followed by people with disabilities (21%), the elderly (13%), and chronically-ill adults (6%). Elderly people account for the fastest growing segment of MA beneficiaries, with an increase of 12% from 2003 to 2005. In 2004, the MA program expenditures accounted for $14 billion, of which approximately 55% was covered by federal contribution. Although the elderly and those with disabilities represent a small proportion of the MA recipients, they account for the largest share of the costs; in 2004, they accounted for 33% and 42% of the MA expenditures, respectively. The increasing enrollment and associated costs of the MA program are challenging the state to maintain affordable and broad coverage to beneficiaries.

The MA network consists of 68,000 providers, including close to 900 hospitals, approximately 45,000 physicians, more than 2,000 pharmacies, and some 800 nursing homes. License and registration by the appropriate state agency are needed by practitioners to be eligible to enroll in the MA network. The administrative and operational burden borne by the MA program to maintain and provide assistance to the MA network is substantial. To increase efficiency of the system, in 2004 the MA program launched a new Internet-based claims processing and management information system called PROMISe™ (Provider Reimbursement and Operations Management Information System). The main goal is to help providers speed up their routine activities and to resolve issues in reasonable time. For example, from any point connected to the World Wide Web, PROMISe™ allows providers to electronically file claims and view the status of any claim, as well as to quickly retrieve updated information on recipients' eligibility. More details about this initiative may be found at: http://www.dpw.state.pa.us/omap/promise/omappromise.asp

## Study/Discussion Questions

1. What were the main stimuli for the establishment of the Medicare and Medicaid programs?

2. Describe and discuss the main components of Medicare. How many parts constitute Medicare and what benefits do each offer?

3. Examine the Medicaid provisions. Propose activities that the states could adopt to monitor expenditures while preserving access and quality of care provided.

4. What differences exist between government financing of Medicare and Medicaid? What are the implications for providers?

5. Access the Medicaid program website in your state. Describe its component and identify ongoing strategies to control costs and improve quality.

## Suggested Readings/Websites

Cassel CK, ed. *Medicare Matters: What Geriatric Medicine Can Teach American Health Care.* Berkeley, CA: California/Milbank Books on Health and the Public; 2005.

The Centers for Medicare and Medicaid Services Website. http://www.cms.hhs.gov/.

Shi L, Singh DA. *Delivering Health Care in America: A Systems Approach.* Boston, MA: Jones & Bartlett; 2003.

Hoffman ED, Klees BS, Curtis CA. *Brief summaries of Medicare & Medicaid.* Office of the Actuary, CMS – Baltimore, MD: Department of Health and Human Services, November 2005.

*Medicare Chart Book.* HJKF Foundation – Menlo Park, CA: Kaiser Family Foundation, July 2005.

*Medicare Fact Sheet: Medicare Spending and Financing.* HJKF Foundation – Menlo Park, CA: Kaiser Family Foundation, April 2005.

The Henry J. Kaiser Family Foundation Web Site (2006). The Kaiser Commission on Medicaid and the Uninsured. Available at: http://www.kff.org/about/kcmu.cfm.

*The Medicare Prescription Drug Benefit.* HJKF Foundation – Menlo Park, CA: Kaiser Family Foundation, 2005.

## References

1. The Centers for Medicare and Medicaid Services. Available at: http://www.cms.hhs.gov/. Accessed May 19, 2006.

2. Hoffman ED, Klees BS, Curtis CA. *Brief summaries of Medicare & Medicaid.* Office of the Actuary, CMS – Baltimore, MD: Department of Health and Human Services, November 2005.

3. *Medicare Chart Book.* HJKF Foundation – Menlo Park, CA: Kaiser Family Foundation, July 2005.

4. Moran DW. Whence and whither health insurance? A revisionist history. *Health Affairs.* 2005;24:1415-1425.

5. *Medicare Prescription Model Guidelines Version 2.0.* USP – Rockland, MD: United States Pharmacopeial Convention, February 2006.

6. *The Medicare Prescription Drug Benefit.* HJKF Foundation – Menlo Park, CA: Kaiser Family Foundation, 2005.

7. *Medicare Fact Sheet: Medicare Spending and Financing.* HJKF Foundation – Menlo Park, CA: Kaiser Family Foundation, April 2005.

8. Newhouse JP. Financing Medicare in the next administration. *N Engl J Med.* 2004; 351:1714-1716.

9. Heffler S, Smith S, Keehan S, Borger C, Clemens MK, Truffer C. U.S. health spending projections for 2004-2014. *Health Affairs.* 2005 Jan-Jun;Suppl Web Exclusives:W5-74-W5-85.

10. Scarrow AM. Physician reimbursement under Medicare. *Neurosurg Focus.* 2002;12:e8.

11. Gellad WF, Huskamp HA, Phillips KA, Haas JS. How the new Medicare drug benefit could affect vulnerable populations. *Health Affairs.* 2006;25:248-255.

12. Kahn CN, Ault T, Isenstein H, Potetz L, Van Gelder S. Snapshot of hospital reporting and pay-for-performance under Medicare. *Health Affairs.* 2006;25:148-162.

13. Holahan J, Ghosh A. Understanding the recent growth in Medicaid spending, 2000-2003. *Health Affairs.* 2005 Jan-Jun;Suppl Web Exclusives:W5-52-W5-62.

14. Holahan J, Rowland D, Feder J, Heslam D. Explaining the recent growth in Medicaid spending. *Health Affairs.* 1993;12:177-193.

15. *The Kaiser Commission on Medicaid and the Uninsured: Financing the Medicaid Program: The Many Roles of Federal and State Matching Funds.* HJKF Foundation – Menlo Park, CA: Kaiser Family Foundation, January 2004.

16. Zuckerman S, McFeeters J, Cunningham P, Nichols L. Changes in Medicaid physician fees, 1998-2003: Implications for physician participation. *Health Affairs.* 2004 Jan-Jun;Suppl Web Exclusives:W4-374-84.

17. Davidoff A, Kenney G, Dubay L. Effects of the State Children's Health Insurance Program expansions on children with chronic health conditions. *Pediatrics.* 2005;116:e34-42. Epub 2005 Jun 15.

# Chapter 12

## Medical Malpractice Protection

David G. Halpern, JD and Jose L. Gonzalez, MD, JD, MSEd

### Executive Summary

Innovations in health care technology have improved our quality of life and increased both patients' and physicians' expectations for successful health outcomes. Yet the practice of medicine remains an art and inexact science where unexpected events and adverse outcomes, despite the best of care, continue to be a reality. When unwanted outcomes occur, the patient or family may blame one or more providers, or the health care system itself, and a lawsuit may follow.

Personal injury law, of which medical practice is a subset, requires the existence of a legal relationship and a duty that is owed a plaintiff by a defendant. In medicine, this duty is described as the standard of care. The standard of care that is owed depends upon the nature of the relationship and the circumstances in which the care is provided. In a malpractice claim, a plaintiff must prove that a health care provider has violated the applicable standard of care and thereby caused him injury.

The incidence of adverse events or bad outcomes is higher in medicine than in other settings for the simple reason that physician-patient relationships often begin with a patient who is already ill or injured. Medical care is also frequently provided under conditions that are less than optimal and often time pressured. Effective communication with patients and family can do much to reduce anxieties, to develop a sense of trust in the provider and the treatment process, and to promote a better understanding and commitment to the treatment plan and its outcomes. Successful communication, verbal and written, can mean the difference between reactive lawsuits and non-litigious responses.

This chapter is designed to introduce physicians to the current medico-legal landscape, the effects it has on them, as well as other health care providers, and how to equip themselves to deal with current issues and challenges.

## Learning Objectives

1. Review the history and current status of medical malpractice liability and litigation in the U.S. system of health care delivery.

2. Understand the extent of medical errors and avoidable adverse patient outcomes within the U.S. system of health care delivery.

3. Define the types of documentation and communication techniques that maximize protection from medical malpractice claims.

4. Discuss the importance and ethical appropriateness of truth-telling in medical error and avoidable patient outcomes disclosure.

## Keywords

adverse medical events; interpersonal communications; legal duty; medical malpractice; medical record documentation; physician-patient relationship; truth-telling

## Introduction

In recent years, physicians and other health care providers throughout the United States have come to know and, to some extent, to fear a rising tide of malpractice claims. Taken as a whole, the United States is widely considered to be among the most litigious of societies. The United States is among the best educated and equipped countries on Earth in terms of technological and scientific innovation. Advances in science have brought tremendous opportunities, including a longer and better quality of life for many. These same advantages, however, have wrought tremendous challenges to health care and its delivery. Longer lives have resulted in an aging population with a shifting of the demands on resources, not the least of which involves an expanded and more taxing role for all providers in the field of health care.

Americans, by and large, are living longer and most are living better. Innovations in medical care have improved our quality of life and created heightened, if not new, expectations by the recipients of health care. Historically, physicians have been among the most respected of professionals, and their rewards, personal as well as monetary, have been commensurate with the recognition. Still, when outcomes are unanticipated and adverse, patient and family expectations can be shattered. Adverse outcomes are commonly accompanied by a host of patient and family emotions and actions which present important personal and professional challenges to practitioners, including the possibility of defending themselves in litigation. This chapter is designed to introduce the practicing physician to the current medico-legal landscape in America, what effects it has had on physicians and other health care providers, and what can be done to better equip physicians and others to deal with the current issues and challenges before them.

Recent government reports indicate that there were over 14,000 claims against U.S. health physicians in 2004.[1] Total payments in 2003 reached $4.45 billion.[2] The costs for insuring physicians, other health care providers and hospitals were estimated at $11 million in 2003.[2] Concern that the rising costs of health care are due to a growing number of lawsuits is now a major, nationwide issue. President George W. Bush and others have proposed legislation to restructure the medical liability system in America. Outside the Capital Beltway, various state legislatures have responded in similar fashion, enacting medical malpractice tort reform provisions that limit provider liability and establish caps on monetary damages.[3]

Critics of medical malpractice reform argue that the medical malpractice crisis is more myth than truth. In his book, *The Medical Malpractice Myth*, Tom Baker, professor at the University of Connecticut School of Law, posits that the average malpractice insurance premium in 2004 was $12,000 per physician, hardly a crisis.[4] Others have argued similarly that the medical liability system is not out of control and not in need of repair.[4] These contentions notwithstanding, it is clear that the current state of medical malpractice litigation, regardless of locale, practice type and the immediate political landscape, poses a real and present danger to physicians and other health care providers.[5]

## Medical Malpractice Litigation

A medical malpractice claim falls into a broader category of litigation generally described as personal injury or tort law, common to which are the following legal elements that the aggrieved or injured person(s) (plaintiffs) must prove to establish a legal right to remedy:

1. The existence of a legally recognized relationship between the injured person(s) and the party who is alleged to have caused the injury (the tortfeasor, in legal terms). This is commonly referred to as the legal duty that is owed by the tortfeasor.

2. The allegation that the tortfeasor, by act or omission, breached the duty that he owes to the injured person(s).

3. The allegation that the injury or damages resulted from the violation of the duty.

The element of legal duty is generally established when a physician or other health care provider commits to providing treatment or care to a patient. The concept of duty, well established in law, is seldom heard in a clinic or a hospital. "Standard of care" has become the alternate term of art, which describes the relative legal duty that is owed by a health care provider in a medical malpractice action. The duty, or standard of care, that is owed will depend upon the nature of the relationship. For example, the duty owed by a physician will generally demand a greater level of responsibility and expertise than the duty owed by a physician's assistant or nurse. Similarly, the greater the applicable level of expertise of the provider, the greater the duty that is owed. This is illustrated in a patient suffering from a disease of the heart. The duty that is owed by the patient's primary care physician will, generally, be less than that owed by the cardiologist or cardiovascular surgeon, at least for purposes of treating the heart condition.

The standard of care is also determined by the circumstances in which the physician-patient relationship develops. The standard that is applicable in any given scenario depends not only upon the level of the provider's expertise, but also upon the conditions which define the interaction between the patient and provider, (e.g., the physical location where a patient demonstrates symptoms may define different standards of care for the very same provider). For example, the standard of care owed by a surgeon in a clinic setting may be to promptly diagnose and transfer the patient to a properly equipped surgical center; the same event occurring in a hospital would likely require this same physician to initiate surgical intervention. It is notable that although much of the focus on patient safety and adverse events has come from the hospital setting, the overwhelming majority of health care in the United States is in fact delivered outside of hospitals.[5] A provider's failure to act as would a reasonably prudent, similarly trained physician in the same or similar circumstances is medical negligence. The providers' failure to meet the applicable standard of care establishes the necessary breach element in a medical malpractice action.

Finally, once the first two elements are established, the injury or damages element must flow from the health care provider's breach of the applicable standard of care. The critical, often insurmountable, hurdle in many medical malpractice cases is establishing that the medical negligence that is alleged is actually the cause of the injury or damages incurred.

## When Bad Outcomes Happen

Common to most personal injury lawsuits is the existence of a discrete injurious event, such as a motor vehicle accident or workplace mishap. This is often, but by no means always, the case in the world of medical malpractice. More typical is a bad outcome or adverse event following either a discrete modality of treatment or a longer term course of treatment and care. Unlike a vehicular accident or slip and fall, the medical malpractice plaintiff frequently enters the provider's realm *because he is already injured or ill*. In and of itself, an adverse outcome is not necessarily a reflection on the experience or competence of the care giver. Bad things can happen to anyone. But for the injured and ill, the likelihood of a bad outcome can only be expected to increase as these individuals are, after all, less than whole when they seek treatment.

Although risks in providing treatment may differ in severity, they are always inherent in delivering medical care. The risks may be small, such as in caring for a common cold, or may be great, as when a patient's entire immune system is "destroyed" to perform bone marrow transplantation. Medical management of the injured and ill is undeniably prospective. It is also deductive. Symptoms may, but often do not, point to a definitive diagnosis. Modalities of treatment may or may not be efficacious, despite the most reassuring literature and best of care. The intellectual challenge as well as the clinical responsibility for providers is to arrive at a plan of care that is most appropriate under the circumstances.

Circumstances for care are seldom optimal. Health care resources, though vast in the abstract, may be limited in application and are increasingly being taxed by demands from an aging and more medically sophisticated patient population. Health care staff and the necessary medical expertise may also be in short supply, especially in time-sensitive situations. Increasingly complex diagnostic tools often entail increased costs, and current payment and reimbursement schemes only serve to add pressure to the diagnostician's ability to make the best and most appropriate decisions. As a result, providers are repeatedly faced with the challenge of trying to do more with less.

In spite of these constraints, health care today can be provided in less time thanks to various technical and therapeutic advances. Although often blamed on cost-saving pressures, the trend to shorter hospital stays[6] can also be credited to better medicine. Regardless, the consequences of these changes are that interactions among different and complementary disciplines are often rushed and shortened, with less time for consultation. Much more important, the resulting time pressures lead to less time with patients and less time to document their health management and clinical course. In fact, the success or failure of a plan of care may have nearly as much to do with the manner in which the provider communicates the risks facing the patient, as in providing the actual care itself.

## Communication: The Good, The Bad, and The Rest

Patients or family, by virtue of their need or desire for a change in a health condition, entrust themselves or their loved ones to a physician or other provider. In so doing, health care providers frequently are afforded an opportunity to develop and cultivate the physician-patient relationship prior to implementing treatment. It is here that the path of an alleged medical malpractice tortfeasor takes a sharp turn from the road on which other alleged wrongdoers travel. Effective communication — where the provider details the patient's condition, the treatment options (including the option of no treatment) and the risks of the proposed management to the patient — entails much more than a well-articulated and legally sound consent form. Providers who give this interaction short shrift may in fact shortchange both the patients and themselves.

Time is but one obstacle to effective physician-patient communication by busy providers. Even an earnest and diligent communicator can find his best efforts thwarted in the setting of a busy clinic, hospital ward or emergency room. Under given circumstances, patients may not hear or understand what is being said to them or be willing to process or accept information, much less to question what they are told. Patients may also perceive and present their condition quite differently from that described in the medical literature and may have different expectations for care and different thresholds for seeking it.[7] And, increasingly, cultural differences may create communication barriers that may be overtly obvious or so subtle as to be imperceptible to providers.

Communication that invites the patient and family to consider medical care as a collaborative team effort is likely to result in a number of positive attributes to the physician-patient relationship:

1. **Trust.** The patient and family often enter the physician-patient relationship with heightened emotions, including anxiety, fear, and possibly skepticism or even cynicism. They are emotionally vulnerable and more sensitive to interactions with providers. Taking the time to engage the patient and thoroughly explain a situation can do much to alleviate fear and to nurture a feeling of trust in the provider and in the treatment process itself.[8]

2. **Understanding.** Effective communication during a course of medical treatment requires a commitment of time and attention to ensure that the patient and family understand the possible eventualities and are prepared to respond to them. However, this commitment can pay dividends in facilitating more effective and timely treatment. Furthermore, such understanding can make the difference between an outcome that is perceived as wholly and legitimately unexpected; one that is unexpected, yet should have been foreseen; and one that is clearly

adverse, but nonetheless expected as a possible result of the treatment provided.

3. **Commitment.** When the patient and family consider themselves to be active participants in the treatment plan, they become invested rather than isolated and uninformed in the management decisions and the possible outcomes. They share the good and the bad, the successes and the failures.

Trust, understanding and commitment, or the lack thereof, can in turn mean the difference between a litigious reaction to an adverse outcome and a non-litigious response. Anecdotal evidence supports the proposition that litigation is more likely to occur in situations where the provider's care is:

— episodic rather than continuous; or

— continuous, but insensitive to the vulnerabilities of the patient and family.

Stated another way, when an adverse outcome has occurred, the patient may suffer not only from the treatment itself, but also from the manner in which the adverse event is revealed to the patient or family and responded to by the health care providers.[8]

## Charting: Friend and Foe

"If it's not in the chart, it didn't happen." Ask most health care providers today to respond to this old saw and you are likely to learn how misleading it is, if not downright false. Alternatively, ask an experienced medical malpractice attorney, and the response is likely to be quite different. Litigation generally occurs months, and sometimes years, after a bad outcome. Memories fade. Providers come and go. Often the best, and at times the only, evidence remaining is the documentation of the care that ensued from the health care physician-patient relationship. All providers are steeped in the tradition that good documentation, whether in the outpatient clinic or the in-hospital setting, makes for good medicine, and that effective continuity of care depends upon an accurate, if not wholly complete, medical record.

Yet mistakes in charting occur, as do mistakes in clinical care. The medical challenge and malpractice sanctuary for the health care provider lies in minimizing both. Difficulty in establishing and implementing an appropriate and successful treatment plan, however defined, is inherent to the medical profession. The difficulties in accurately documenting a proposed and provided plan of care are minor by comparison. Since time is at a premium, care must come first and charting necessarily follows, often as a distant second. However, serious problems follow when charting is neglected, and while time constraints may explain poor documentation, they can never excuse it. Important information can be omitted or misstated, and ambiguous or vague terminology can lead to medication and other management errors, with devastating outcomes.

In the hospital setting, nurses and other non-physician providers are the backbone of care. As compared to attending physicians, they spend more time in direct contact with patients, deliver more of the actual care, communicate more medical and diagnostic information, and generally interact more frequently and in greater depth with the patients and their families. Demands on their time require that charting occurs minutes to hours after the fact. As such, entries in the medical record as to the time that care or treatment was provided are seldom precisely accurate. The "plus or minus" of a few minutes, seemingly innocuous during the course of care, can become monumental in a court of law. Hurriedly phrased clinical observations, readily explainable during transfer of care reports, can be interpreted, misinterpreted, and misused in litigation by an experienced attorney. What had been an easily explained slip of the pen can instead be characterized as negligence or misconduct during trial, with serious implications for both the author and the multiple other providers in the reporting chain.

## Problem Solving in the Wake of a Bad Outcome

Mistakes happen and consequences, both immediate and latent, can follow; they are inevitable. Nonetheless, the myth that the physician can do no wrong persists in the minds of many lay persons. It is understandable why patients would choose to believe this, but it is much less clear how and why this perception continues to be perpetuated in our medical schools. Perhaps, in an environment where precision and expertise predominates, medical learners find it difficult to accept their fallibility and to accept the "emotional consequences of mistakes."[9]

A marked rise in medical malpractice litigation over the past ten to twenty years has had predictable consequences. Although the debate on their merit continues unabated, recent legislative changes in the name of tort reform have brought economic damages caps and narrowly applied limits on providers' medical malpractice liability. Most medical schools now incorporate risk management and medical malpractice litigation training into their curricula. Hospitals, already well-versed in these affairs, similarly continue to improve their policies and procedures for avoiding medical errors and responding to adverse outcomes. Despite these strides, silent or guarded responses by providers to questions posed by patients or families on the heels of an unexpected or adverse outcome occur daily in medical settings across the country. Fear of litigation, concern for compromising statements, and avoidance of possibly inculpatory admissions all drive the understandable instinct by the "challenged" health care providers to stonewall. Yet, it is this very same wall that establishes the dynamic where litigation is more likely to follow "…regardless of the actual level of medical care employed in a case, a malpractice suit flows from the malignant synergy of a bad outcome, an injury or death, and bad feelings such as patient guilt, grief, rage, surprise, and abandonment."[10]

When an adverse outcome occurs, patients and families find themselves in a difficult and awkward situation: having entrusted their care to a physician or health care team, they now want to understand what happened; how it happened; and why it happened. They have the right to question. To the extent that there has been good communication throughout the course of treatment, many of these questions will already have been answered. To the extent that they have not, the incidence of litigation will be a function not only of how the families perceive the care, but also on the credibility and sincerity of the caregivers.

## The Apology in Truth-Telling

A growing sensitivity to the skills of effective and truthful communication in medical care suggests that a new paradigm may be on the horizon. Where treatment is followed by an adverse outcome, an appropriately phrased apology can do much to address patient and family concerns and to allay a sense of bitterness. It is difficult to overemphasize the importance of identifying what is appropriate from what is not. Where no medical error is apparent, an expression of regret for the outcome may be all that is needed to keep the physician-patient relationship intact.[10] In circumstances where a medical error has occurred, the proper form of communication is the subject of considerable debate. Legal counselors are prone to argue for nothing more than an expression of sympathy to best guard against a compromised defense. In contrast, many more counsel for an apology that contains both a sincere expression of regret for the outcome and an expression of accountability for that outcome. Some have, in fact, observed that an apology that lacks accountability in the face of a preventable adverse outcome may do more harm than good.[11]

Recognition of both the value and the entrenched fear of the consequences of an accountability-based apology have prompted legislative changes in various states across the country.[11] In 1986, Massachusetts was the first state to demonstrate the political wisdom of legislating protections for providers who are willing to offer expressions of sympathy. From Florida to Texas to California, other states have followed with laws that preclude statements of regret from being used as evidence of liability in civil actions.[12] In 2003, Colorado went a step further, showing the political courage to protect a care giver's expression of fault from being used against him or her in a civil action.[12]

Although study after study has shown that a sincere and truthful apology following a bad outcome will reduce the likelihood that a lawsuit will be filed, health care providers should never forget what Harvard Medical School's Thomas G. Gutheil observed nearly twenty years ago: "To assume that an apology is any kind of solution to a bad or even tragic outcome is overly optimistic. Realistically, an apology as an admission of error only works within a well established, enduring atmosphere of frank collaboration which dates back to the earliest stages of the [provider] patient relationship."[10]

Reflecting on the various elements necessary to establish and support a medical malpractice claim, consider the following case study. As you respond to the circumstances of the case history, keep in mind the preventive value of effective and compassionate communication, both verbal and written.

## Conclusion

Physicians today continue to practice in a litigious environment. Heightened expectations based upon medical advances and increased demands on limited resources present challenges to all providers in the delivery of quality, safe, and cost-effective health care. Despite a growing trend toward limiting legal liability, the threat of malpractice looms large and should serve as a powerful stimulant for physicians and other providers to limit their liability exposure.

The importance of the physician-patient relationship in mitigating this exposure cannot be overemphasized. Within the context of this relationship, effective, interpersonal communication skills, accurate and complete record documentation, and truth-telling after an adverse event are each key to both medical malpractice protection and quality, safe health care delivery. Mastering these competencies, along with medical knowledge and technical proficiency, may be the best antidote for the rising tide of medical malpractice litigation.

## Case Study

Patient Baby J is the newborn daughter of a married couple in their early 20s. Parents and grandparents are well educated and from upper-middle income households. Baby J was diagnosed in-utero with a congenital heart defect. Shortly after delivery, she was transferred to a large pediatric medical center where successful repair of a coarctation of the aorta was performed on day three of life. Following an uneventful recovery, Baby J was transferred to the general cardiac floor where her care was directed by a team of resident physicians, nurses and cardiology faculty. Throughout the next few days, the infant displayed symptoms that included fussiness and feeding difficulties. Attributing them to routine post-cardiac surgical course, Baby J's providers addressed these symptoms by complementing the mother's breastfeeding with enteral feedings. Over the same period, the nurses' daily progress records reflected an excess, rapid weight gain despite continued fussiness and difficulty feeding. Recorded daily fluid "ins and outs" were, however, inconsistent with the infant's clinical findings and course. The nursing records also reported a steadily increasing anxiety from the child's parents and grandparents with frequent and repeated interactions between the nurses, physicians and the family, typically in response to the family's request to revisit and revise the plan of care.

### Questions

1. What could have been done to address the inconsistencies between the nursing record and the patient's clinical course?

2. As the principal provider, how could you ensure effective communication between all care givers and accurate and complementary documentation?

3. What could have been done to proactively address the family's questions and concerns?

On day thirteen of life, continued expressions of concern by the family prompted one of the residents to revisit Baby J's plan of care with the cardiology attending. That same day, the patient's clinical status decompensated rapidly, with acute respiratory distress, pleural effusion, central hypoxia, and kidney failure. Following successful resuscitation, the child's symptoms were diagnosed secondary to low cardiac output syndrome.

### Questions

1. How and when would you have approached the patient's cardiology attending with your questions and concerns as to the patient's clinical course?

2. Could this patient's acute deterioration have been avoided?

Once stabilized, specialists were consulted, including a genetics consult and genetic screening that identified the patient as having Turner's syndrome. A pediatric neurologist was also consulted to determine what, if any, brain damage Baby J suffered during the period of respiratory decompensation. A series of CT-scans suggested a global CNS ischemic insult that would likely leave Baby J with permanent neurological damage and little hope of meaningful quality of life. A second pediatric neurology consult requested by the family was consistent with the first. The parents responded to the prognosis with appropriate grief and requested that their daughter's chest and feeding tubes be withdrawn. In disagreement, the cardiology faculty convened an ethics conference to address the family's request to withdraw care. The conference was difficult and emotional for all participants. Sadness without admission of guilt for Baby J's adverse outcomes was related to the parents by the health care givers. At the conclusion of the meeting, the parents relented in their decision to withdraw Baby J's care and she resumed her convalescent care.

At age two, Baby J had approximated several major developmental milestones but retained significant spatial motor difficulties as well as moderately severe cognitive and verbal deficits. Within the year following these events, the parents filed suit seeking claims for alleged negligence against the cardiology team, the hospital and the medical school which staffs the hospital with faculty and resident physicians. After months of intensive litigation, the case was resolved through an arbitrated settlement.

### Questions

1. How did this patient's delayed diagnosis of Turner's Syndrome affect the physician-patient relationship?

2. Was the ethics conference necessary? Could it have been prevented?

3. Was the physicians' apology to the family indicated? Would you have expressed it differently?

4. Any final thoughts on the negligence suit and its prevention?

## Discussion

### Documentation

Review of the medical record failed to establish that the patient's daily weights were taken on a consistent basis. The arbitrator subsequently determined that the substandard documentation likely delayed awareness of Baby J's changing clinical picture and progressive cardiac dysfunction and impaired venous return. Nurse charting during ward care also described the pedal pulses as "abnormally decreased" on several occasions, albeit without other physical indicators suggestive of abnormal peripheral perfusion, such as delayed capillary refill or peripheral cyanosis. The record, however, did not contain any subsequent documentation as to an acknowledgement or response to these nurse findings by the medical staff. The apparent absence of communication between the nursing and medical staff, including the physicians' failure to read or address the contents of the nurses' notes section of the chart, further influenced the arbitrator's eventual negligence determination.

A nurse progress note on the afternoon of Baby J's acute clinical deterioration observed signs suggestive of low cardiac output syndrome including, among others, mottled skin on the legs and mild sub-costal retractions. More pointedly, the note suggested but did not clearly state that these symptoms were observed in the presence of a resident physician. In deposition, the nurse confirmed her uncertainty as to the actual meaning of these physical signs, while the resident physician testified that he was unaware of and not present when the nurse observed the described findings.

Finally, the charting of the consulting pediatric neurologists articulated a prognosis that was so specific and so bleak that it drew skepticism from other providers involved in Baby J's care. This, in turn, triggered a series of events which divided the medical staff, creating tensions between care givers in the ICU and on the floor, doctors and nurses, and resident physicians and cardiology faculty.

**Communication**

During Baby J's post-operative convalescence, she was cared for in two settings: the hospital's intensive care unit and the general cardiac floor. During Baby J's stay in the ICU, the parents observed and appreciated the level of care provided. As a consequence, the family developed a high degree of comfort and confidence in the ICU care givers and, as frequently seen, came to expect prompt, often immediate responses to their perceived needs. Upon transfer to the general cardiac hospital ward, the differences in the level of care provided therein, with an increased patients-to-nurse ratio and a greater proportion of first contact care delivered by resident physicians and students, was not lost on the family.

Evidence developed in litigation showed that following transfer, a significant communication gap developed between the family and the health care providers. The evidence clearly reflected an unambiguous and growing schism between the care givers, who felt that the family had become extraordinarily demanding of their time, i.e., "high maintenance," and the family, who came to feel as if their pleas for assistance were given insufficient attention, if not outright ignored. Specifically, the family grew increasingly frustrated at their inability to obtain timely updates on their daughter's clinical course, changes in management plan and overall status in spite of multiple requests. In this context, the cardiology health care team's daily visits frequently occurred early in the day and seldom intersected with the family's inquiries and requests.

Expectedly, the family's negligence suit distinctly alleged that multiple attempts to engage nurses and physicians were repeatedly ignored in disregard of the family's increasing frustration with their daughter's feeding difficulties, fussiness and perceived decline in her overall clinical appearance throughout the hospital stay, and that this disregard directly contributed to their daughter's adverse outcome.

As may be surmised, the alleged negligent health care, while largely defensible from a legal standard of care perspective, entailed mostly charting and communication issues. Issues which, as stated above, are likely to increase the probability that a family will seek redress through the courts and that the ensuing litigation will avail in their favor.

## Suggested Readings/Websites

Marchev M. The Medical Malpractice Insurance Crisis: Opportunity for State Action. National Academy for State Health Policy Website. July 2002: http://www.nashp.org/Files/gnl48_medical_malpractice.PDF.

National Center for Health Statistics: http://www.cdc.gov/nchs/hus.htm.

Vincent C. Understanding and responding to adverse events. *New Engl J Med.* 2003;348:1051-1056.

Hilfiker D. Facing our mistakes. *New Engl J Med.* 1984;310:118-122.

Gutheil TG. On apologizing to patients. Risk Management Foundation. *Forum.* 1987;8:3-4.

Wu AW. Removing Insult from Injury – Disclosing Adverse Events. AHRQ Web M&M. Perspectives on Safety, February 2006: http://www.webmm.ahrq.gov/perspectives.aspx.

Sparkman C. Legislating Apology in the context of medical mistakes. *AORN J.* 2005;82:263-266, 269-272.

Committee on Medical Liability and Risk Management, Berger JE, Deitschel C, eds. *Medical Liability for Pediatricians*, 6ᵗʰ ed. Elk Grove Village, IL: American Academy of Pediatrics; 2004.

## References

1. National Practitioner Data Bank 2004 Annual Report. U.S. Department of Health and Human Services. Health Resources and Services Administration. Available at: http://www.npdb-hipdb.hrsa.gov/pubs/stats/2004_NPDB_Annual_Report.pdf. Accessed July 10, 2006.

2. National Practitioner Data Bank. Public Data Files. Available at: http://www.npdb-hipdb.hrsa.gov/publicdata.html. Accessed September 21, 2006.

3. Marchev M. The Medical Malpractice Insurance Crisis: Opportunity for State Action. National Academy for State Health Policy Website. July 2002. Available at: http://www.nashp.org/Files/gnl48_medical_malpractice.PDF. Accessed July 9, 2006.

4. Baker T. *The Medical Malpractice Myth.* Chicago, Illinois: University of Chicago Press; 2005.

5. Phillips RL Jr, Bartholomew LA, Dovey SM, Fryer GE Jr, Miyoshi TJ, Green LA. Learning from malpractice claims about negligent adverse events in primary care in the United States. *Qual Saf Health Care.* 2004;13:121-126.

6. National Center for Health Statistics. Available at: http://www.cdc.gov/nchs/hus.htm. Accessed August 1, 2006.

7. Betancourt JR. Cultural competence — marginal or mainstream movement? *New Engl J Med.* 2004;351:953-955.

8. Vincent C. Understanding and responding to adverse events. *New Engl J Med.* 2003;348:1051-1056.

9. Hilfiker D. Facing our mistakes. *New Engl J Med.* 1984;310:118-122.

10. Gutheil TG. On apologizing to patients. Risk Management Foundation. *Forum.* 1987;8:3-4.

11. Wu AW. Removing Insult from Injury – Disclosing Adverse Events. AHRQ Web M&M. Perspectives on Safety, February 2006. Available at: http://www.webmm.ahrq.gov/perspectives.aspx. Accessed July 8, 2006.

12. Sparkman C. Legislating apology in the context of medical mistakes. *AORN J.* 2005;82:263-266, 269-272.

# Chapter 13

## Dealing or Succeeding with Disease Management

Harry L. Leider, MD, MBA, FACPE, Raymond L. Wedgeworth, MA, and Laurie Russell, MS, RN, CCM

### Executive Summary

Historically, physicians regarded disease management (DM) programs as an intrusion to their practices and of limited value. As a result, many DM programs had limited success at engaging physicians as partners in the DM process and instead focused their efforts on educating patients about self-managing their chronic disease. This situation was largely driven by the cumbersome nature of many early DM programs, physicians' inherent bias for professional autonomy, and the lack of aligned financial incentives to reward physicians for collaborating with the DM program.

This chapter describes an emerging new dynamic, due largely to the following: DM programs are improving in their "ease of use" for physicians; financial incentives are being introduced (by Medicare and the private sector) that reward physicians for supporting DM programs; and physician leaders are becoming increasingly supportive of DM programs that improve quality of care and reduce costs. Finally, this chapter provides a set of case studies that demonstrate the potential for DM programs to offer value to both patients and physicians by using new technologies and care management strategies. It is the authors' belief that within the next 5 to 10 years physicians will no longer feel that they need to "deal" with DM programs – but instead will truly believe that they will be more successful and improve the quality of patient care by collaborating with these initiatives.

### Learning Objectives

1. To understand the historic relationship among physicians and disease management (DM) programs.

2. To understand how evolving private payor and public sector initiatives measure and reward physicians for positive clinical outcomes that DM programs can positively impact.

3. To explore successful models for physician collaboration with DM programs.

4. To examine new tools, tactics, and technologies that facilitate physician participation in DM programs.

**Keywords**

disease management ; pay for performance; physician buy-in

## Introduction

Despite the fact that they have existed for more than 20 years, many physicians regard disease management (DM) programs as a nuisance or burden. This view is rapidly changing due to new technologies that make DM programs less intrusive, and the development of programs that reward physicians for improvements in quality of care. In the near future, it is likely that a growing majority of physicians will embrace disease management as a means to improve patient care and, as a result, to achieve higher levels of reimbursement.

This chapter will review the factors that created the historically negative dynamic among physicians and disease management initiatives, as well as emerging forces that are encouraging physicians to support disease management. This chapter will also present examples that illustrate how DM programs and physicians can work together in a manner that improves health outcomes for patients and, ultimately, could also improve the income of physicians.[1] In the end, physician leaders will play a key role in developing DM programs and engaging other physicians in supporting these initiatives.[2]

## Definition of Disease Management

There are many definitions of disease management. A common and practical definition was created by the Disease Management Association of America:[3]

"Disease management is a system of coordinated health care interventions and communications for populations with conditions in which patient self-care efforts are significant. Disease management:

• Supports the physician or practitioner/patient relationship and plan of care;

• Emphasizes prevention of exacerbations and complications utilizing evidence-based practice guidelines and patient empowerment strategies; and

• Evaluates clinical, humanistic, and economic outcomes on an ongoing basis with the goal of improving overall health."

The definition goes on to delineate the specific elements that usually serve as the building blocks of effective DM programs.

"Disease management components include:

- Population identification processes;

- Evidence-based practice guidelines;

- Collaborative practice models to include physician and support-service providers;

- Patient self-management education (may include primary prevention, behavior modification programs, and compliance/surveillance);

- Process and outcomes measurement, evaluation, and management;  and

- Routine reporting/feedback loop (may include communication with patient, physician, health plan and ancillary providers, and practice profiling)."

In general, nurses and other non-physician health care providers (e.g., respiratory therapists, dieticians) conduct most DM interventions, such as patient education and monitoring.  For example, a typical DM program for heart failure will provide a patient with a personal nurse who will call the patient periodically to provide support and guidance.  This support includes intensive education about medication compliance, adhering to a low-sodium diet, monitoring daily dry weights, and self-monitoring for symptoms of heart failure.  Some DM programs will also contact a patient's primary care physician if "optimal" therapies (according to evidence-based guidelines) have not been prescribed.  For example, the physician of a patient with heart failure who has not been prescribed an ACE inhibitor or beta-blocker—medications recommended by the American College of Cardiology/American Heart Association because they have been shown to decrease mortality—might be contacted by a representative of the DM program.[4,5,6]  The combined impact of these interventions provides the patient with the tools to self-manage his or her risk of heart failure, and the knowledge to call his or her doctor or DM nurse before an episode might emerge that would require a hospitalization. Typically, heart failure DM programs have reduced hospitalizations by 40% to 50% for patients with moderate to severe disease.[7,8,9]

Prior to the recent advent of several large, government-sponsored pilot programs, most DM programs have been sponsored by managed care organizations.  These programs generally targeted heart failure, asthma, diabetes, cardiovascular disease, high-risk maternity, and, more recently, emphysema and rarer diseases such as sickle-cell anemia, multiple sclerosis, and rheumatoid arthritis.  These conditions were generally chosen because they cause frequent hospitalizations that can often be prevented, or because DM programs can improve the quality measures that health plans report to their clients (e.g., diabetes or asthma). These measures, called the Health Employer Data Information Set (HEDIS)[10] are used by large employers to select health plans. Organizations, such as the National Committee on Quality Assurance (NCQA),[11] also use these measures during their accreditation process for health plans.

Health plans have two basic options when implementing DM programs. They can outsource these programs to an independent DM vendor or develop the capacity to provide these programs themselves. The latter course generally involves building or purchasing specialized software to collect clinical data, create a care plan for each patient, and report program outcomes. Nurses are then hired to directly interact with patients, usually by telephone, and, occasionally, in their homes or in physicians' offices. Conversely, a DM vendor will generally already have these capabilities in place, and will sometimes "guarantee" improved clinical and financial outcomes for the targeted population.[12]

## Historical Context of Physicians and DM

Although DM programs historically focused most of their efforts on patients rather than physicians, almost all programs recognize the critical importance of ensuring that patients take the proper medications and that physicians support the efforts of the DM program's nurses. To achieve these goals, DM programs will typically send "updates," "report cards," or "care plans" to the primary care doctor after interacting with patients. Since virtually all physicians participate in multiple health plans, and each plan has one or more DM programs, it is not uncommon for physicians to receive many different types of communications, each one requesting different actions or follow-up — even for the same disease. These varied and frequent communications represent one of the major sources of discontent for physicians, as they can be very time-consuming to review and respond to appropriately.

Until recently, health plans typically provided no additional reimbursement to physicians for time spent reviewing and responding to these DM communications. In the typical fee-for-service primary care practice, income is dependent on seeing a high volume of patients. Therefore, most physicians took a negative view of any DM communication or activity that had the potential to either reduce the number of patients that could be seen or increase the time spent per patient.

Physicians often perceive DM programs as infringing on their autonomy, creating a major source of tension.[13] DM programs routinely attempt to improve patient care and outcomes by encouraging patients and physicians to follow evidence-based guidelines. It is well-documented that physicians frequently do not follow guidelines for a variety of reasons, such as a lack of knowledge, inability to perform the requirements of the guideline, or a belief that the required actions won't affect the outcome.[14] Therefore, the efforts of DM staff to influence physicians can create dissonance and, at times, antipathy.

Furthermore, many physicians inherently believe that they should be "in the driver's seat" when it comes to managing disease. Since they manage patient care, many physicians don't see the need for "external" DM programs. Even if they do understand the value in supporting patients between office visits and hospitalizations, physicians believe they should be the ones providing DM, and resent the fact that payors generally won't compensate them for building the necessary infrastructure to provide these services. This tension is particularly common when trying to engage specialists to support DM programs; primary care physicians are often more likely to acknowledge the benefit of these programs.[15]

## New Dynamics Between Physicians and DM

The American health care system has produced the most advanced medical technologies and procedures in the world. In addition, and partially as a result of these advances, our population enjoys an extended average life span. Nonetheless, major studies continue to drive a national debate on the quality of care in our country. [16,17] As a result of these studies, and the increasing amount of money spent on health care, public concern is beginning to force fundamental changes in the health care system.

The rapid growth in health care spending and concerns over quality of care also impact the way physicians negotiate contracts and practice medicine. Innovations such as pay for performance models (P4P), quality report cards, "tiered" provider networks, and the development of health information technology (HIT) solutions such as electronic medical records (EMRs) are significantly changing the way physicians work. In this new environment, physicians are increasingly being held responsible not only for the time spent in direct contact with their patients but for the entire spectrum of care a patient receives – even between office visits or hospitalizations. Incentives and new support infrastructures are being created to shift the focus of health care from coping with acute exacerbations of illness to keeping patients well. This shift in focus has created greater opportunities for physicians and DM programs to collaborate on a deeper, more supportive level than they have in the past.

## Pay for Performance Models

### New Public Initiatives

The Centers for Medicare and Medicaid Services (CMS) is the federal agency responsible for oversight of the Medicare, Medicaid, and State Children's Health Insurance Programs (SCHIP). One in four Americans receives health care from one of the programs that CMS administers.[18] In 2005, CMS spent $484.3 billion in health care payments.[18] Medicare is the principal Social Health Insurance (SHI) program in the United States serving persons 65 and older, disabled individuals who are entitled to Social Security benefits, and those with end-stage renal disease, and is increasingly involved in the national debate on the quality of care. Given the weight of the Medicare program on the national health care system, this involvement is driving significant changes in both the public and private sectors. For this reason, we will focus primarily on the Medicare initiatives in this section on the government-sponsored, DM programs.

Various Medicare initiatives have been developed to encourage improved quality of care in virtually all settings where Medicare beneficiaries receive services, including physicians' offices, ambulatory care facilities, hospitals, nursing homes, and home health care agencies. To create these new incentive systems, CMS is working with public agencies and private organizations that share a common goal of improving quality and reducing unnecessary health care costs. These include the National Quality Forum (NQF), the Joint Commission on Accreditation of Healthcare Organizations (JCAHO), NCQA, the Agency for Healthcare Research and Quality (AHRQ), the American Medical Association (AMA), and many other organizations. CMS is also providing technical assistance to a wide range of health care providers through its Quality Improvement Organizations (QIOs).

The primary goal of these efforts is to improve the quality of care for Medicare beneficiaries. In addition to specific initiatives for hospitals, physicians, and physician groups, CMS is pursuing pay for performance initiatives to support better care coordination for patients with chronic illnesses, such as the Medicare Health Support program and the Care Management for High-Cost Beneficiaries Demonstration. A few of these initiatives are described in further detail below:[19, 20.21]

### *Physician Group Practice Demonstration[19]*

Mandated by Medicare, Medicaid, and the Benefits Improvement and Protection Act of 2000 (BIPA), this demonstration is the first pay for performance initiative specifically for physicians under the Medicare program. The program rewards physicians for improving the quality and efficiency of services delivered to Medicare fee-for-service beneficiaries. The demonstration seeks to encourage coordination of Part A and Part B services, promote efficiency through investment in administrative structure and process, and reward physicians for improving health outcomes. Ten very large (200+ physicians) group practices across the country are participating in this demonstration, which became operational in April 2005. The physician group practices can earn performance-based payments after achieving savings in medical costs in comparison to a control group. The performance payment is largely based on various quality results.

### Medicare Health Support Program (formerly the Chronic Care Improvement Program)[20] (MMA 2003, section 721)

This pilot program is testing a population-based model of disease management. The participating organizations are paid a monthly per-beneficiary fee for managing a population of chronically ill beneficiaries with advanced congestive heart failure and/or complex diabetes. These organizations, which include DM vendors and insurance companies, must guarantee CMS a savings of at least 5% plus the cost of the monthly fees compared to a similar population of beneficiaries. Payment of fees is also contingent upon performance on quality measures and satisfaction of both beneficiaries and providers. Eight sites have been selected for the pilot phase: Humana in South and Central Florida, XLHealth in Tennessee, Aetna in Illinois, LifeMasters in Oklahoma, McKesson in Mississippi, CIGNA in Georgia, Health Dialog in Pennsylvania, and American Healthways in Washington, DC, and Maryland. After two years, pending successful interim results, this pilot may be expanded more broadly, possibly nationwide. Many of these programs have made it a priority to incorporate information exchange and continued feedback with physicians as a means to manage the beneficiaries' health.

### Care Management for High-Cost Beneficiaries[21]

This demonstration will test models of care management in a Medicare fee-for-service population. The demonstration will target beneficiaries who are both high-cost and high-risk. Six organizations were selected to operate the three-year demonstration. The payment methodology and performance monitoring will be similar to that implemented in the Medicare Health Support Program, with participating providers required to meet relevant clinical quality standards and to guarantee savings to the Medicare program.

In summary, as one of the largest purchasers of health care in the world, CMS' interest in advancing quality, and its cost-saving initiatives will have profound effects on disease management companies, physicians, and the American health care system.

### Private Initiatives

The private sector is also actively pursuing quality and cost-saving initiatives. Baker, in a 2006 eWeek story, reported that the first national Pay for Performance Summit attracted representatives from software vendors, pharmaceutical companies, physician groups, health insurance companies, and patient advocacy groups.[22] The goal of the Summit was to change reimbursement models, basing doctors' pay less on seeing patients and more on keeping patients healthy. Integrated Healthcare Association (IHA), the conference sponsor, had expected about 300 attendees, largely from California. Total attendance far outstripped their expectation, with 750 registrants drawn from 35 states and several countries.

According to Baker, some attendees believe that P4P is finally becoming practical, particularly because the IHA performance showed that health plans could agree on performance measures. "It's always been a changing target. Now there are starting to be common criteria with health plans doing the same thing," said Farid Hassanpours, a medical director at the non-profit Inland Empire Health Plan in California.

### Tiered Networks

As employers continue to struggle with health care costs, they often revisit old concepts. One such concept is that of tiered networks, the process of offering employers a package of limited "preferred" provider networks, as well as an option for broader provider networks. Like tiered pharmaceutical benefits that set different co-payments for generic, brand name, and non-formulary drugs, tiered networks offer patients financial incentives for choosing the preferred (and theoretically more cost-effective) doctors and hospitals.[23]

When first introduced, the concept of tiered networks was based primarily on the willingness of physicians to accept deep discounts. This has evolved so that health plans are now selecting physicians based on cost-effectiveness and clinical quality indicators.[23] Although measuring costs and quality are still somewhat imprecise, performance measurements have improved enough to support cost and quality initiatives. Through IT advances, and deployment of technologies such as EMRs, it will become easier to adequately measure outcomes and solidify the movement to P4P.

### EMRs

Even as tiered networks and P4P programs put new demands on health care providers, EMRs are making it easier for doctors to follow guidelines, measure results, and identify patients who will benefit from disease management programs. As David Brailer, MD, the former National Coordinator of Health Information Technology, stated, "we cannot switch from years of paying for volume to paying for value unless we can give doctors the tools to do so." Efforts are underway to help physicians obtain and use HIT. In addition, P4P could provide a financial incentive to encourage doctors to adopt technology for collecting and tracking needed information.

An IT infrastructure is needed to support the quality and cost initiatives already in process. One way to expedite the implementation of P4P is for disease management companies and physician's offices to collaborate on data exchange, allowing them to fully leverage the IT platforms that already exist.

### Conclusion to New Dynamics

As public concerns about health care costs and quality continue, public and private initiatives around quality and costs will grow. Physicians will have to grapple with P4P, tiered networks, and other initiatives that increase the focus on cost and quality. Fortunately, reducing unnecessary health care costs and improving quality of care are also goals of DM programs. As a means to stay in preferred networks and achieve P4P bonuses, physicians will have increased incentives to collaborate with DM programs in the next few years.

How would this work from the physicians' perspective? One emerging model is the use of EMRs and other health information technologies to identify patients who qualify for DM programs. These same technologies enable physicians to share clinical data with DM programs. These programs can aggregate the data, collect additional information from patients via their interaction with DM care managers, and provide useful feedback to the physician. In this way, physicians and DM programs can work together to meet their shared goals for performance and outcome measurement.

## Care Collaboration

In its June 2006 Report to Congress, the Medicare Payment Advisory Commission (MedPAC) devoted an entire chapter to discussion of "care coordination," citing its potential to improve value in the Medicare program.[24] Experts and organizations interviewed for the report considered two functions essential: 1) a care manager, (usually a nurse) to assist the patient in self management and to monitor patient progress, and 2) an information system to identify eligible patients, store, and retrieve patient information, and share information with those who need it.

Interviewees for the report also stated that programs were more effective when the beneficiary's primary care physician was involved.  At least one study has shown that family and general practitioners are more likely to report awareness of disease management programs, and to use them. Of note is the fact that they also find these programs more useful than do specialists.[15]

Although successful DM program models are well-described in the literature, what qualifies as success is very different depending on the perspective of the stakeholder. In order for a DM program to be successful from a physician's point of view, it must generally include the following basic prerequisites:

• Clinically sound and effective;

• Helpful to patients;

• Supportive of the patient-physician relationship;

• Helpful to physicians by providing the physician with useful data;

• Limited in terms of physician time commitment;

• Endorsed by a trusted physician "champion" who remains involved; and

• Supported by aligned financial incentives.

In general, new DM programs are typically viewed with initial skepticism even if a physician group has a successful existing relationship with the DM vendor or health plan.  To summarize, physicians will only consider participation if they are convinced that the new program will support improved outcomes for their patients and that the planned interventions are based on sound medical principles.

Fortunately, the challenges are not as significant when in comes to engaging patients — and this fact can often be used to also engage physicians. Patients will embrace a program that is easily accessed and can provide tangible help. Based on their positive experiences, patients who participate in DM programs often encourage their physicians to consider supporting a program. Physicians will generally endorse enrollment if the patient wants to try a well-conceived program that does not stray from evidence-based medicine.

Programs that support the patient-physician relationship and provide useful information to the physician are regarded as helpful. In particular, additional data that the DM program is able to collect are often welcomed by the physician. Examples include notification of recent hospital Emergency Department visits and admissions, prescription refill records, and physical measurements collected at home (e.g., daily dry weights for the heart failure patient, home blood pressure readings and blood sugar measurements for the high-risk maternity patient).

This type of data is only useful if the actual values or measurements are supplied. For example, providing a simple count of admissions without the hospital names, dates of admission/discharge, and discharge diagnoses is not useful. Similarly, instead of alerting a physician that a blood pressure reading or weight is out of range, the specific values must be provided. This allows for comparison between DM-reported patient data to similar information that was measured in the office. Some leading-edge DM programs utilize technologies such as electronic weight scales that transmit information over the phone directly to providers.

Many DM programs interact with physicians by pointing out simple gaps in care. Missing vaccinations, patient self-reported non-adherence to prescribed medications, medications recommended by national guidelines but not prescribed (or prescribed but refused by the patient), and untreated depression are examples of common gaps in care that can have serious implications in terms of morbidity, mortality, and quality of life. By alerting the physician and providing relevant evidence-based references, DM programs can support physicians in improving quality of care.

A related strategy is to empower the patient to "ask your doctor" about various topics, including identified gaps in care. Armed with suggested questions in simple non-threatening language, the patient is encouraged to have an effective discussion with the physician. Such suggestions may occasionally be interpreted by the physician as interference, but more typically they are viewed as helpful reminders.

In addition to providing actionable data, a DM program must visibly support the patient-physician relationship. Effective programs follow the principle that the physician's plan of care is of primary importance. Therefore, DM staff must always strive to seek physician input on any planned interventions and must communicate effectively with the physician's office. One effective model that supports DM-physician collaboration places a nurse directly within the physician's practice. Such models naturally encourage ongoing communication, present a coordinated approach to the patient, and generally function as an extension of the physician practice.

Effective programs also recognize that physicians have limited time for additional activities during their daily practice of medicine. Physicians will be more likely to collaborate with DM programs if there are incentives for time associated with "routine" activities requested of physicians — such as reviewing reports, providing patient data (such as labs) to the DM program, and returning phone calls to care managers. Some DM programs reimburse physicians a monthly "participation fee," which compensates the practice for their time, regardless of clinical outcomes.

Finally, DM programs cannot be successful without a trusted physician executive at the helm. A competent Medical Director, with an appropriate clinical and executive background, provides credibility for the program and ensures that it is operating to the benefit of both patients and physicians. Typically the Medical Director provides the connection between practicing physicians in the field and the DM program. This individual must remain accessible and available to answer questions and receive feedback from doctors interacting with care managers and patients enrolled in the program.

The size of a practice is a key factor in how programs are best implemented to maximize physician engagement. Practices with large numbers of patients are often of sufficient size to warrant an "internal" program with imbedded nurses, and dedicated software or an EMR (to identify and track enrolled patients). Practices with only a small number of patients eligible for enrollment (e.g., less than 20) cannot economically support an internal program. Bringing DM tools and approaches to small practices remains a challenge for DM programs.

## Conclusion

In summary, DM programs were traditionally implemented by managed care organizations, and although they achieved some success, their efforts were routinely met with resistance and hostility by many physicians. The "hassle factor" inherent in paper-based communications, lack of aligned financial incentives, and physicians' innate need for autonomy reinforced this tension. However, as described in this chapter, a growing set of information technologies and economic incentives is creating and reinforcing a new dynamic where the interests of physicians, health plans, the government, and patients are more closely aligned. The case studies provided in this chapter provide some emerging models of how physicians can productively participate in DM programs and also be rewarded for contributing to improvements in patient outcomes. With strong physician-leadership within DM firms, health plans, and medical groups, and the alignment of financial incentives, it should be possible to achieve an environment where physicians more routinely embrace and are rewarded for supporting DM programs.[12]

## Case Studies

Despite the challenges and constraints discussed above, there are a growing number of examples where DM programs have successfully engaged physicians and implemented tools and approaches that have been seen as beneficial to patients.

### TeleWatch™ Telemonitoring System

Remote patient monitoring allows various biometric values (e.g., weight, blood pressure, blood glucose) captured in the patient's home to be transmitted over a phone line to care managers or physicians. These tools are often used by DM programs for patients with more severe disease. One such technology, the TeleWatch™ Patient Monitoring System, was designed by the Johns Hopkins Applied Physics Laboratory in collaboration with the Johns Hopkins Division of Cardiology. TeleWatch™, a telephone-based system, is useful for managing outpatients with chronic illnesses, such as heart failure and diabetes. The system was successfully used in the outpatient cardiology clinics at the Johns Hopkins Hospital and within comprehensive heart failure clinics at Johns Hopkins Bayview Medical Center.

Later, through collaboration with Johns Hopkins HealthCare (a managed care organization affiliated with Johns Hopkins Medicine) the technology was extended to the Medicaid, commercial, and retired military populations. A major advantage of TeleWatch™ is that it does not require high-tech equipment, only a telephone, bathroom scale, glucometer, and home blood pressure monitor. Skilled nurses meet face-to-face with patients to educate them about their disease and how to use the TeleWatch™ system. Patients call in to the system by phone to self-report key symptoms and clinical data, such as shortness of breath, fatigue, weight, blood sugar, and blood pressure. This reporting is conducted using the telephone's regular keypad.[25]

Patients can also leave a message for the nurse or request a return phone call. Using sophisticated clinical branching algorithms and predictive modeling, the system will alert the nurse if the patient-reported information is outside custom-set parameters, or if the patient fails to call in. Nurses monitor the system, 24 hours a day, 7 days a week. Routine reports are generated for the primary care physician, who also receives an urgent phone call if a patient's condition worsens. The TeleWatch™ system was readily accepted by patients and physicians, and is currently being modified for use with patients suffering from COPD and those in a high-risk pregnancy.

### Vanderbilt Medical Group: DM within the physician practice and use of an EMR

The Vanderbilt Medical Group in Nashville developed its own internal DM program under the auspices of a grant from BlueCross BlueShield of Tennessee (BCBS). *StarTracker* (the DM component of the *StarPanel* EMR system) was implemented within the Primary Care Center, which has a strong focus on managing patients with chronic disease. Using diagnosis codes, medication lists, and test-result ranges, Vanderbilt nurses query the system to find groups of patients with specific diseases. Because StarTracker is a component of the EMR used within the practice, retrieval of relevant information from paper records is not necessary, saving considerable time.

"Practicing preventative medicine can take more than 7 hours per day in a busy practice," according to Dr. Jim Jirjis, assistant professor of medicine and director of the Adult Primary Care Center.[26] "This is impossible to accomplish within the standard 15-minute problem-oriented office visit."

In StarTracker, DM population-based rules are formulated to automatically prompt the DM team. Every time a medical record is accessed, a color-coded (red, yellow, and green) "patient dashboard" flags problems. For example, a missing HgbA1c test or LDL cholesterol results >100 will result in flags. Also using StarTracker, staff members assist doctors by ensuring that tests and treatments are timely, and that patients are adequately engaged and knowledgeable about their condition. "This is important, because you cannot count on an entire population to get all of the monitoring and care they need solely on the basis of periodic 15-minute office visits," Jirjis says.

He elaborates, "You need a population tracking system that monitors even patients who do not follow up or come to appointments. That system needs to be able to identify gaps in care and execute on them either by calling patients in for testing, education patients, adjusting medicines, or setting up visits." Doctors receive periodic reports on the status of these patient groups. "StarTracker is an extension of the physician's office, equivalent to having another nurse just to monitor chronic disease," Jirjis said. Furthermore, Jirjis reported that outcomes included an increase in diabetic foot exams of 63% and diabetic testing of 35%.

Because this DM program is internal to the practice, it was readily embraced by physicians. "It's very important not to have an external entity doing this," according to Jirjis. One key advantage is that Vanderbilt nurses inform patients they are calling from their doctor's office and communicate that they are following protocols approved by their physicians. Although there is not yet an algorithm to adjust medications, physicians are requesting it. Development of algorithms, referrals and formal patient education are also in process.

Jirgis and William M. Gregg, MD, (co-developers of StarTracker) comment that developing their own IT System/DM Infrastructure requires significant funding as the components are very expensive. Regardless of clinical outcomes, payors typically do not want to fund a system for a particular physician or hospital which will be used by patients other than their own. Such is the case with StarTracker. The original BCBS investment has expired, and Vanderbilt is seeking new sources of reimbursement.

**XLHealth DM programs:**
**Educating patients to self-manage and addressing "Gaps in Care"**

XLHealth was founded as Diabetex in 1998 by a group of doctors and health care professionals who wanted to help bridge the gaps that exist between diabetic patients, health plans, and physicians in today's complex health care system. In 2004, the company adopted the XLHealth name and expanded its services to include a broad range of related chronic illnesses, including congestive heart failure, cardiovascular disease, chronic kidney failure, and end-stage renal disease (ESRD).

The hallmark of XLHealth's program is a network of local DM "assessment centers" (currently in New York, Tennessee, Texas, and Maryland) that are operated by registered nurses in collaboration with physician partners. Enrollment in XLHealth's DM programs is voluntary. Nurses are trained in population management with the goal of predicting and preventing recurrence of chronic disease complications such as amputations due to diabetic ulcers, hospital admissions for pulmonary edema, or recurrent cardiac events. Patients are encouraged to visit the assessment centers for an initial visit, which includes: a physical examination, health risk questionnaire, screening for depression, a "brown bag" medication inventory (i.e., the patient brings in all of their prescription and OTC medications for review by a nurse), and disease-specific health education. In some states, local pharmacists are utilized for medication assessment and education.

The program varies somewhat depending on the chronic condition. Using diabetes as an example: the physical examination includes a dilated retinal examination using an advanced digital retinal camera (Eyetel™ digital technology), an extensive lower extremity examination, including ankle-brachial index pressure measurements and vibration sensation testing. All patients with neuropathy or peripheral vascular disease receive free diabetic shoes and inserts, as well as a temperature probe to self-monitor for foot inflammation and prevent development of infection.

Regardless of the chronic condition, the patient's primary physician receives the assessment results and subsequent data collected in the center or made available to the program by the health plan, such as lab and pharmacy. Patients receive continuing education and coaching via the telephone or through follow-up visits in an assessment center. Group education sessions are provided on common self management topics, such as depression and nutrition, for patients with diabetes and heart failure. A hallmark of the program is the regular communication between nurses and primary physicians. To ensure that this communication is effective, the program maintains a Medical Advisory Board of local physicians in every state to review program interventions and results.

### Philips Motiva™: Disease management platform

The Motiva™ system delivers automated, yet personalized, educational content, health care reminders and feedback to chronically ill patients at home using a secure broadband connection to the television. Optional Bluetooth measurement devices send biometric data (e.g., blood pressure, weight) to a remote caregiver, such as a family member, physician, or nurse. Designed with the older patient in mind, the system is accessed via a remote control, similar to one used to change TV channels.

The content is completely customized to the patient's needs, and delivers brief motivational educational sessions, incorporating behavioral health strategies and guideline-based disease management activities. For example, a patient with hyper-cholesterolemia could watch a video that explains the condition, complete a questionnaire that assesses the individual's risk of developing a heart attack, and then go on to complete one or more activities that would support adherence to both lifestyle (e.g., diet and exercise) and medications prescribed by the physician.

In addition, various vital sign monitoring devices, such as scales for measuring daily weights in heart failure, blood pressure cuffs and glucometers, can be added to Motiva™ at the discretion of the provider. These actionable data are monitored via an Internet-based DM platform by the physician or nurse. The Motiva™ system was a winner of a Medical Design Excellence Award and named "One of the Top 5 Disease Management Ideas of 2005." Philips Motiva™ was released commercially in the United States in May 2006.

### InforMedix: Med-eMonitor™

Attention to medication adherence is an essential element of DM programs. The Med-eMonitor™ solution was designed for use in the home and addresses adherence by offering a combined medication organization, reminder and education system, and an "e-health diary." The compact system can be mailed to the patient and programmed remotely via the Internet. Up to five medications are placed into a portable compartmentalized device that prompts the patient for each of their medications and automatically tracks adherence. Once the compartment is opened, health information and questions can be displayed as determined by the clinical protocol and physician. Adherence data are downloaded on a daily basis and available to the clinical team via the web. The Med-eMonitor™ System was successfully piloted in patients with diabetes, heart failure, and schizophrenia.[27,28]

## Study Questions

1. Which of the following is not one of the reasons why physician support has historically been lacking for DM programs?

    a. Lack of financial incentives

    b. A need for professional autonomy

    c. Too few patients in their practices with chronic disease

    d. Cumbersome DM programs

    e. Resistance to following clinical guidelines

    Answer (c)


2. Typical DM programs utilize all of the following EXCEPT:

    a. Evidence based guidelines

    b. Patient education on self-management

    c. Outcomes measurement

    d. Programs that substitute for usual doctor's care and visits

    e. Population identification processes

    Answer (d)


3. Care Coordination was cited by the Medicare Payment Advisory Commission (MedPAC) in its June 2006 Report to Congress as having the potential to improve value in the Medicare program. True or False?

    Answer (True)


4. Which of the following characteristics are necessary for a successful DM program in terms of physician acceptance?

    a. Clinically sound and effective

    b. Attractive and helpful to patients

    c. Supportive of the patient-physician relationship

    d. Helpful to the physician/ provide useful data

    e. Limited in terms of a physician time commitment

    f. Endorsed by a trusted physician "champion" who remains involved

    g. Supported by aligned financial incentives

    h. All of the above

    Answer (h)

5. Most DM programs are designed to outreach directly to:

a. Patients

b. Physicians

c. Caregivers

d. Hospital staff

Answer (a)

6. Why has pay for performance become center stage in health care delivery?

a. Advances in technology that allow for the measurement of results

b. Rising health care costs

c. Public concern about the quality of health care

d. All of the above

Answer (d)

7. What is the goal of tiered networks?

a. To increase the revenue of health plans

b. To direct patients to cost-effective physicians that provide quality health care

c. To reduce physician salaries

d. All of the above

Answer (b)

8. Electronic Medical Records (EMRs) make it easier to:

a. Follow recommended medical guidelines

b. Measure clinical results

c. Identify patients that would benefit from disease management

d. All of the above

Answer (d)

## References

1. Mechanic D. Physician discontent: challenges and opportunities. JAMA. 2003;290:941-946.

2. Leider HL. Gaining physician buy-in for disease management initiatives. *Dis Management and Health Outcomes*. 1999;6:327-333.

3. www.DMAA.org

4. McMurray JJ, Ostergren J, Swedberg K, et al. Effects of candesartan in patients with chronic heart failure and reduced left-ventricular systolic function taking angiotensin-converting-enzyme inhibitors: the CHARM-Added trial. *Lancet*. 2003;362:767-771.

5. MERIT-HF Study Group. Effect of metoprolol CR/XL in chronic heart failure: Metoprolol CR/XL Randomised Intervention Trial in Congestive Heart Failure (MERIT-HF) *Lancet*. 1999;353:2001-2007.

6. Effect of enalapril on survival in patients with reduced left ventricular ejection fractions and congestive heart failure. SOLVD Investigators. *N Engl J Med*. 1991;325:293-302.

7. Clarke JL, Nash DB. The effectiveness of heart failure disease management: initial findings from a comprehensive program. *Dis Manag*. 2002;5:215-223.

8. Krumholz HM, Amatruda J, Smith GL, et al. Randomized controlled trial of an education and support interventions to prevent readmission of patients with heart failure. *J Am Coll Cardiol*. 2002;39:83-89.

9. Vaccaro J, Cherry J, Harper A. Utilization reduction, cost savings, and return on investment for the PacifiCare Chronic Heart Failure Program. *Dis Manag*. 2001;4:131-142.

10. http://www.ncqa.org/PROGRAMS/HEDIS/index.htm

11. www.NCQA.org

12. Leider HL. Selecting a vendor for disease management programs. *Dis Management and Health Outcomes*. 1999;6:131-139.

13. Leider HL. Influencing physicians: the three critical elements of a successful strategy. *Am J Manag Care*. 1998;4:583-588.

14. Cabana MD, Rand CS, Powe NR, et al. Why don't physicians follow guidelines: a framework for improvement. JAMA. 1999;282:1458-1465.

15. Wholey D, Michail N, Christainson J, et al. Physician use of disease management programs. *Dis Manag*. 2005;8:26-34.

16. Kohn LT, Corrigan JM, Donaldson MS, eds. The Committee on Quality of Healthcare in America and the Institute of Medicine. *To Err is Human: Building a Safer Healthcare System*. Washington, DC: National Academies Press; 2000.

17. The Committee on Quality of Healthcare in America and the Institute of Medicine. *Crossing the Quality Chasm: A New Health System for the 21st Century*. Washington, DC: National Academies Press; 2001.

18. Centers for Medicare and Medicaid Services. CMS Financial Report for Fiscal Year 2005. Available at: http://www.cms.hhs.gov/CFOReport/Downloads/2005_CMS_Financial_Report.pdf. Accessed August 21, 2006.

19. Centers for Medicare and Medicaid Services. Medicare "Pay for Performance (P4P)" Initiatives. CMS Office of Public Affairs, January 31, 2005. Available at: http://www.cms.hhs.gov/apps/media/press/release.asp?Counter=1343. Accessed August 21, 2006.

20. Centers for Medicare and Medicaid Services. Medican to award contracts for demonstration projects to improve care for beneficiaries with high medical costs. Office of Public Affairs, July 1, 2005. Available at: http://www.cms.hhs.gov/apps/media/press/release.asp?Counter=1499. Accessed August 21, 2006.

21. Centers for Medicare and Medicaid Services. CMS Announces Demonstration Projects for Beneficiaries with High Medical Costs. October 1, 2004. Available at: http://www.cms.hhs.gov/DemoProjectsEvalRpts/downloads/CMHCB_press_release_10_2004.pdf. Accessed September 22, 2006.

22. Baker ML. Pay-for-performance programs spark debate. *eWeek*. February 7, 2006.

23. Terry K. What "Tiered Networks" will mean to you with strong growth among private firms. *Medical Economics*. September 17, 2004.

24. Medicare payment advisory commission. Report to the congress: increasing the value of Medicare. Washington, DC: MedPAC; 2006, 32.

25. Palmer J, Spaeder J. Outpatient management of disease using the TeleWatch patient monitoring system. *Johns Hopkins APL Technical Digest*. 2004;25:253-259.

26. Yarnall KS, Pollack K, Ostbye O, Krause KM, Michener JL. Primary care: is there enough time for prevention? *Am J Publ Health*. 2003;93:635-641.

27. Ruskin P, Van Der Wende J, Clark C, et al. Feasibility of using the Med-eMonitor system in the treatment of schizophrenia: a pilot study. *Drug Information Journal*. 2003;37:283-291.

28. Artinian N, Harden J. Kronenberg M, et al. Pilot study of a web-based compliance monitoring device for patients with congestive heart failure. *Heart Lung*. 2003;32:226-233.

# Section 4
# Practice Administration

# Chapter 14

## The Practice Setting: Office, Hospitals, and Others

Theodore D. Fraker, Jr., MD, FACC and
Alan P. Marco, MD, MMM, CPE, FACPE

### Executive Summary

There are many ways to structure a practice. Options include private practice, academics, governmental, individual practioners, single-specialty groups, multi-specialty groups, hospital-based, office-based, or any combination of these. Each type has unique advantages and disadvantages, but they all have the common need to address the primary issues of access to care and communications. In this era of patient-centered care, customer service is key. Effectively contracting for payments, especially with the rise of prospective payment systems, is critical to support the practice, and volume helps.

Because of patient safety, outcomes, and cost-containment initiatives, collaboration between physicians and hospitals is more important than ever. Understanding the roles and obligations in credentialing and privileging will help the physician to be successful. Participation in Medical Staff affairs will help hospital-based physicians, as well as those who also see patients in other settings.

### Learning Objectives

1. Identify key issues in building a practice.

2. Describe essential elements in maintaining a practice.

3. Recognize regulatory issues that relate to current medical practice.

4. Outline issues that pertain to hospital-based practices and the organized medical staff.

### Keywords

academic practice; access; accreditation; communication; credentialing; hospital-based practice; hospitalist; lean health care; medical staff organization (MSO); military medicine; pay for performance

## Introduction

The practice of medicine has never been more exciting or more challenging. Today's health care environment is a complex system within which patients and physicians find themselves mutually dependent. The explosion of medical knowledge and technological advances, combined with changing demographics of American society and escalating fiscal concerns contribute to the unique medicolegal climate of the 21ˢᵗ century. While many physicians will find challenging careers in management or medical imaging, the fundamental basis for the practice of medicine is still the encounter between an individual patient and a physician. In this chapter, we will try to define many of the issues intrinsic to the encounter between patients and physicians.

Modern medical practice offers many options, including academic multi-specialty settings, solo or small-group private practices, or large-group models. Among the newer models are employed physician arrangements, such as hospitalist practices.

Academic practices typically are based at academic medical centers. However, depending on the specialty, you might be office-based or in other arrangements. The distinguishing characteristic of an academic practice is its commitment to education and research.[1] While many other practices may support education, usually there is not a direct tie to the academic mission. In a traditional academic practice, the old maxim of "publish or perish" still exists; however, over the past decade, clinical productivity has also become an important issue. Seeing patients won't get you promoted, but it will serve to renew your contract. Often, the faculty practice in a group-practice model (faculty practice plan) is indistinguishable from a private practice, with the expectation of clinical activity (and therefore compensation) altered to allow for academic productivity.

Private practices, while emphasizing clinical care, are focused on earning a living in an increasingly difficult environment. Physicians may be solo practitioners, in a single-specialty group, or a multi-specialty group. Groups focusing on primary care may have fewer factions to deal with than those that combine primary care with specialty physicians. There are many questions to ask before joining a multi-specialty practice.[2] Solo practitioners have issues such as finding call coverage and staffing the office.[3] Presumably, a larger practice would have some economies of scale in call coverage, hospital coverage of admitted patients, and practice management, as well as affording greater leverage in negotiating with third-party payors.

Group models tend to be large practices that employ physicians and other providers. They may be part of an integrated delivery system such as Kaiser, Mayo Clinic, or the Cleveland Clinic. These models benefit from economies of scale and, if in an integrated system, cut out much of the tension between the hospital and the physicians.

## Building a Practice

Today's health care organizations have adopted a philosophy of patient-centered care. This focus on customer service has evolved from lessons taken from the manufacturing and service industries. Regardless of the type of practice that interests the physician, the two key concepts that are most important in building a client base are access and communication.

### Access

From the patient's point of view, the ideal physician would be available 24 hours a day, 365 days per year to deal with medical emergencies, health care concerns or the need for information. Patients understand that this is an unrealistic expectation. Physicians understand that medical emergencies know no schedule; so, elaborate systems have been developed to handle medical emergencies. These include hospital emergency departments, urgent care centers, and coverage arrangements with other physicians or other physician groups. Still, better access to physician services is the key to building a successful practice.

Typically, a physician who opens a new practice (either alone or with other physicians) does some market research to assess the need for services in a given geographic area. Underserved areas will offer an immediate patient base, while communities with an overabundance of providers will not enjoy rapid growth unless the new providers offer better service. Easier access is part of better service. It entails offering appointments on the same day of the request, with times available in early mornings, evenings, or weekends, depending upon the community's needs. Because there is an insatiable public demand for physician services, practices will grow; the only issue is the pace of growth.

New practices grow by an infusion of patients, either from an influx of people into a new or growing community, or from migration of patients from other, established practices. As the population of new patients in the practice grows, there is a steady increase in return visits as patients come back to the office for follow-up. In many practices, the steady growth in return visits eventually fills available appointment slots so that new patients cannot be seen in a timely fashion. This poses a dilemma for the practice: new patients provide more revenue per visit, but returning patients are easier to see and provide financial stability for the practice.

### The "No-show" Problem

All practices struggle with the problem of patients who fail to arrive for a scheduled appointment. The "no-show" rate will vary based upon the demographics of the community and other factors, such as the time of year. Most practices keep careful data on these absentee rates, since practice revenue is so adversely affected. All practices have fixed costs (e.g., rent, water, electricity, heating, taxes, and salaries) that must be paid whether or not there are patients to see. Many practices call to remind patients the day before a scheduled visit, but this can be labor-intensive and costly. Some practices overbook patients (just like the airline industry overbooks passengers), but this can lead to delays in patient flow, which may adversely affect customer satisfaction. Most practices track the absentee rate by patient and will then discharge the patient from the practice if there is a repetitive pattern of absenteeism. A practice cannot survive with a high rate of unkept appointments.

One potential solution to reduce the no-show rate is "open access scheduling" in which the practice strives to see patients when they want or need to be seen, usually the same day of the request or within one business day.[4-7] Open access scheduling cuts down on the no-show rate because appointments are scheduled when the patient wants or needs to be seen. The office staff spends less time booking and rebooking cancelled appointments. The downside of open access scheduling is that it requires flexibility on the part of both the office staff and the physician. Chapter 15 has more detailed information on this scheduling strategy.

### Customer Service Training: For Your Staff and You

Health care is a service industry, not unlike the restaurant or tourist business. Most patients have a difficult time assessing the quality of the medical decision making because they lack the requisite knowledge. However, patients are acutely aware of the way they are treated by the office staff and by their physician. The success of the practice will hinge upon the least courteous member of the practice team. The physician is judged by a combination of medical skills and bedside manner, but the office staff is judged almost solely by courtesy, listening skills, empathy, and willingness to provide information. These "soft" skills, which are so important to a practice, are not intrinsic to all office staff members, and must be taught. The physician or business manager who runs the practice needs to be constantly assessing customer satisfaction. Superior customer service must be a core value of the practice, and will need to be reinforced with periodic staff training.

### Quality in an Office Practice: The Need for Continuous Improvement

While patients will likely judge the quality of the office practice based largely upon access and courtesy, the payors (i.e., private insurance carriers, CMS, etc.), regulators (local, state, and federal), and referral sources will judge quality based upon more stringent criteria. The current buzzwords for health care are safe, effective, patient-centered, timely, efficient, and equitable,[8] but federal policy makers and the insurance industry are very worried about the ever-escalating cost of health care in the United States. Thus far, there have been no effective means for controlling over-utilization of health care resources, and there are no solutions in sight. By 2011, a large number of baby boomers will be eligible for Medicare, shifting a huge burden of health care coverage from the private to the public sector. Baby boomers not only comprise a large segment of the U.S. population, they also have high expectations, large accumulated wealth, and considerable political clout.

### Communication in Health Care

If access is the foundation for building a successful practice, communication is the infrastructure that will hold the practice together. First and foremost, physicians and their staff have an obligation to communicate with patients. The availability of information over the Internet has contributed to patients becoming more informed consumers. Patients are desperately seeking more information about their diagnosis, prognosis, and any risks associated with diagnostic or therapeutic procedures. Physicians must be prepared to embrace this desire for knowledge, recognizing that few patients will ever understand their own medical issues as well as their physician understands the problems. Successful practices will be proactive in providing patients with up-to-date information and authoritative resources to help them understand that body of medical knowledge that pertains to their individual needs. The office staff can help enormously in educating patients about common medical problems but, ultimately, the physician has a fiduciary (or trust-based) responsibility to inform patients about their health status.

Even more challenging, though just as important, is the need for more effective communication between physicians. Except for the most rural or underserved parts of America, patients who have access to health care rarely see just one doctor. Modern medicine is far too complex. Primary care providers are expected to be familiar with a large body of general medical knowledge, and subspecialty physicians are expected to be familiar with incredible details within their specialty. The result of this complexity is that physicians rely upon each other in the care of patients who have anything other than the most straightforward medical problems.

As if the complexity of medicine itself were not enough, patients often see multiple physicians, each with a different perspective, a different assessment, and probably a different plan of care. Each interaction with a different doctor raises the likelihood of an unintended drug or procedural complication. Physicians understand this problem and have developed a tightly scripted method for succinct communication amongst providers. The essential elements of this communication are the problem list, the procedures, the medication list, and the plan of care. While more complete information about each patient is highly desirable, time-pressured and harried physicians resort to this brief compendium of information in the transfer of care from one provider to the next. Thus the accuracy of this limited amount of information about the "whole person" is crucial to effective medical care. Here again, the electronic medical record can assist physicians in compiling and tracking this crucial information.

Lastly, physicians have certain limited obligations to communicate about patients to insurance companies (i.e., the payors), the government (i.e., Medicaid and Medicare), and to certain regulatory agencies (e.g., the Bureau of Motor Vehicles for a disability parking tag). All medical information should be considered confidential and strictly "owned" by the patient. Thus, the transfer of medical information to any agency or person must be approved, in writing, by the patient or the patient's legal representative. All communications must be compliant with federal Health Insurance Portability and Accountability Act (HIPAA) regulations to protect the privacy of patients. Chapter 9 offers more information about HIPAA and its requirements.

### Maintaining the Practice — No Margin, No Mission

In the past, physicians were paid in anything from promissory notes to barter to cash according to the prices they set for themselves. In current practice, fee schedules may be set by the payor with various fees for specific services, or the payor may use multiples of the Medicare fee schedule. The advantage to the payor is that it is relatively straightforward to negotiate a rate, such as 125% of the Medicare allowable, but negotiating many individual fees is costly and time-consuming. However, depending on the field, there may be advantages to either method. In many primary care fields, Medicare multiples are a reasonable way to set fees, since Medicare pays about 80% of the average commercial rate. However, in procedure-oriented specialties, there may be a significant difference, especially if there are key procedures that are not widely available in the area, such as transplant surgery.

The pay for performance (P4P) reimbursement design is based on the concept that higher-performing physicians should be rewarded for providing better care. However, defining good performance can be problematic. According to the American Medical Association (AMA), a P4P plan should: ensure quality of care, foster the relationship between patient and physician, offer voluntary physician participation, use accurate data and fair reporting, and provide fair and equitable program incentives.[9] A performance measure should be quantifiable, reproducible, directly tied to a desired outcome, and under the control of the physician. Many of the proposed measures do not meet these guidelines. For example, even as straightforward a measure as the number of diabetics in your practice that get foot exams fails. While it is measurable, it is tied to a clinical process rather than a clinical outcome. The outcome is that fewer diabetics should have complications such as foot ulcers. In this example, the patient may have an exam, but early signs could be missed (a physician issue), or the patient may not follow the recommended course of action, resulting in complications. Some physicians feel that credit should be given for offering the foot exam, but this is also a process measure rather than an outcome measure, since it only indirectly relates to the incidence of complications.

In the past, P4P has relied on "withholds" that hold back some payment and are returned when performance criteria are met. Current systems appear to give additional money for better performance, but many are based on smaller base payments, so the "performance bonus" just brings the physician up to current levels. It is possible that P4P programs may not improve actual patient care, but merely recognize those who are already high performers.[10]

## Hospital-based Practice

The changing nature of reimbursement has made hospital-based practice very challenging. In the mid 1980s, the Health Care Financing Administration (now known as the Centers for Medicare and Medicaid Services, or CMS) implemented a change in the way hospitals were reimbursed, moving from a cost-based system to a prospective reimbursement system based upon Diagnosis Related Groups or DRGs. Prior to this change, hospitals charged Medicare for services based upon cost plus a small margin. However, as a result of wide regional variations in cost for hospital services (coupled with double-digit increases in the rates of health care cost), CMS transitioned to a system of prospective reimbursement based upon the principal diagnosis.[11] While hospitals do receive additional compensation for complicated cases, the money that a hospital receives from CMS for a Medicare-covered patient is pre-determined by what the admitting physician documents as the principal diagnosis. Many private insurance companies soon followed suit, so that today most hospital reimbursement is fixed, DRG-based, and indexed to CMS payment schedules. This fundamental change in reimbursement to hospitals has had profound effects upon the practice of medicine in the hospital setting, and upon the relationship between hospitals and the physicians who work there.

Hospitals and their associated medical staffs exist in an environment of mutual dependence. Hospitals need physicians to admit and care for patients, and physicians need the rooms, nursing and ancillary staff, and diagnostic services provided by hospitals to render that care. Prior to DRG-based reimbursement, hospitals had little incentive to control costs, since the more diagnostic and therapeutic services the physician ordered, the more the hospital was paid. This is no longer true. Under DRG-based reimbursement, services rendered during the hospital stay now represent costs that detract from net profits. Hospitals have responded to this decreased reimbursement by closely scrutinizing their workforce, improving management of their supply chain, and consolidating services to achieve economies of scale. They have also aggressively pursued better-paying contracts from their commercial insurers, since most hospitals barely break even on Medicare reimbursement. The greatest challenge facing hospital administrators now is convincing physicians to assist in controlling utilization of inpatient hospital services and reducing lengths of stay. Both strategies are crucial for hospitals to remain profitable. Hospitals do best with increased number of admissions, a short length of stay, and rapid turnover. While hospitals thrive in an environment of rapid turnover of inpatients, this change in the practice climate has put increased pressure on clinicians to provide nearly constant monitoring of the patient's hospital course. This has led to the development of specialists in inpatient care, such as "hospitalists."[12]

### The Medical Staff Organization

The medical staff organization (MSO) is an entity integral to the hospital, yet separate from it. The medical staff is composed of physicians and other licensed independent practitioners who decide collectively how medicine will be practiced within the confines of the hospital. The medical staff is organized around a set of bylaws, rules, regulations, policies, and procedures. Medical staff bylaws represent fundamental principles regarding medical staff participation, credentialing, privileges, and obligations. The medical staff bylaws typically are approved by the hospital's governing body (usually a board of trustees), and can be amended only with board approval. Medical staff policies and procedures, however, deal with day-to-day operations, including items such as the code of conduct for practitioners, patient safety, and continuous performance improvement. Medical staff policies and procedures can be amended with the approval of the medical staff executive committee, the elected body that governs medical staff activities.

The MSO typically elects officers including a Chief of Staff, a Vice Chief of Staff, a treasurer, and a secretary to lead the organization. The members of the medical staff elect an executive committee to oversee and assist the leadership in establishing relevant policies and procedures for the organization as a whole. The central functions of the medical staff leadership include: 1) establishing criteria for practitioners to join the medical staff, and thereby practice within the hospital; 2) verifying the credentials of practitioners joining the medical staff; 3) granting privileges for practitioners to perform specific functions within the hospital based upon documentation of appropriate training and experience; and 4) re-credentialing practitioners at periodic intervals based upon evidence of continued high-quality care. The medical staff bylaws typically define how these four functions will be carried out. The bylaws also define how officers are selected, how the executive committee is elected, and the frequency of meetings, as well as the mechanism for amending the bylaws. Verification of training and experience, and making recommendations to grant specific privileges requested by the medical staff member is one of the most important functions of the medical staff leadership.

Physicians who wish to work in the hospital environment need to understand the credentialing and privileging process. Medical school and post-graduate medical education prepares physicians for a career in medical practice. However, training programs differ in the types of experience that they offer, and MSOs often have very different criteria for obtaining specific hospital privileges. Many hospitals require board certification in a primary specialty as a prerequisite for obtaining hospital admitting privileges. Physicians may be required to show documentation that they have performed a sufficient volume of specific procedures. Completion of an approved residency training program does not necessarily guarantee that privileges will be granted for specific procedures. To facilitate the privileging process, it is important for physicians in training to keep accurate records of all their experiences, including the volumes of invasive or noninvasive procedures.

MSOs struggle with privileging for procedures performed by physicians with different training backgrounds. Examples include vascular interventional procedures (which are done by interventional radiologists, cardiologists and/or vascular surgeons) and spine surgery (which may be done by both neurosurgeons and orthopedic surgeons). The credentialing committee is obligated to develop fair and objective criteria for privileges that assure patient safety while still recognizing that physicians can have varied pathways to clinical competence.

In addition to the central functions of the medical staff leadership, members of the medical staff are encouraged, and often expected, to participate in hospital activities directed toward patient safety, clinical efficiency, and continuous quality improvement. The care rendered by a hospital or health care system is intrinsically linked to the quality of its medical staff, so physician participation in hospital quality initiatives is crucial to the success of the whole organization. All hospitals have committees composed of nursing staff, hospital personnel, and medical staff members whose charge is to oversee various aspects of hospital care. For example, all hospitals have a committee that reviews tissues removed at surgery to be assured that the pre-operative diagnosis and the specimen removed are consistent. Most hospitals have a utilization review committee, which is responsible for assuring that admissions to the hospital and the use of hospital resources are appropriate. Hospitals have a safety committee responsible for tracking medication and procedural errors, and most have a separate committee that looks specifically at hospital-acquired infections (surveillance, preventions, and control). All hospitals struggle with managing the volume, accuracy, and complexity of information contained in medical records. Hospitals form "medical records" or "medical information management" committees to deal with record completion (especially by physicians), standardized abbreviations, standardized record formatting, and information distribution. While the bureaucracy of the hospital committee structure may seem complex and foreboding, physician participation is crucial.

## Hospital Accreditation

Physician involvement in hospital quality assurance activities is essential for the mission of any health care organization, but it is also mandatory for hospital accreditation. All health care organizations must undergo periodic independent accreditation to be eligible for Medicare funding, as well as for participation in most private insurance plans. The largest accrediting organization in the United States is the Joint Commission on Accreditation of Healthcare Organizations, or JCAHO.[13] JCAHO conducts periodic site visits to hospitals and health care organizations to verify that appropriate standards of care are being met, and to assure continuous improvement in the safety and quality of care provided. The organization evaluates the whole spectrum of health care organizations, including ambulatory care sites, home health care organizations, laboratories, long-term care facilities, health care networks, and preferred provider organizations. Formerly, JCAHO scheduled regular site visit evaluations about every three years. As of 2006, the organization switched to unannounced site visits that can occur at any time. This change requires health care organizations to be in a state of perpetual readiness for the rigorous evaluative process for which JCAHO is famous. These site visits are expensive, stressful, and labor-intensive for the health care organizations, but essential for assuring the public that national standards of care are being met in the local community. A key component of the JCAHO evaluation is the relationship between the hospital and the medical staff.

## Hospital-based Physicians

There are a number of traditionally hospital-based physician practices. In the past, these have included pathologists, emergency medicine physicians, anesthesiologists, and radiologists. Current additions to these ranks include hospitalists and critical care physicians. These physicians may be practicing as individual practitioners, in single or multi-specialty groups, or in an employment model with the hospital. The biggest difference between these groups and others in an office-based practice is the potential for the use of an exclusive contract. In an exclusive contract, the group obtains the right to be the sole provider of certain agreed-upon services to the hospital or health care organization. The group gets the stability of not having to compete with others for patients, and the hospital gets the benefit of a stable group of providers that can offer emergency call coverage, quality care initiatives, and other benefits. At first blush, this may seem to violate the Sherman Act in that it ties the purchase of one service (for example, anesthesia services) to the purchase of another (such as surgical services). However, since there is a clear benefit to the system overall in the form of improved patient care, these sorts of arrangements are allowed.[14]

These physicians are frequently involved in hospital committees and other functions, in part because of their proximity and availability for meetings compared to physicians that practice outside the hospital. However, these groups of physicians may have less power and influence over hospital policy because the administration does not view them as "bringing patients to the hospital." Since they infrequently have admitting privileges, this is technically true, but short-sighted. Importantly, the public may think that these groups of physicians are employed by the hospital, since patients rarely choose a hospital based on its anesthesiologist or radiologist. Depending on the state, this may place the hospital at risk for suits under the argument of vicarious liability based on the theory of apparent or ostensible agency (the physician appears to be the hospital's agent to the laymen). While this argument has been struck down in Virginia,[15] it has been upheld in Illinois.[16]

Anesthesiologists may practice as solo, independent providers, or in groups (or occasionally employed by the hospitals themselves), with or without mid-level providers, such as Certified Registered Nurse Anesthetists (CRNAs) or Anesthesiologist Assistants (AAs). These two mid-level providers are Master's prepared and specifically trained in the technical aspect of anesthesiology. Some hospitals employ CRNAs (or contract with CRNA groups) for anesthesia services. Except in the few cases where states have opted-out of the CMS requirement, CRNAs must be supervised by a physician, who can be an anesthesiologist or the operating physician.[17] Not all states license AAs, but those that do typically require that they be medically-directed by an anesthesiologist. While CRNAs and AAs are important members of the health care team trained to administer anesthesia, only physicians are trained to practice the medical specialty of anesthesiology, which encompasses a wide range of care from pre-operative evaluations to consultations in Pain Medicine to post-operative care in the Post-Anesthesia Care Unit and Critical Care Units.

While radiologists typically practice in the hospital because of the capital investment needed for imaging equipment, there are frequently independent offices and joint ventures where complex imaging modalities are available in free-standing centers. In this situation, the radiologist (or group) provides the capital and then can capture the facility fee, which may be considerably more than the professional fee for reading the images. Of course, they would have to pay for the building, equipment, and staff out of this money, but since a free-standing center does not have to deal with uninsured patients and emergency cases, they may have lower total costs, thus enabling higher profit margins. Image processing and handling technologies may revolutionize radiology practice. There are some groups that station members in Europe so that they are reading electronically-transmitted images during their day while it is night in the United States. Having group members rotate through helps deal with issues, such as credentialing in telemedicine.

While pathologists may run laboratories in hospitals, they may also have off-site centers where they may process specimens from offices or small hospitals, as well as from their primary affiliation. Besides interpreting tissue slides and results from analysis of body fluids and other specimens, most pathologists have significant administrative roles in supervising the plethora of staff that are required for high-functioning laboratories and blood banks. Their expertise is necessary to navigate the increasingly complex regulatory world.

Emergency Medicine is one of the newest medical specialties, recognized as the 23ʳᵈ medical specialty by the American Board of Medical Specialties (ABMS) in 1979, and as a primary board in 1989. Practice sites are typically hospitals, but can vary widely. Small, critical-access hospitals may staff their Emergency Departments with residency-trained Emergency Physicians, but those practices are quite different from the large urban trauma centers. The biggest difference is the amount of back-up from the other medical specialties, since an acute myocardial infarction patient can walk into either setting. Most Emergency Physicians are employed by groups that provide coverage to hospitals, but they can also be independent contractors or even employees.

Hospitalists, as their names implies, work in the hospital. They offer the advantage of having dedicated staff who are focused on the acute episode of care, yet are experienced in navigating the complexities of discharge planning and coordination of care. While some group practices shy away from hospitalists, many small groups or independent practitioners welcome the idea that someone will be looking out for their patients without the outpatient physician having to lose valuable patient contact time driving to and from the hospital. Hospitalists may be employed by (most common to least common): hospitals; managed care organizations; local medical groups (usually large multi-specialty groups); geographically diverse, for-profit, hospitalist companies; academic hospitalist practices; or, they may be self-employed.[12] Similarly, critical care physicians practice in hospitals, and come from a variety of backgrounds including surgery, anesthesiology, and pulmonary medicine. They, too, can be solo practitioners, in group practices, or employees. Use of critical care physicians improves outcomes for ICU patients.[18] There are inroads being made in telemedicine that allow critical care physicians to consult on patients remotely. This model allows for their specialized knowledge to be applied to more patients, especially those at smaller hospitals that would not otherwise be able to support a critical care service.[19] In the setting of critical care telemedicine, there still must be "boots on the ground" to take care of the physical needs of the patients.

## Military Medicine

The Uniformed Services provide excellent medical training and an extraordinary practice environment for those interested in military medicine. Several pathways are available for medical training. Those individuals selected for undergraduate education in the nation's military academies can apply to the Uniformed Services Medical School in Bethesda, or to any of the 125 medical schools in the United States. The government provides a salary stipend and covers all the costs of a medical school education. Alternatively, individuals can enlist in the military and attend the college of their choice with salary support and full coverage of all college expenses. Residency training is provided in military facilities, except for those subspecialties for which there is no approved military training program. The government "sponsors" residency and/or fellowship training in certain specialties by providing salary support for the trainee, as well as educational support (i.e., money) for the training program. The payback for obtaining medical training in the military is five years of service for those attending the military academies, four years of service for those supported though undergraduate colleges, four years of service for the medical school education, and one year of service for every year of sponsored residency/fellowship training. The time spent in military residencies does not count toward the service commitment. Military salaries for physicians are generally lower than those in the private sector, but physicians trained at government expense have had salary support during their education and they accrue no indebtedness from undergraduate and/or postgraduate education. Military physicians can expect to be deployed overseas multiple times during their career, offering the opportunity for unparalleled travel and cultural experiences.

## "Lean" Health Care

The United States spends more money on health care, both in total and per capita, than any other nation in the world, approaching 16% of gross domestic product with health care cost inflation over 8% in 2004, and about 46% of all health care expenditures being financed through federal, state and local public sources.[20] Yet despite tremendous technological achievements unique to the U.S. health care system, there is no guarantee of universal coverage for every citizen, infant mortality rates and longevity are worse than any other industrialized countries, and recent studies have shown that only about 50% of people who have had an encounter with the health care system (this excludes persons with no access) receive appropriate care based upon accepted national guidelines. In 2011, the "baby boomers" will be eligible for Medicare benefits, thus shifting more cost to the public sector. This combination of rising cost, unrestrained societal expectations, and relatively poor outcomes for the money spent will force health care policy makers to rethink the basic structure of American medicine. We are going to have to do better with fewer financial resources.

In the past several years more and more health care thinkers are talking about "lean" health care, an adaptation of the principles of the famed Toyota production system to the perceived problems of cost and quality in health care.[20] Central to the lean concept is the relentless elimination of waste, or *muda*, in Japanese. Eliminating waste is more than just trying to eliminate monetary expense; it is about eliminating wasted time, wasted steps, wasted supplies, or any other activity that adds no value to the final product or process. Many policymakers believe that there is waste in health care expenditures and that systems of the future will need to be much leaner. What physicians should expect is downward pressure on hospital reimbursement, on physician reimbursement, and escalating activities to control utilization of health care resources. Whether these activities can also improve the quality of care remains to be seen.

## Conclusion

While there are many different practice models, they have key components in common. Focusing on patient safety and quality improvement will give a physician the ability to compete in today's market. This competition will be beneficial for patients as quality measures become increasingly available to the public, and for cost containment as pay for performance gains a toehold. Knowledge of the economic and regulatory environments will be essential for new physicians.

## Case Study

You are Dr. Sue Prior, Vice President for Medical Affairs at Bedlam Air Medical Center, one of the three hospitals in town. One of the physicians in the area wishes to apply for medical staff privileges as a hospitalist at your facility. Dr. Mi D'Ochre moved to the area several years ago and has practiced at the other two hospitals in town, Pourries General Hospital and Sisters of South Orlando Hospital (SOSO).

Before sending him an application for medical staff privileges, you invite Dr. D'Ochre to your office for a brief interview. What issues would you address? How does the role of a hospitalist fit in with your hospital's plans?

You agree that he would potentially serve a need in the hospital. What information would the Credentialing Committee wish to look at? What do you need to find out about his performance at the other hospitals? What is the best way to accomplish this? He asks for privileges in sedation and anesthesia so that he can perform procedures in the critical care units. How would you respond?

The hospital agrees to hire Dr. D'Ochre and he will report to you as VPMA. You meet to discuss compensation, since he will be an employed physician. Are there any legal issues to be concerned about? What performance measures can you link to his compensation? Are there other roles in the organization in which it can be reasonably expected for him to participate?

## Study/Discussion Questions

1. How can a practice maintain access for patients while reducing the "no show" problem?

2. What are some factors that are important for success in a practice? How do these factors vary among physicians, non-physician providers, and staff?

3. Describe how pay for performance (P4P) could apply to a practice in your specialty.

4. Accreditation issues are important in hospital practices. How does the individual physician's involvement play a role in hospital accreditation?

5. Many physicians work primarily in hospitals. What kinds of practice arrangements are possible, and how might this help the hospital provide services to its physician staff and patients?

## Suggested Readings/Websites

American Medical Association Organized Medical Staff Section:
http://www.ama-assn.org/ama/pub/category/375.html
Resources for policies, white papers and other information for MSOs.

Petersen LA, Woodard LD, Utrech T, Daw C, Sookanan S. Does pay for performance improve the quality of health care? *Ann Intern Med.* 2006;145:265-272.

Joint Commission on Accreditation of Healthcare Organizations. *Doing More with Less: Lean Thinking and Patient Safety in Health Care.* Oakbrook Terrace, IL: Joint Commission Resources, Inc.; 2006.

Medical Economics® Magazine, Young Doctors' Resource Center:
http://www.memag.com/memag/static/staticHtml.jsp?id=112051
This specialized section of the magazine's website provides newsletters and various resources for practice management.

## References

1. Levinson W, Linzer M. What is an academic general internist? Career options and training pathways. JAMA. 2002;288:2045-2048.

2. Terry K. Questions to ask before joining a multispecialty group. Med Econ. 2002;9:124.

3. Rice B. Do you have the right stuff to go solo? Med Econ. 2001;1:121.

4. Murray M, Berwick DM. Advanced Access: Reducing waiting and delays in primary care. JAMA. 2003;289:1035-1040.

5. Valko GP. Open access scheduling: a medical director's view from the trenches. Health Policy Newsletter. 2003;16. Available at: http://jdc.jefferson.edu/hpn/vol16/iss2/7/. Accessed August 18, 2006.

6. Berry LL, Selders K, Wilder SS. Innovations in access to care: A patient-centered approach. Ann Intern Med. 2003;139:568-574.

7. The Committee on Quality of Healthcare in America and the Institute of Medicine. Crossing the Quality Chasm: A New Health System for the 21st Century. Washington, DC: National Academies Press; 2001.

8. Bodenheimer T. Innovations in primary care in the United States. BMJ. 2003;326:796-799.

9. Rosenthal MB, Frank RG, Li Z, Epstein AM. Early experience with pay-for-performance. JAMA. 2005;294:1788-1793.

10. National Center for Health Statistics. Health, United States, 2005 With Chartbook on Trends in the Health of Americans. Hyattsville, MD; 2005. Available at: http://www.cdc.gov/nchs/data/hus/hus05.pdf#executivesummary. Accessed August 18, 2006.

11. Nelson JR. Hospitalist Practice. American College of Physicians. Available at: http://www.acponline.org/counseling/hosps.htm. Accessed August 16, 2006.

12. Joint Commission on Accreditation of Healthcare Organizations. 2002 Hospital Accreditation Standards. Oakbrook Terrace, IL: Joint Commission Resources, Inc.; 2002.

13. Jefferson Parish Hosp. Dist. No. 2 v. Hyde, 466 U.S. 2 (1984)

14. Hancock, Daniel, Johnson & Nagle, PC. Apparent Agency? Apparently Not. October 26, 2005. Available at: http://www.hdjn.com/pdfs/Client%20Advisory%20-%20Apparent%20Agency102605.pdf. Accessed August 15, 2006.

15. Gilbert v. Sycamore Municipal Hospital, 156 Ill. 2d 511, 523, 622 N.E.2d 788, 795 (1993).

16. American Society of Anesthesiologists. CMS Supervision Rules for Nurse Anesthetists. Available at: http://www.asahq.org/Washington/narules.htm. Accessed August 16. 2006.

17. Rothschild JM. Chapter 38. "Closed" intensive care units and other models of care for critically ill patients. AHRQ. Available at: http://www.ahrq.gov/clinic/ptsafety/chap38.htm. Accessed August 16, 2006

18. Breslow MJ, Rosenfeld BA, Doerfler M, et al. Effect of a multiple-site intensive care unit telemedicine program on clinical and economic outcomes: An alternative paradigm for intensivist staffing. *Crit Care Med.* 2004;32:31-38.

19. Centers for Medicare and Medicaid Services. National Health Expenditures Data. Available at: http://www.cms.hhs.gov/NationalHealthExpendData/downloads/tables.pdf. Accessed August 18, 2006.

20. Joint Commission on Accreditation of Healthcare Organizations. *Doing More with Less: Lean Thinking and Patient Safety in Health Care.* Oakbrook Terrace, IL: Joint Commission Resources, Inc.; 2006.

# Chapter 15

## *Open Access Scheduling*

George P. Valko, MD

### Executive Summary

Open or advanced access scheduling is a key process to improve patient access to care. This process is but one part of a major initiative by the Institute for Healthcare Improvement (IHI) called the Idealized Design of Clinical Office Practices (IDCOP). Rather than measuring the success of a practice by how far ahead a schedule is booked, the new gauge of success is the amount of open appointments that are available to allow patients to be seen when they want or need to be seen, for either routine or urgent visits. The benefits to a practice can be substantial in terms of financial, patient satisfaction and other outcome measurements.

Implementing open access scheduling requires leadership, education, and planning. Leadership is needed to guide the clinicians, staff and patients through change and to stay the course through difficulties. Education is key to help all understand why change must occur and how to deal effectively with an entirely new way of thinking about scheduling. Proper planning establishes goals, allows the implementation to proceed smoothly, and helps to monitor and measure the progress of the change.

Seminars, literature and consultants are readily available to help with the implementation of open access scheduling or other office redesign initiatives. It is paramount to remember that each practice—whether private or academic, solo or group, primary or specialty care—is unique. Open access scheduling can be modified to fit each practice type for the benefit of clinicians, patients and staff.

### Learning Objectives

1. Understand the concept of open access scheduling and its objectives.

2. Implement open access scheduling.

3. Evaluate the effectiveness of open access scheduling through appropriate metrics.

4. Identify problem areas and take appropriate steps to resolve them.

## Keywords

access; advanced access scheduling; Institute for Healthcare Improvement (IHI); Idealized Design of Clinical Office Practices (IDCOP); open access scheduling

## Introduction

A longtime tenet of a successful medical practice has been to adhere to the three "As": availability, affability and ability. Availability, or access, to medical care or a clinician has become increasingly more important, as witnessed by the advent of nurse-practitioner driven medical offices in large retail outlets. Although access is also demanded in the inpatient setting and systems must be in place for after hours care, such as phone- or e-medicine, the office visit remains the *sine qua non* of a medical practice.

For years, the hallmark of a successful practice has been appointments that have been booked months in advance. However, if a patient missed (or cancelled) an appointment or the clinician cancelled office hours, that patient would have to wait weeks or months for another appointment. For patients who are ill or for other reasons need to be seen urgently, the wait is less but usually at the expense of other patients' appointments or the clinicians' time, i.e., they are "squeezed" into an already busy schedule. To try to maintain a full schedule, office staff would double- and triple-book appointment slots in anticipation that a certain percentage of patients would cancel or not keep their appointment.

Other barriers to access imposed by archaic scheduling systems such as multiple visit types, (new/established physical, new/established sick, follow-up short, follow-up extended and prescription refill, to name just a few) keep patients from being seen in a timely fashion. If a patient visit didn't fit into one of the established categories, the individuals would have to be seen on a different day. Managing this type of scheduling system, based on the clinicians' needs, wastes staff time and effort and benefits no one—especially not the patient.

Open or advanced access appointment scheduling was developed by the Institute for Healthcare Improvement (IHI) as a key process to improve patient access to care in the office setting and to allow a better office experience for the clinician. The process is but one part of a major initiative by IHI called the Idealized Design of Clinical Office Practices (IDCOP). One of their working mantras is to "give the patient what they want and need when they want or need it"; another is to "do today's work today." With open access scheduling, the new hallmark of a successful practice is to have the bulk of the patient appointments available for the same or next day. Together with the elimination of the barrier of multiple visit types, open access scheduling allows patients to be seen at their convenience, desire or need—whether it is for a well exam or sick visit—and leads to improved patient satisfaction. By having appointments available every day for months in advance, there is an increase in patients who arrive for a visit and a decrease in those who miss appointments. This results in a healthier bottom line, since more receipts are generated and staff can be used for other office duties rather than to schedule and reschedule patients.

Open access scheduling requires a complete change in the way clinicians, staff and patients think about scheduling. Although not easy, by following a few guidelines any office can achieve the goal of open access scheduling and other aspects of redesigning the clinical office.

## Characteristics and Benefits of Open Access

It is well documented that open or advanced access scheduling enables patients to be seen on a timely basis. But open access scheduling is more than just a "no booking" or carve-out model of scheduling. Characteristics of an open access scheduling system include:

• Capacity and demand are in equilibrium on a daily basis, enabling patients to be seen when they want to be seen. Since most of the appointments are available every day, patients may call any time for an appointment and be accommodated. Because the number of clinicians is already matched to the demand, all patients who call can be seen that day, or within the next few days.

• Elimination of the distinction between urgent and routine care. Under open access scheduling, most, if not all, barriers to access are removed, including multiple appointment types; a patient can be seen for a well visit just as easily as having to be "fit in" for a sick visit under the traditional scheduling system.

• Hidden capacity is discovered. Since patients are seen close to the time that appointments are made, no-shows and cancellations are decreased and arrival rates are increased.

• Work is complete at the end of the day. Under the traditional method of scheduling, work is always put off for the future since the appointments are booked months in advance. Also, there is time in the schedule to complete phone calls and paperwork, since patients aren't double- or triple-booked.

The primary benefits of open access scheduling accrue to both the patient and the physician; patients are afforded greater ease in obtaining appointments and physicians enjoy increased productivity. Other benefits include:

- Improved patient satisfaction as a result of receiving same-day appointments;

- Improved timeliness of patient care, (including accommodating the patients of colleagues who are out of the office);

- Increased number of patients who arrive for a scheduled visit, largely due to increased availability;

- Decreased patient no-shows and cancellations;

- Decreased physician cancellations;

- Improved office efficiency due to reduced need to reschedule patients; and

- Improved bottom line resulting from full schedules.

If all these benefits exist, then why don't more practices move to open access scheduling? Part of the answer: change is difficult. Other reasons may be the lack of impetus for change. Traditional scheduling systems are clinician-centered practices that are booked well into the future. To get out of that comfort zone is difficult and usually requires a drastic set of circumstances to precipitate change. Many clinicians feel the motivation to change when they discover that they are working harder to maintain the same level of patient satisfaction and financial rewards, or that those rewards even have decreased. Open access scheduling is a patient-centric system that not only allows the patient to be seen when they want or need to be seen, but also allows the physician more flexibility. However the decision is made, changing to an open access scheduling system requires leadership, planning, and education.

## Leadership

Strong leadership is fundamental to implement change in any organization, especially when the process is applied to a core practice operation, like appointment scheduling. The leader can be the department chair, medical director, administrator or practice manager, or whoever is in charge of the practice. Leadership must be totally committed to implementing open access scheduling and understand that it may not be a popular decision, especially among older clinicians, who are accustomed to and invested in the traditional scheduling system. The change may also disturb patients, who want to have the comfort of a future appointment in hand when they leave the office. Many reasons have been cited as to why a clinician will not want the change: his schedule is booked and they have a good show rate; her patients need an appointment in order to schedule time off from work; his patients need to make transportation or baby-sitting arrangements. It is these same patients who often clamor for sooner appointments when they are sick or have an urgent deadline for a medical form to be completed.

Beyond the practice leadership, another crucial role needed to successfully implement open access scheduling is that of a champion. This person will be the one to rally the staff and clinicians, handle the day-to-day details, and field the concerns and criticisms to deliver the product. The champion will need the support of the leadership and should work with a core group of people who are equally committed to move forward with open access scheduling. The core group must be able to meet on a regular basis and have decision-making authority; they must also be transparent in decision making and able to share information. Above all, they must be diplomatic in their dealings with the rest of the practice.

## Planning

Planning involves setting goals and objectives, creating methods of measuring progress towards those goals, and developing contingency plans. One goal of the open access scheduling system may be to insure that every patient is seen when they need or want to be seen within the hours of operation. Another goal may be to achieve a high rate of continuity of care. These goals are more easily achieved if the main mission of the practice is patient care and clinicians see patients on a full-time schedule. If it is an academic practice with additional missions of research and teaching, both the faculty and residents may have less patient time, making these goals more difficult to achieve. Academic practices have other obstacles, such as resident work-hour restrictions and out-of-office rotations that make continuity of care more challenging.

Additional practice goals for open access scheduling may be to insure that the third next available appointment (the industry standard of measurement of availability) is within one to two days for each clinician; that there is a reduction in the number of no-shows; an increase in the arrival rate; and improvement in overall practice receipts.

Another part of the plan must be to decide exactly how much open access is right for the practice. Usually 100% open access is not practical. A more mature open access, sometimes referred to as "advanced access" is based on "good backlog," in which a percentage of future appointments are made for specific reasons. Such reasons include a clinician's need to see a patient on a certain date (for example, a warfarin check or suture removal), or a patient's desire to have an appointment on a certain date because of transportation issues. This is in keeping with the tenet to give patients what they want or need, when they want or need it. Therefore, a practice may decide that 75% of all patients should be seen on the same day or within 24 hours, with the remainder held for future appointments. Another practice may decide to have 60% of all appointments available within 24 hours of calling, 20% available within the next week, and 20% available within the next six to twelve months. There is no hard and fast rule, and each practice may design the advanced access to meet their needs and characteristics.

The practice must also plan for an increase in phone calls to the schedulers, especially in the morning. This increase is generally offset by a decrease in the amount of calls for rescheduling under the old system, so there is no increase in staff time. Indeed, there may be a decrease in staff time for scheduling because if a clinician must cancel a session, there are fewer patients to reschedule and most patients can be accommodated when the clinician has his next office hours.

There are additional methods of ensuring continuity of care that can be balanced with the need to have all practice patients seen and clinicians' schedules filled. This can be accomplished by having a fixed time during which only clinicians' personal patients will be able to make an appointment with their clinician; after that time, any practice patient may be scheduled. For example, Clinician X has office hours on Monday, Wednesday, and Friday. The practice protocol is to have 20% of open access appointments available to be made at anytime during the year, 20% available for the next week on a rolling basis, and 60% open for the next day. Only Clinician X's patients will be able to make an appointment with Clinician X for the future advanced access appointments, and only Clinician X's patients will be able to make an appointment for the next day if they call during the hours of 8:00 am – 10:00 am. If after 10:00 am Clinician X still has available appointment slots for the next day, or if a patient on Clinician X's schedule cancels their appointment for the next day, any practice patient will be able to be scheduled into those open appointment slots.

Finally, the practice must decrease the number of visit types to just a few. An example may be to have only three types of visits, such as "new patient physical," "new patient sick," and "established patient." The times allotted for the types of visits should be uniform. For example, allot 15 minutes for any visit type except for a "new patient physical" (30 minutes) with the theory that all visits will even out over time. This will eliminate the distinction between urgent and routine care, as it won't matter whether an appointment is filled with an ill patient or a patient with a follow-up or physical exam. Along with this practice, each clinician should do as much as possible for the patient in each visit, maximizing their visit, so a patient does not have to come back soon for a different problem, and each visit can be billed at a higher level.

Contingency plans should also be considered. For example, how will the practice handle patient demand when several clinicians are away at once at peak vacation time or during a busy flu season? Also, the leadership must be aware of some of the potential pitfalls of open access scheduling and plan for them. The most common are the "black market" or "underground economy" — clinicians and staff that secretly hold a patient list and schedule them the morning of a patient session. For example, Clinician X has 14 appointments available for the next day, but directed a staff member to put in 10 patients as soon as the open access schedule opens for that day. Therefore, only four slots are now open for any patient of Clinician X who calls to be seen. If 10 patients call in, six cannot be accommodated in Clinician X's schedule. This hurts the patients who try to play by the rules but are now shut off from an appointment. It also leads to patient and physician complaints that open access is not working. In reality, open access will work well if everyone follows the plan.

Another possible pitfall arises when patients become aware that it is easy to get another appointment if they miss their original one, and therefore, are constantly substituting appointments. The practice must decide if it is better for patient care and the bottom line to let this continue or to penalize a patient by not giving a first-available appointment.

## Outcome Measures

The next step of the plan is to gather measurements of the practice's effectiveness. This is a great time to take the pulse of the practice, not only from a total management perspective, but also to look at specific items needed for the change to open access scheduling. Obviously, a computerized scheduling system will greatly aid in this process; an electronic medical record is a huge plus for total redesign of the office.

For each individual clinician, and the practice as a whole, measure the total number of patients who were: 1) scheduled, 2) arrived, 3) no-shows (did not show and did not call to cancel, or called to cancel immediately before or after the scheduled appointment time), 4) cancelled, or 5) bumped (cancelled by the clinician). This should be done each month to determine whether open access is making any improvement in those areas, as well as to gather details of each clinician's practice statistics. It also would be helpful for future measurement of continuity of care to note if those categories of patients were scheduled to see their own or another clinician. Another important measurement is how long it is until the third next available appointment, for each clinician and the practice as a whole, for both well and sick visits. As a standard industry measurement of patient access, rates can be used to track quality improvement.

The next items to measure are the total numbers of patients scheduled for each day, week, month, quarter, and year. This will give the practice a better understanding of the peak times for patient visits.  In addition, track the number of phone calls for each day, especially those that ask for an appointment; this will provide a measurement of demand.  For example, are Mondays busier and more popular compared to Wednesdays? Are the winter months busier than summer months? If so, are these a constant?

As a prelude to matching capacity to demand, measure each clinician's work hours, along with their productivity and days in the office. This includes the number of patient sessions per clinician, as well as the number of patients per session. If there is a mismatch between the capacity of the clinicians and the patient demand on certain days or months, part of the plan to correct this would include changing office schedules accordingly.

Lastly, it is a good idea to initiate some form of patient and clinician satisfaction survey to measure operational items, such as availability of appointment times, how long it takes to get an appointment with an individual clinician (or anyone in the practice), timing of return phone calls, etc. This information can be valuable for determining the success of open access scheduling.

## Education

Stakeholder education is crucial to the acceptance and ultimate success of open access scheduling implementation. Appropriate education for patients, staff, and the clinicians must be developed and disseminated.  The most basic (but most difficult) concept for everyone to grasp is that instead of a patient making an appointment now for a future date, the patient will call at a future date when they want an appointment. The importance of this concept cannot be overemphasized, because patients and clinicians alike are accustomed to making appointments for the future. It is helpful to have brochures made for each patient that show the usual weekly schedules of clinicians. If the practice uses a web site, it is helpful to post that information there also.  If the practice uses voice mail, clinicians should incorporate their weekly patient schedule into their individual greeting.

The personnel designated to answer phones for triage or scheduling should receive in-depth instruction about open access.  They should offer each patient an appointment when they expect it, but emphasize open access as the main option.  Flyers with FAQs (frequently asked questions), signage boasting open access and word of mouth are other ways to get the message out. Except for the "wow" factor that will happen when a patient gets an appointment the same day, when they expected it would be weeks from now, there is no substitute for ample time to prepare and inform everyone involved. That will help them become comfortable with the change, and to accept the notion that open access will work—and work better—than the old way of scheduling.

## Implementation

There are several documented methods to implement open access scheduling. One method involves a plan to work down the backlog of patients—patients who already have appointments in the future—and another would be to start anew at some point in the future. As with other aspects of open access scheduling, there are no hard and fast rules, and a hybrid model can be made to suit the needs of each practice. In addition, some practices may prefer to pilot new programs with a few clinicians to get the bugs worked out, while other practices may opt to have the all the clinicians go through the change together and adjust as needed.

Whichever implementation method is chosen, the practice must first determine the demand for patient appointments and the capacity to meet those appointments. This will allow the practice to make any needed adjustments to accommodate all patients who may want to be seen. Demand is calculated by the number of appointments already scheduled by day of the week plus the number of requests for appointments the practice receives for those days by phone or walk-ins. Demand is different for individual days of the week; a Monday may be busier than a Wednesday, or the Tuesday after a 3-day weekend may be busier than any other day of the week. Demand may be also greater during peak flu seasons or during traditional back-to-school physical times. For example, if 100 patients are already scheduled for a Wednesday, but 20 more patients call for an appointment that day and another 20 patients walk in hoping to be seen, then the demand is for 140 appointments.

Next, the practice should calculate how much clinician time it would need to see those 140 patients. If the practice has reduced the number of visits types, and if every visit was 15 minutes in length, then it would take 2,100 minutes (140 patients x 15 minutes/patient) or 35 hours of clinician time to see those patients.

Following this, the practice must determine its capacity to see those patients. Capacity is based on how many patients per hour each clinician can see, and how many and what hours they work. For example, if a clinician can see four patients per hour and has eight 3-hour sessions, then that clinician can see 12 patients per session or 96 patients in a week. The capacity of the practice is the total number of patients able to be seen by all clinicians in the practice during a certain time period. For example, if there are five clinicians and they can see a total of 12 patients per hour and have two 3-hour sessions per day, then 72 patients can be seen in one day. Using these calculations, the core group can determine when the demand would be greatest, allowing them to match capacity to demand by changing schedules, if necessary.

If the practice decides that it will implement open access scheduling by working down the backlog, then the backlog must be calculated. The backlog is the total number of appointments already made for the year divided by the average number of patients the clinicians see per day. For example, if there are 504 appointments already scheduled and the clinicians have been averaging 72 patients per day, then there are 7 days of backlog (504 divided by 72). To meet the new demand, the practice can now make plans to work down this backlog by temporarily increasing capacity through 1) increasing the number of patients a clinician should see per hour; 2) increasing the number of hours or days a clinician should see patients; or 3) hiring additional clinicians. For example, by adding two patients per day to each of the five clinicians, 10 more patients could be seen. At this rate, it would take 50 working days (504 patients/10 patients per day) to eliminate the backlog, at which time the practice would go to fully open access scheduling and return to its usual capacity.

Another method to implement open access scheduling is to plan for a start date at some point in the future. Determine the percentage of open access versus advance access appointments that would fit the practice style and comfort levels. For several months leading up to the start date, do not make any appointments except for the advanced access appointments. After the start date, fully implement open access scheduling. Education of the patients is the key to the success of this method and must be started early, and continued throughout the implementation phase. This method may be better suited to academic or other practices in which the clinicians do not have a full-time clinical load.

## Assessment

The champion and core group must do ongoing assessments to gauge the success of the implementation and to determine if anything needs to be changed based on hard data. However, it is well worth it to allow the system to work itself out over a given period of time rather than to constantly make changes. The group should regularly present any and all data to the practice to allow for constructive criticism and comment, but the bottom line is that each practice can adjust the open access scheduling to fit its style and personality.

## Conclusion

Most patients who make a traditionally-scheduled appointment with their clinician can expect a wait of weeks or months. Indeed, the hallmark of a successful practice has been to have a long waiting list of booked appointments. For patients who are ill or who need to be seen urgently, the wait is usually less—but at the expense of other patients' appointments or the clinician's time.

The promise of open or advanced access scheduling is that a patient can call for any type of appointment, routine or urgent, and be told to come in the same day or the next, without overloading the schedule or the clinician. Developed by the Institute for Healthcare Improvement, open access scheduling is a major change in the way patients are scheduled for appointments in that most of the appointments are kept open until that day or the next. Instead of the clinician having an empty visit slot because a patient forgot or cancelled the appointment, all slots are full with patients who showed because their appointment was made when they needed it. Instead of staff wasting time scheduling and rescheduling patients who have forgotten appointments, they are freed up to do other duties. This has a positive effect on patient, clinician and staff satisfaction as well as the bottom line.

Although seemingly onerous to begin, open access scheduling can be implemented successfully in any practice setting, large or small, private or academic. It takes a combination of leadership, planning, education and the will to make change happen.

## Case Study

After several months of debate and planning, The Department of Family and Community Medicine of Jefferson Medical College in Philadelphia (a large, urban academic family practice) decided to implement open access scheduling in July 2002. Many reasons led to this decision, including the desire to improve patient satisfaction with access to the clinical office and to decrease the rate of patients who did not show for or cancelled their appointments. There was also a need to increase clinical productivity and income, while maintaining the ability of the faculty to pursue their academic mission of teaching and research.

By analyzing patient visit data over the last five years, it was apparent that these were intertwined. For example, for regular patient hours, only 57% of patients who were scheduled for a visit actually arrived for that visit despite a costly phone reminder system. Contrasted to this were the 85% of patients who arrived for sick or urgent visits when the appointment was made the day before, what the Institute for Healthcare Improvement termed "hidden capacity." A 10% increase in arrived patients for regular office hours would mean a large increase in productivity for the faculty, as well as less time taken away from their other academic pursuits.

Numerous obstacles were confronted both during planning and initial implementation. Chief among those obstacles was that of all the practices in the country that were using open access scheduling, none was an academic institution with a residency program, so there was no blueprint to follow. Obtaining buy-in from busy clinicians and mandating this drastic change was another obstacle which was overcome through education and the initial phase-in of an only 50% open access system. Since it had worked so well, the current scheduling is more of an advanced access model with 60% appointments open within 24 hours, 20% appointments open a week in advance, and 20% open months in advance to accommodate all types of patients.

The results from the start and now four years later have been dramatic and sustained. The faculty have an average of 67% arrived visits, up from the 57% before open access scheduling, with a decrease in no-shows from 19% to 13% with similar results for the residents. This led to an improved bottom line with charges and receipts. And although busy during patient hours, the clinicians did not have to use research or teaching time to keep their patient total at the expected level and indeed became more productive. Based on information culled from independent surveys, their level of satisfaction with the system is excellent.

Since continuity of care is so important to family medicine and is an RRC requirement, results of the continuity studies have shown that the residents and faculty have preserved their continuity patients with about 69% continuity for residents and 86% continuity for faculty for the current year.

Open access scheduling is serving the patients well, as shown by an independent satisfaction survey. The majority of the patients have both a favorable rating of open access scheduling and think it is better that the traditional scheduling that exists in other offices. In addition, patient complaints about their inability to get an appointment have dropped considerably.

In all, open access scheduling has been a success for the Department of Family and Community Medicine of Jefferson Medical College.

## Study/Discussion Questions

1. How does open access scheduling differ from traditional scheduling systems with same day appointments?

2. Do all appointments have to be scheduled the same day?

3. What if a patient doesn't want to use open access?

4. What are the benefits to open access scheduling?

5. How does a practice measure success?

## Suggested Readings/Websites

### ARTICLES:

Berwick DM. *Escape Fire: Lessons for the Future of Health Care.* New York, NY: The Commonwealth Fund; 2002.

Kennedy JG, Hsu JT. Implementation of an open access sheduling system in a residency training program. *Fam Med.* 2003;35:666-670.

Maeseneer JM, DePrins L, Gosset C, Heyerick J. Provider continuity in family medicine. *Ann Fam Med.* 2003;1:144-148.

Murray M, Tantau C. Same-day appointments: exploding the access paradigm. *Fam Pract Manag.* 2000;7:45-50.

Murray M. Answers to your questions about same-day scheduling. *Fam Pract Manag.* 2005;12:59-64.

Murray M, Berwick, DM. Advanced access: reducing waiting and delays in primary care. *JAMA.* 2003;289:1035-1040.

Nutting PA, Goodwin MA, Flocke SA, Zyzanski SJ, Stange KC. Continuity of primary care: to whom does it matter and when? *Ann Fam Med.* 2003;1:149-155.

O'Hare CD, Corlett J. The outcomes of open-access scheduling. *Fam Pract Manag.* 2004;11:35-38.

Scherger JE. The end of the beginning: The redesign imperative in family medicine. *Fam Med.* 2005;37:513-516.

Steinbauer JR, Korell K, Erdin J, Spann SJ. Implementing open access scheduling in an academic practice. *Fam Pract Manag.* 2006;13:59-64.

### WEBSITE:

Institute for Healthcare Improvement: www.ihi.org

### MEETINGS:

Institute for Healthcare Improvement (IHI) Annual International Summit on Redesigning the Clinical Office Practice. (An excellent meeting for all aspects of clinical office design with a chance to talk to those who have done it. See website above).

# Chapter 16

## Understanding the Referral Process

Stephen E. Whitney, MD, MBA, BCM
and Jerald L. Zarin, MD, MBA, FAAP

### Executive Summary

No one physician can possibly have all the knowledge or expertise necessary to care for patients in the 21st century, necessitating the occasional consultation with other experts. The nature of our health care system requires physicians to develop referral networks. It is the responsibility of the physician to refer patients to competent providers in the approved network of their patients' insurance plans. The courts have held that physicians have a duty to know that the practices and facilities to which they refer patients are safe and competent.[1] Physicians who do not develop good networks of specialty providers will not reap the benefits of increased patient satisfaction and communication with the specialists, and will incur additional administrative hassle and expense.

Referrals to specialists that provide clarity as to the service requested will save your staff a great deal of time, effort, and frustration. Letting the specialist know your expectations will also build stronger, long-term relationships. Establishing systems to facilitate referrals smoothly is a wise investment in time and effort. Training the practice staff to do referrals properly will save the practice time and money, and will likely lead to happier and satisfied patients. It is important to have a system in place to manage the information gained from referrals so that critical information is seen and dealt with in a timely manner.

Even when all the rules of the insurer are followed, managed care companies will not approve all the referrals. There are several levels of appeal for denials. Time spent learning the appeal process, and developing a relationship with the medical directors of the two or three largest insurers of your patients, will yield substantial benefits in reduced denial rates and faster resolution of disputes, and may also help to build patient satisfaction and loyalty.

## Learning Objectives

1. Understand the importance of clear communication in the referral process.

2. Understand the importance of having adequate systems in place in their practice to ensure appropriate referrals are made and tracked.

3. Understand how the referral process can fit in with other practice management skills and priorities, such as quality improvement, marketing, risk management, and customer service.

## Keywords

appeal; authorization; balance bill; communication; consultation; covered benefit; demand management; denial; health maintenance organization (HMO); independent review organization (IRO); managed care organization (MCO); medical necessity; National Committee for Quality Assurance (NCQA); negligent referral; Point of Service (POS); Preferred Provider Organization (PPO); prior authorization; reconsideration; referral; utilization management

## Introduction

Regardless of one's opinion of the current state of the U.S. health care system, managed care is, and will continue to be, the predominant form of payment for health care services. In the Houston area for example, traditional "indemnity" type of health insurance accounts for less than 5% of the market. Although Health Maintenance Organizations (HMOs) are less popular than in the 1990s, they still have a significant percentage of the insured market in some areas. Preferred Provider Organizations (PPOs) and Point of Service (POS) option plans are very common. Governmental programs, such as Medicare, Medicaid, and the State Children's Health Insurance Programs (SCHIPs), increasingly are administered through managed care plans. Each of these systems, and the individual insurers in each type, has different requirements for the referral process. Wise physicians will structure their practices in ways that facilitate working within all the systems. Those who do so will find their physician partners/employees, staff, and patients are all better served and happier. Time spent at the front end will pay off handsomely in terms of reducing denials, appeals, and unhappy patients and specialists.

There is an increasing body of literature examining how physicians communicate. Most physicians consider themselves good communicators, but many of their patients and colleagues may not agree! In large surveys of patient satisfaction, many complaints relate to a perception that the physician doesn't listen to the patient or really care deeply about their welfare.[2] In one study, 91% of "mishaps" that occurred in one teaching hospital were related to communication issues.[3] Establishing systems that encourage good communication may help physicians avoid these negative perceptions and clinical problems.

This chapter will examine separate aspects of the referral process: the communication between the referring physician and the specialist or other health care entity, and the insurance process and requirement for submitting requests; getting authorization and payment from the patient and insurer; and dealing with the system when things don't go as planned.

## Why Require an Approval Process for Referrals?

Many physicians see managed care as an unnecessary intrusion into the physician-patient relationship. They see little good and much harm in the insurance "middleman." Why should MCOs require physicians to notify them of referrals, much less ask permission from the company to send a patient to a specialist?

The referral process falls under the basic category of *utilization management*. Somewhere between 70% and 90% of the premiums paid by members (patients) go to pay the costs of medical care, with the rest going to overhead and profit. Companies have two basic ways to control costs. Basic economics tells us that expense = (volume of services) x (unit price). The unit price is controlled through discounts from physicians, hospitals, pharmaceutical companies, and ancillary providers, usually obtained in exchange for the promise to direct the flow of patients to those providers and products. Control of the volume of services is where the referral management process falls.

Numerous studies have shown a considerable variation in how much care (and its associated cost) is delivered to similar patient populations.[4] There are wide variations in rates of a selection of surgical procedures, such as coronary artery bypass and hysterectomy, based on geography and local practice patterns for the same severity of disease. This would imply that physicians do not always agree when a surgical procedure is medically necessary versus other means of treating an illness. Likewise, for most conditions, there is a variety of medications that have similar efficacy. These variations led to attempts to define and publish guidelines for determining when something is "medically necessary," and for the creation of formularies of preferred drugs. Milliman® Care Guidelines®[5] and InterQual®[6] are two of the most commonly used sets of guidelines to help insurers review the necessity and appropriateness of care. There are also services that evaluate new medications and technologies to determine when something should be considered appropriate therapy (covered) versus experimental therapy (not covered). How aggressively a company decides to manage utilization determines what is on prior authorization lists and the percentage of services that are denied for payment. They will often set targets for such things as inpatient bed days per 1,000 plan members per year, or referral rate per 1,000 members per year. Insurers set premiums based on: expected medical costs + expected administrative costs + desired profit.

In a competitive market, insurers work to offer the most comprehensive benefits for the most reasonable premium possible. Employers might demand a less expensive product, or limitations on the increase in the cost of insuring their workforce in a particular year. The insurers may respond in one of four ways:

- Institute tighter controls.

- Reduce benefits and services that are covered under the plans.

- Design in higher co-payments.

- Take a loss that year to build market share.

In addition to the attempt to reduce utilization, some requirements to notify or to obtain authorization are implemented as a way to alert the company that expenses have been incurred, though they will not hit the system or be reported for some period of time. Without that information companies do not know if they are on track with their cost projections. Since decisions on plan design and pricing occur at least six months before the start date of new members, such advance warning is critical to the insurers.

Several studies have questioned the effectiveness of "gatekeeping" in controlling costs for insurers.[7] In recent years there has been a tendency to reduce the number of items that require precertification by the health plan. This is partly a result of the managed care backlash of the late 1990s, but also because an analysis of plan costs versus utilization savings did not show a benefit for low-to-moderate cost services. Some insurers made headlines by announcing the elimination of most precertification requirements. What was not in the press releases was their plan to increase the retrospective analysis of services and potential denial of payment after the services were rendered. The HMO Act of 1973[8] does not allow providers to bill the patient if the service is denied, so the conflict is between the provider and the insurer. This strategy takes the patient out of the fight and the insurer off the front page of the newspapers. Fights between physicians and insurers don't pack the same news punch as a company "denying needed medical care" to some unfortunate patient.

There are several other means to reduce the volume of services members use (*demand management*). These include member education campaigns about what can be done at home to improve health and treat minor illness; workplace health promotion and injury prevention programs; and nursing-staffed phone advice services.

## Referral Etiquette and Communication—Referring Physician

There are a few general concepts that can improve communication with your panel of specialists. To the referring physician, it seems obvious what is being asked for, but if a physician referring patients to the specialist expects something else, the consultant may *assume* the referring physician wants the same service as most of the other physicians he or she works with. The forms required by managed care companies for prior authorization of referrals may not be adequate to convey the information a specialist needs to give the most helpful consultation to your patient. These forms were designed to provide the managed care organization (MCO) with the information it deems necessary to approve or deny payment for the service, not to improve communication between the physicians making and receiving the consult request.

Some of the basics you will want to communicate include:

- The specific service you are requesting;
- The number of visits you are requesting;
- Whether you expect to continue managing the patient with the consultant's help, or whether you want the consultant to take over the care;
- Who will authorize and order any needed studies;
- Who will provide any patient education needed as part of the care;
- How the consultant will communicate his or her findings to you and the patient;
- Whether you expect or want the consultant to educate you about the condition; and
- Your working diagnoses, and visit notes and values from studies you have already done to evaluate the problem.

Many believe that a request for consultation should be a physician-to-physician direct communication. In many cases this is the best way to ensure that the needed information is accurately passed in a timely manner. However, physicians who use the same specialists routinely have developed other lines of communication to convey the information without unduly disrupting the workflow of both physicians.

One commonly used means to deliver information is through a form or checklist designed to insure all the pertinent information is conveyed. This form can be attached to the prior authorization approval form, and sent to the consultant. Others prefer a checklist to make sure that any important information that is not included on that patient's particular insurance authorization request is communicated to the specialist, and also to the insurer. The checklist you design can be specific to the type of practice and types of referrals you make most often. Many denials issued by insurers are issued due to incomplete information. To alleviate this problem, several insurers have moved to online referrals that do not permit the user to proceed until critical fields are completed.

As more practices switch to electronic medical records (EMRs), it may be easier to print certain parts of the chart (such as the last visit note, the medication list, and a problem list) that will include more information. If the referrer and the consultant are part of an integrated system, it may be helpful to mention that laboratory or diagnostic imaging results are available on the main computer system. Bysinger et al. report on a collaborative project in the Pacific Northwest including several hundred providers and major payors; their private intranet system has drastically reduced the number of problem referrals to less than 5%, and simultaneously reduced the staff time dedicated to referrals.[9] At present such a system qualifies as a "best practice." In the foreseeable future most physician offices will have EMR systems. Widespread adoption of electronic communication systems will make web-based referral systems routine.

Sending material that is not pertinent may actually hinder the communication process. Some offices find that installing computer systems just makes it that much easier to find and print information, and that the amount of clutter and paper increases. Avoid the temptation to include extra "stuff" just because you can; it will not benefit you, the consultant, or the patient. This is another reason to use a form or checklist to be sure the right information is being communicated.

## Referral Etiquette and Communication—Consultant

Most consultants depend on referrals from other physicians as much or more than they do on word of mouth referrals from their satisfied patients. Andrea Eliscu states that physicians receive 45% of new patients from referrals. She also states that a new patient that is physician-referred generates three times more in revenue each year than one who is self-referred, and twice the revenue of an existing patient.[10] An internist is unlikely to know a particular surgeon's complication rate for the procedure his patient needs. What he does know is how responsive the consulting physician is to the referrer's desires. Specialists, hospitals or outpatient therapy centers that find out what their referring physicians want, and then meet or exceed their expectations, will likely enjoy more referrals. A survey of your referring physicians is a good method to uncover negative aspects of your practice and procedures that might need changing.

Everybody wants respect. Primary care physicians are no exception. There are several ways a specialist can design his practice to show respect to the referring physicians. Eliscu offers the following list:[10]

- In all activities, respect the referring physician's time;

- Make it easy for referring physicians to reach practice physicians—even on evenings and weekends. If not, they'll simply refer to another practice this time —and probably the next;

- Maintain a dedicated telephone "physician hotline" strictly for referrals—and let referring physicians know about it. If the practice receives referrals from a wide geographic area, provide a toll-free number for inquiries about test results and patient updates;

- Schedule referred patients quickly. Prompt availability is an endearing trait to a primary care physician and concerned patients;

- Conduct a patient satisfaction survey and communicate the results to referrers;

- Set aside a few time slots in the schedule every day to accommodate referrers whose patients need an immediate appointment;

- Prepare and distribute appropriate communications materials, such as a physician referral handbook; and

- Communicate effectively with referrers about the practice's services and the benefits of each. Use physician-to-physician newsletters or case studies to let them know about new procedures, new techniques, strengths of existing services, and services systems that have been created to enhance the relationship; and join with hospitals to partner programs that please primary care physicians, such as continuing medical education (CME), mini internships, and easy-to-use directories.

Jane Oliva offers a well-organized review of issues to consider in moving your office toward securing "preferred referral" status.[11] She observes that members who use health savings accounts and are armed with information from the Internet may have higher expectations of specialists. In addition, the societal trend toward consumers demanding better customer service will create opportunities for practices that can deliver timely service that meets or exceeds patients' expectations.

Conveying the necessary information both ways can be an important patient safety issue. For example, patients often forget to mention some of the medicines they are taking, or problems they have had. Some practices have medication lists for their patients to copy and send with referral information to help the specialist choose treatments. If the patient admits to taking medications that don't match the list sent by the referring physician, there is a chance to explore compliance issues and patient education opportunities.

It is important for the consultant to review the information received and, if it is inadequate, to request additional information. Broken systems do not tend to repair themselves—by informing the referring physician that important information is not being sent, you will help him or her to improve and become partners in the care of the patient. Establishing a good working relationship and good lines of communication can lead to increased referrals in both directions, and help to market your practice to other physicians.

For billing purposes, even when a physician asks you to consult on a patient in a face-to-face conversation, there should be a written note or order for the consultation, specifying the service requested. It would be wise to check with the insurer to make sure that any needed authorization requests have been done. After the consultation, a report must be generated.

## Risk Management for the Referring Physician

Suboptimal communication causes both medico-legal issues and increases the risk of being sued if a mishap occurs. The above practices may help improve communication between physicians.

Another potential problem occurs when the practice does not have a system to monitor visits, and whether the results and recommendations of the specialist make it back to the referring physician for review with the patient's chart. There are numerous cases where physicians have gotten into trouble because a staff member filed an abnormal test report in a chart without the physician having the opportunity to see or act on the result. It is not reasonable to expect a physician to remember that he requested a consultation or ordered a test for a patient, and that he has not yet seen a report or result.

There are many options to address this problem. Those with electronic scheduling systems may have automated reminders to make sure the report of the consultation has been seen by the physician. If there is no report, the staff can call to see if the consultation took place. If not, the referring physician or his designated staff may want to call the patient. If the consultation did take place, the staff can inquire about the report. Specialists who are consistently delinquent in generating reports risk losing the business from their referral base.

A low-tech solution might be to use a non-electronic tickler file. Create an expandable file labeled for each day of the month, and file a copy of the referral form under a date after the referral. As above, assign a staff member the responsibility to clear that day's notes and forms. This does not work as well, however, if the referral is for greater than a month away.

The decision not to file the chart until all lab, radiology, and consultant reports have been received and added creates other problems. Patients who have seen the physician recently are much more likely to call the office in the days shortly after the visit than at other times. Charts not filed will cause additional delays for the staff in trying to locate them.

A relatively new concept, *negligent* referral, has become a potential liability issue.[1,12,13] Physicians have a duty to refer to qualified specialists and facilities, but it is not clear how much the physician has to do to verify their competency; many physicians feel this is an MCO's responsibility. One study reported in *The Journal of the American Medical Association* found that 5% of physicians applying for ambulatory staff privileges falsified their credentials.[14] MCOs do investigate the essential indicators of competence of the specialists, such as primary source verification of licensure, training, and board certification. Once approved, it is more difficult for a health plan or insurance company to remove physicians if they begin to accumulate lawsuits or complaints against them. However, if the patient needs a referral to a specialist that is not in the network of the patient's insurance, the referring physician has an obligation to appeal the decision expeditiously, and the MCO has an obligation to provide an appropriate physician.[1] In general, if the referring physician is uncomfortable, it is worth requesting an exception to the restrictions of the plan, and appealing if the exception is denied. Dealing with medical directors and health plan decisions will be covered in more depth below.

Once the referral is made, there still may be an obligation to continue to evaluate the care given by the specialist.[12] When there are multiple consultants, it is important for the primary care physician or substitute (such as a hospitalist), to continue to be involved in the patient's care, since consultants have an obligation to send reports to the referring physician, but not necessarily to each other. Patient safety experts recite many stories of near misses and tragedies resulting from lapses in communication across multiple physicians caring for a single patient.

When a referral is not approved, the referring physician must document any attempts made to appeal the decision and advocate for appropriate treatment for the patient. Formal appeals may have forms that help document the process, but some appeals may be done with only a call to a health plan medical director. If a patient decides not to follow through with a recommended referral, document your recommendation and their refusal.

## Managed Care Referrals

For many office staff members, managed care referrals are the most tedious and dreaded part of their duties. If a request is denied by the insurance company, the staff must report the denial to the physician, and go through the whole process again when referring to another specialist. Then they must work through the patient confusion as they explain that they should not see their primary physician's first choice, but this new provider instead. Bysinger et al. sums up the down side of referrals, "…in the age of managed health care, no single medical/business process has proven more costly, more frustrating, more impersonal or more damaging to the patient-physician relationship."[9] The Medical Group Management Association (MGMA) states that the average practice operates under the auspices of 16 managed care contracts.[15] It is impossible for a physician to remember which physicians and hospitals are in-network under each of the plans. What can be done to make the process more accurate, more efficient, and less painful?

The single most important step in the referral process occurs when the practice decides to accept a managed care product. It is absolutely imperative that someone, who is knowledgeable in managed care, review the contract before the practice signs on. Most contracts specify that the physician follow the plan's guidelines for referring patients, and for other aspects of the plan's utilization management (UM) and quality management (QM) plans. Not all companies will offer a copy of the UM or QM plans, or even an explanation of what compliance looks like in their system. They definitely won't offer (unless asked) the numbers of complaints they receive from plan members or providers, or the percentage of authorization requests that are approved versus rejected for technical difficulties rather than for lack of medical necessity, or because services are not covered as a benefit under the member's policy. Much of this information is public knowledge and may be obtained by the state agency licensing MCOs. There may be considerable variances as to what each plan requires. Some plans rarely require prior authorizations, and only for services that may not be included in the covered benefits; while others require prior authorization for many radiology studies, expensive laboratory tests, certain pharmaceuticals, and all referrals. Some plans don't require prior authorization, but may have a policy to retroactively review an order, and even deny a service previously rendered based on lack of medical necessity. Ask your colleagues how easy the company is to deal with. Ask the company for statistics, like the percentage of requests that are denied. The importance of doing your homework cannot be overstated.

The company writing a contract will have its own best interest in mind. Since the law states that any ambiguity in a contract will be construed against the drafter of the contract, the contracts tend to include a substantial amount of "boilerplate" clauses that state that anything that can go wrong is not the company's responsibility. Some very troublesome clauses may actually be required by law in an HMO contract. For example, a provider cannot bill a patient for services the HMO refuses to pay for, *balance bill*, unless they have the patient sign a form indicating awareness that the service is not an HMO benefit, but that they want the service anyway and will pay for it. This is not boilerplate, but rather a part of the HMO Act.

A professor of a local business school, recounting her experience as a negotiator for physician independent practice associations in the southeastern United States, told of an insurance company that had a standard contract they internally referred to as their "dumb physician" contract. If a physician objected to *any* clause in the contract before signing, the company would apologize and state that the physician had been given the wrong contract, and then give them a much more reasonable contract that did not have the most unfair provisions.

It is important to get expert advice prior to signing a contract, in order to protect your practice and your partners. Many county medical societies and national professional societies have guides to help their members evaluate contracts. For a small fee, some organizations will even provide a consultant to evaluate standard contracts.

## Issuing the Referral

It is important to develop a quick and easy reference to identify the providers who are in-network for each insurance plan you accept. The bare minimum for practices that accept only a few managed care plans is to have the plan directories of in-network providers together and easily accessible, with the preferred specialists highlighted. In most practices, these provider directories will still be needed for the occasional referral to a seldom-used specialty provider. For the most common plans and most common specialists needed, a printed matrix table with specialties on one axis, insurances accepted on the other, and the names of the specialists the practice prefers to use in the boxes is a quick and easy tool to create and use (Table 1, page 268). For computer-enabled practices, the same table can be created in spreadsheet format, which would also allow for the table to be updated easily. Whether you use a table or spreadsheet, you will find over time what elements are needed to make it the most helpful in your particular situation.

## Table 1: Matrix of Specialists

| Insurer | | | | |
|---|---|---|---|---|
| | HMO 1 | HMO 2 | PPO 3 | Medicare |
| Cardiologist | Dr. Jones | Dr. Smith | Dr. Jones | Dr. Jones |
| Pulmonologist | Dr. Able | Dr. Able | Dr. Po[1] | Dr. Able or Po[1] |
| Nephrologist | Dr. Green[2] | Dr. White | Dr. White | Dr. White |
| Orthopedist | Dr. Wilson | Dr. Wilson[3] | Dr. Wilson | Dr. Wilson |

1 Bilingual    2 Open till 9 PM    3 No Preauthorization required

Besides a form for your staff to use to determine whom you prefer to refer to in each plan, consider a referral checklist to use to make sure everything needed for a referral is included when you send information to the specialist. For example, you might request that patients being referred to a cardiologist have any ECGs done in your office sent with the referral, or that children sent to a gastroenterologist have their growth charts included.

In deciding which specialist you want to use, be sure to consider not only the professional competence, but also the customer service aspects of their practice—your patients will! If they are treated rudely, have to wait a long time in the waiting room, or can't understand the physician, it will reflect badly on you, too. Depending on the nature of your practice and the demographics of your community, you may also want to note in your table which offices are bilingual or offer other special services, hours of operation, or locations.

## The Authorization and Appeal Process

An authorization from the MCO usually is necessary for your patient to receive a service from a provider, be it physician, ancillary practitioner, or facility. Each insurer has different policies as to what services require authorization, and how to request the service. Generally elective hospitalizations, surgery, therapies, and high-dollar items require prior authorization or pre-certification. The payor decides what goes on its required list of services based on the potential for abuse, or the possibility of saving money without an assumed decrease in the quality of care provided to its members. This would also include areas where there may be benefit concerns, i.e., requiring authorization for surgery that may be cosmetic such as scar removal, rhinoplasty, or breast reduction. Many payors do not cover bariatric surgery, and even though a request for this surgery will be denied, the insurer requires a formal request be filed and formally denied.  Most insurers do not cover services deemed to be experimental or investigational.  Benefit policies for many insurers are posted on the Internet and may be viewed by the public.

Authorizations may be requested by fax, mail, online, or by telephone with an "intake" nurse.  Online requests are increasing, and may be completed on secure sites via the Internet, email, and telephone data lines.  When the request is in writing, the MCO may want you to use a specific form that contains patient demographic information and clinical history.  In some areas of the country, as in Houston, Texas, the Medicaid health plans agreed on a standard form produced by the county medical society.  Depending on the payor, requests may be made by any provider or only the patient's primary care physician.  State law and MCO accreditation standards govern the turnaround time for approval or denial of a request for services.  A denial for medical necessity may only be issued by a physician.  A dentist may deny dental services, just as a psychiatrist or PhD-preprared psychologist may deny mental health services.

If a request is denied for lack of medical necessity, the MCO will provide the method to appeal in its notice of denial.  If the denial was because the service requested was not a benefit, one may only register a complaint.  An appeal may be made by the member/patient, a person acting on behalf of the member, or the provider of the service.  The appeal should contain new information that will show why the denial should be overturned.  There may be a deadline for submitting an appeal.  Law, accreditation standards, and company policy govern the turnaround time.  If a denial is for a current inpatient, or a service deemed urgent, an expedited appeal may be submitted for a quick turnaround.  Initially, the appeal is reviewed by the physician who made the original denial, in a process called "reconsideration."  If there is new information, this physician may overturn the denial and approve the service.  If the denial is upheld, another physician must review the appeal.  This "first level" appeal can generally be performed by a physician of any specialty.  The National Committee for Quality Assurance (NCQA) standards require that all appeal reviewers used as consultants by the health plan be board certified.[16]  If the second physician upholds the denial and the health plan policies allow for a "second level" appeal, the MCO will notify the appealing physician of how to request a second appeal.  Sometimes this may only be requested by the patient or the provider of the service.  This second appeal usually will be performed by a board certified physician from a specialty similar to that of the requesting practitioner.  A same-specialty reviewer may be requested at any time in the appeals process.

If the second level appeal is upheld, there are different options for the patient and practitioner depending on state law and health plan policy. An appeals board, composed of a fourth physician, health plan member or patient advocate, and a health plan employee, who was not involved in any decision making for this member, may be convened to review the case. An alternative that has become very common is the external review by an independent review organization (IRO). As of 2004, 44 states required this type of review for medical necessity denials.[17] These IROs have become the ultimate authority for MCOs, and their decision is final. Generally the cost is borne by the health plan. The reviews are performed by board certified physicians in a specialty similar to that of the original requesting practitioner. In Texas, the state with the longest use of IROs, the overturn rate for the first six years was approximately 51% totally overturned and 8% partially overturned.[18]

## Referrals as Opportunities

Most futurists state that the health care industry will become more consumer-driven in the 21ˢᵗ century. In some respects, health care providers are regarded as a commodity rather than as a medical home, where the patient has a long-term continuing relationship with their personal physician. This has occurred partly because of aspects of our society entirely external to medicine, and partly due to external forces relating to health care issues, such as shorter average employment with one company, and the change of employer-sponsored insurance with each move. But many of the changes are a result of how we practice medicine. When solo practice was the norm, patients chose their physician, and all of their interactions were with that one trusted provider. With the rise of group practice, larger on-call groups, nurse call lines, and managed care, chances are that patients choose a physician because he or she participates in their insurance plan. If patients call after hours it likely will not be their physician they speak with, and they may not see the same provider if they have to be seen in the office for an urgent problem.

All physicians' offices have diplomas and licenses hanging on the walls, and most have automated telephone answering systems instructing patients to "listen carefully as our options have changed." In the modern marketplace, it is more important than ever that you stand out from the crowd in good ways. Michael Porter, of Harvard Business School, speaks of the importance of having a "sustainable competitive advantage." The organization and customer service you provide around the referral process may make you, and all those associated with you, shine, or they may cast doubt on your level of caring and competency. Certainly a system that is as "broken" as our current health care system is provides lots of opportunity for an efficient office to distinguish itself. Start by asking yourself, from the patient's perspective, what you want when you need a referral. Does the patient really want to know what you think of MCOs in general, and their insurer in particular, when the physician you prefer to recommend is not in-network? Do they want to deal with bills from an out-of-network provider, because you didn't send them to one that was in-network? Do they really believe that none of the 25 specialists listed in their insurance member guidebook are competent? What they want is to be treated courteously, referred to good physicians who treat them well, and not to have to deal with any hassle. While the *Wall Street Journal* found in an online interactive poll that half of Americans would consider going to a physician not covered by their insurance if they were "highly recommended by a source that you trust," only 1 in 6 have actually done so.[19] Most likely, many of those respondents could have found equally good expertise and service within the plan's network. Your question then is "How can I provide my patients what they want?"

Several groups with an eye to customer service have asked just that question, and have come up with a variety of answers. A group in the Pacific Northwest advertises an "Automatically Authorized Referral Process" for referrals for most services, including admissions and diagnostic testing, that occur within their integrated system. A consulting company states in one of its monographs on managed care that the member (patient) should not have to be responsible for making the system work, nor should they have to (needlessly) pay for anything "ordered by someone in authority."[20] A variety of consumer advocacy groups have posted downloadable guides for navigating the process, raising the expectation that physicians will do what the advocacy groups expect them to do. Many states, and some large health purchasing cooperatives such as the Pacific Business Group on Health, list how well health plans and medical groups do in a variety of areas, including quality of care and communication. While they have not yet posted the ratings for individual physicians, that may be only a matter of time. NCQA, an organization that measures and rates health plan quality, has posted online a number of case studies of plans that had excessive complaints about their referral process, and the steps they took to fix the process. If a plan for which you are a provider has a similar problem, you could discuss these steps with the plan's director of quality improvement, and suggest the MCO undertake a similar project.

However you address the process, it will be helpful if you can measure satisfaction with your processes and systems before you start and track improvement over time. Not only will this help to determine which interventions have the biggest "bang for the buck," but may help improve customer service through the "Hawthorne Effect."[21] Elton Mayo found that employees' performance changed when they knew that management was watching. If your staff knows that you care how patients are treated during their referral transaction, your staff members may change their behavior, consciously or subconsciously. Make sure you ask the people actually doing the job for help in designing the solution. It will increase buy-in to the improvement process and may lead to a superior solution. Spend more time and effort thinking about what you want to measure and what you want to ask your patients, as surveys can be time-consuming and a bit expensive. You will want to make sure you are getting as much value from the surveys as you can. Whether you end up with a private intranet system with a large number of physicians, hospitals, and insurers in your area, or a one-office improvement in your system, monitor the solution to be sure it continues to meet the needs of your patients. Beware of unintended consequences of your changes, and make sure your new system fix doesn't break something else. Once you have begun to approach quality improvement and customer service in a systematic way, you will find that subsequent projects are easier to sell to the staff and physicians.

Health plans are rated on a number of things, but the majority of items on the report cards actually deal with member satisfaction with their physicians, and the services the physicians provide. If your practice is able to ease your patients through the managed care system with few problems, and this assistance results in high patient satisfaction, the MCOs will like you. It may be possible to use good patient satisfaction scores as a bargaining tool when contracting with MCOs. Since you have proven you routinely do things the right way, the company may allow your office to bypass certain prior authorization requirements, perhaps substituting "notification only" for prior authorization. Assuming you want more of their members as patients, they may steer more patients your way. If they are considering instituting pay for performance policies, they may consider rewarding you for an excellent job in the area of patient satisfaction.

## Conclusion

The current systems of practice and payment have created a complex practice environment. Understanding the referral process and implementing appropriate processes will ensure that patients can safely and smoothly pass through the system, receive the care they need, reduce errors and administrative hassle and expense, and improve patient satisfaction. The transition to EMRs and integrated front and back office systems will provide opportunities to more easily create systems that automate and ease the referral process. Having excellent systems may serve as a potential marketing tool for your practice.

## Case Study

Kimberly is a 17-year-old female with a history of congenital nevus syndrome. When she was 18 months of age, she was diagnosed with cat scratch disease by tissue biopsy. At the site where this biopsy was taken she subsequently developed an ugly scar and she requests scar revision and treatment of her congenital nevus. Her PCP refers her to an in-network dermatologist who recommends removal of the congenital nevus and scar revision for cosmetic improvement. The authorization for the congenital nevus was approved; however, scar revision was denied for lack of medical necessity as it was considered cosmetic. The family sought a second opinion from another dermatologist who was not a participating provider in her health plan (out-of-network provider) who recommended removal of both lesions. In his appeal, he provided additional information that the scar removal was not just for cosmetic purposes but was causing her pain and it was being abraded by the constant rubbing from her clothes. Choice Care, her insurance carrier, received the appeal and overturned the denial paying not only for the removal of her nevus, but also the scar revision as it was symptomatic.

## Study/Discussion Questions

1. What does this case teach us?

- *Typically cosmetic procedures are not covered expenses payable by the insurance plan.*
- *The patient has the right to go elsewhere if they choose to pay for it.*
- *The patient has the right to appeal denied medical services (it is important to remember that only a physician can deny medical services, although other specified health care providers can authorize hospitalizations, medical visits and procedures). They also have the right to a timely process in this appeal.*

2. Did this patient have to pay the bill for her 2nd opinion dermatology visit?

*Yes, because the dermatologist was not a network provider in this HMO. Even though a patient can go elsewhere if they don't like the answers they get from their HMO, they will be required to pay for the services rendered even if their denial is overturned. However, the patient can return to the in-network dermatologist for further care.*

3. How does a physician advocate for the patient when services have been denied if he/she truly believes services are medically necessary?

*Remember, the PCP and specialist physician are the patient's advocate. However, at any time if a patient feels they have been wrongly denied needed services they may appeal their case directly and have the right to be heard in a timely manner. When services have been denied most managed care organizations will send a letter to the patient and/or physician explaining why the services have been denied and numbers to call or an address to send a letter if the physician or member feels the decision was in error. The appeal process is a multi-tiered procedure in which only a licensed physician may*

*deny services. Physicians have a duty to exhaust all appeal steps and to request exter-
nal review if necessary. This review of disputed decisions must be performed by physicians who are not plan employees. It is best to review the denial letter and provide
medical evidence as to why the appeal should be overturned. Clear, concise communication is often all that is needed between the medical director of the managed health care
plan and the physician to resolve the majority of these issues. Initial appeals are handled
within the organization, but the final appeal is always completed outside the managed
care organization.*

## Suggested Readings/Websites

### Readings

Currey, Wesley and Linney, Barbara. *Essentials of Medical Management.* ACPE: Tampa, FL;
2003.

Kaufman, Ronald P. *The Business Side of Medicine: A Survival Primer for Medical Students and
Residents.* ACPE: Tampa, FL; 1999.

Nelson, Richard, ed. *A Pediatrician's Guide to Managed Care.* 2nd Ed. AAP: Elk Grove
Village, IL; 2001.

American Medical Association. *Managing Managed Care, 2nd Ed.* American Medical
Association: Chicago, IL.

Peter R. Kongstvedt. *Essentials of Managed Health Care, 5th ed.* Sudbury, MA: Jones &
Bartlett Publishers, Inc. 2007.

### Websites

American College of Physician Executives:  www.acpe.org

National Association of Managed Care Physicians:  www.namcp.org

American Academy of Family Physicians:  www.aafp.org

American Academy of Pediatrics:  www.aap.org

Aetna Medical Policy:  www.aetna.com/cpb/cpb_alpha.html

Blue Cross Blue Shield Technology Center: www.bcbs.com/tec/

National Guidelines Center – AHRQ: www.guidelines.gov/

Humana Coverage Issues:  http://apps.humana.com/TAD/TAD_New/home.asp

Unicare Medical Policy:  http://medpolicy.unicare.com/index.asp

## References

1.  Estate of Tranor v. The Bloomsburg Hospital, No. CV-96-0327 (M.D. Pa. Mar. 15, 1999)

2.  Internal Medicine Center to Advance Research and Education (IMCARE). *Anatomy of Patient Satisfaction: A Primer.* Washington, DC: American Society of Internal Medicine; 1997, 6.

3.  Sutcliffe KM, Lewton E, Rosenthal MM. Communication failures: an insidious contributor to medical mishaps. *Acad Med.* 2004;79:186-194.

4.  Wennberg JE, Freeman JL, Shelton RM, Bubloz TA. Hospital use and mortality among Medicare beneficiaries in Boston and New Haven. *New Engl J Med.* 1989;321:1168-1173.

5.  Milliman Care Guidelines. Available at: http://www.careguidelines.com/. Accessed October 2, 2006.

6.  Interqual. Available at: http://www.interqual.com/IQSite/. Accessed October 2, 2006.

7.  Pati S, Shea S, Rabinowitz D, Carrasquillo O. Does gatekeeping control costs for privately insured children? Findings from the 1996 medical expenditure panel survey. *Pediatrics.* 2003;111:456-460.

8.  Health Maintenance Organization Act of 1973. Title 42 – Public Health, Chapter 6A, Subchapter XI – Health Maintenance Organizations. Available at: http://www.harp.org/hmoa1973.htm. Accessed October 2, 2006.

9.  Bysinger W, Carli T, O'Connor J. Painless referrals. *Med Group Manage J.* 2000;47:32-34,36,38-39.

10. Eliscu AT. Physician referrals important in new environment. *MGM Update.* 1995;34:11.

11. Oliva J .Standing out in the crowd: Securing preferred referral status. *Physician Exec.* 2005;31:54-57.

12. The Physician and Sportsmedicine. 2000;28.

13. California Medical Association, "Liability Considerations with the Use of Hospitalists." 1998. Quoted in Norcal Risk Management, Hospital Rx, The Hospitalist Model: Consider the Benefits, Recognize the Risks.

14. Schaffer WA, Rollo FD, Holt CA. Falsification of clinical credentials by physicians applying for ambulatory staff privileges. *New Engl J Med.* 1988;318:356-358.

15. Spicer J. Making patient care easier under multiple managed care plans. *Fam Pract Manag.* 1998;5:38-42,45.

16. NCQA. UM 4. Timeliness of UM Decisions. Available at : http://www.ncqa.org/publications/umcertpubs.htm Accessed August 16, 2006.

17. Kaiser Family Foundation. Available at:
   http://statehealthfacts.org/cgi-bin/healthfacts.cgi?action=compare&category=Managed+Care+%26+Health+Insurance&subcategory=Patients%27+Rights+Requirements&topic=External+Review. Accessed July 26, 2006.

18. Borges W. After further review: Texas IRO system can reverse bad calls by insurance companies. *Tex Med*. 2003;99:28-33.

19. The Wall Street Journal Online, Aug 30, 2005.

20. Morales E. *Referral Management and Authorization*. From the Medical Management "Signature Series" Burr Ridge, IL: Managed Care Resources, Inc.; 1998.

21. The Hawthorne Effect. Available at:
   http://www.skagit.com/~donclark/hrd/history/hawthorne.html. Accessed October 2, 2006.

# Chapter 17

## Practice Innovation

Michael S. Barr, MD, MBA, FACP

**Executive Summary**

The practice of medicine in the 21$^{st}$ century is challenging for many reasons. Physicians are being pressured to enhance the quality of care, reduce costs, and manage a plethora of administrative processes that often add little value to the delivery of excellent health care. While policy debates and reform efforts are ongoing, practices must address the day-to-day complexities of practicing medicine. Few physicians have sufficient time to generate and implement creative solutions for those processes within their control.

This chapter provides basic guidance on practice innovation, including three principles to help assure efforts will meet the needs of the practice. The use of Michael Porter's Value Chain as well as suggestions to help identify, prioritize, filter, and analyze potential innovations are illustrated using one common practice issue.

**Learning Objectives**

1. Define innovation and how it applies to practicing health care in the 21$^{st}$ century.

2. Understand the importance of using innovative approaches to redesigning the practice of medicine.

3. Identify existing models of innovation and understand how they apply to health care.

4. Apply and implement models of change and innovation without negatively impacting performance.

**Keywords**

innovation; primary activities; supporting activities; value chain; value equation

## Introduction

### What is Innovation?

Innovation has many components. Innovation requires creativity and the ability to see things differently. It's identifying opportunities to enhance the delivery or characteristics of a service, refine the manufacturing of a product, or create a novel way to satisfy an unmet need—or to satisfy that need in a better manner. Innovation is about translating and applying ideas from one industry to another. Innovation is not always "thinking outside the box"—sometimes, it's working within the box with just a few incremental changes.

### Why Innovate?

"Innovate or die" is a common mantra in business circles. This is an extreme statement that is more about revolutionary change as opposed to the evolutionary and incremental change advanced in this chapter. However, the motivation to change implied by this catchphrase also has merit in health care; without innovation at all levels of the health care system, we are destined to achieve the same mediocre health outcomes nationally, and perpetuate the frustrations that many patients and physicians currently experience.

### What Innovation is Not

Innovation is not necessarily expensive, dramatic, or hard. Seemingly small changes can result in significant improvements. Think of the cardboard sleeve that insulates and protects your hand when picking up your favorite double mocha cappuccino. How about the little arrow on your dashboard that reminds you which side of the car the fuel cap is on (particularly important when refueling a rental car)? And think of the rumble strip, now commonplace on most highways, helping to wake up sleepy drivers as they begin to drift off the road — hopefully scaring them enough to pull over and get some rest. None of these innovative solutions were technically challenging, particularly expensive, or hard to accomplish. Are there parallel solutions in the practice of medicine?

Innovation is not synonymous with technology, though we are used to seeing technological innovation. Think back to your last visit to your favorite electronics outlet, and try to recall the endless variety of MP3 players, DVD players and recorders, and digital cameras. It wasn't very long ago that portable CD players, VHS camcorders, and disposable cameras were the latest and greatest innovations. What about innovations in the service industries? Years ago it was shopping carts for groceries (1937), McDonald's and fast food (1955), drive-up windows, and no-frills flying on People Express Airlines (1981). Service innovation now is often technologically-based (e.g., online banking, virtual meetings, web-based commerce). But improvements in "low-tech" customer service are still highly valued. Think of Nordstrom's, luxury car showrooms, and high-priced restaurants.

### What Does Innovation Look Like in Health Care?

During a casual stroll through just about any moderately-sized hospital, one can find many examples of applied technology, redesigned patient care areas, and improved workflow processes. Examples include bar-coded patient identification bracelets, automated prescription delivery systems, and sophisticated remote monitoring of patients. A walk through most physician offices may feel like you are still in the 1950s. Patients wait in chair-filled rooms and complete poor-quality copies of forms that haven't been updated in years. Doctors write in paper charts that are stored on packed shelves—when not stacked on desks along with messages, labs, consult reports, and insurance forms awaiting completion or signature. Wall racks teem with outdated magazines and marginally effective educational material. Experienced staff members train new personnel on workflows that require workarounds just to get through the day.

Of course, these are stereotypical descriptions; there are paper-based and technology-enabled practices that function extremely well. However, many practices have precious little time for what most entrepreneurs in other businesses think about – how to grow, prosper, and improve the customer experience and quality of service. Most offices are challenged with the day-to-day economic imperative of survival, especially the small practices where the majority of Americans receive their health care (see Table 1, below).[1]

## Table 1: Ambulatory Visits Distributed by Size of Practice

| Practice Size | Number of Ambulatory Visits (in thousands)* | National Percent Distribution of Ambulatory Visits According to Size of Physician Office |
|:---:|:---:|:---:|
| Solo | 320,042 | 35.1% |
| 2-4 | 286,980 | 31.5% |
| 5-9 | 194,200 | 21.3% |
| >10 | 109,635 | 12.0% |

Source: *Advance Data from Vital & Health Statistics, Number 374, June 23, 2006

## Innovation in Practice is Essential

Paradoxically, the burdens of practice that limit physicians' ability to devote time for innovation are precisely why innovation is essential. Without change, innovation, and initiative, the costs of health care will continue to escalate; regional variations in cost and quality will persist; safety and security will continue to be major issues for patients; and health outcomes across the United States will continue to be less than satisfactory. Without physician leadership, payor and employer-driven reimbursement models will escalate the pressure to reduce costs and may negatively impact quality and access to health care—particularly primary care—across the United States. Further, many more payors will categorize physicians based on performance assessments, create tiered networks, and tie an increasing amount of payment to process, outcome, and efficiency metrics.

Perhaps it seems naïve to propose that improvements in office-based practices, using standard quality improvement principles to innovate and change, will mitigate some of these macroeconomic pressures. However, we do know that "systems are perfectly designed to achieve the results they get" (Don Berwick), whether at the micro-level (practice) or macro-level (regional and national health care outcomes). The challenge is for physicians to acknowledge and accept responsibility for elements of change within their control, while advocating for the policy and macro-system changes needed to support innovation on a broader, national scale.

## A Framework for Innovation in Practice

"Overwhelmed" was the word used by one physician after an assessment of his practice during an American College of Physicians (ACP) Center for Practice Innovation[2] site visit. It was not our intent to provoke that reaction—but it was understandable. Even a casual, but objective, observational study of most practices will typically reveal significant issues, such as a high volume of phone calls; stacks of messages; difficulty tracking laboratory tests and referrals to consultants; safety and privacy breaches; and gaps in clinical documentation that could leave patients vulnerable to medical errors and physicians liable for malpractice claims. Office staff and physicians typically (and temporarily) overcome the complexities inherent in their office workflow—but at considerable expense with respect to time, frustration, and the opportunity cost of using this energy for potentially more productive purposes. From a patient perspective, these issues are often not readily apparent until a critical need occurs and the system, or lack thereof, reveals its flaws.

Ask any physician or office manager what processes need improvement and most will respond quickly with a list of concerns that they would like to address. However, many will not have a defined process for evaluating or resolving these challenges.

The ancient Chinese war strategist Sun Tzu stated, "Strategy without tactics is the slowest route to victory. Tactics without strategy is the noise before defeat."[3] Identifying objectives, in the absence of a process for prioritization and categorization, is like preparing for war without tactics or strategy. Looking at a report, such as the one prepared for the physician mentioned above, without a roadmap can be frustrating and can de-motivate even the most enthusiastic practice. A framework to deconstruct the complex processes would be highly desirable. Fortunately, Michael Porter's "value chain" provides an excellent model that can be adapted for our purposes. The value chain, described in his 1985 book, *Competitive Advantage*,[4] was originally developed to help corporations identify discrete activities in designing, producing, marketing, delivering, and supporting their products. The model is easily adaptable to health systems seeking insight related to improving operations for the benefit of clinical care—the so-called "microsystem"—a functioning small unit of care delivery.

The value chain includes five primary activities and four supporting activities. The primary activities are inbound logistics, operations, outbound logistics, marketing and sales, and service. The value chain focuses on the complexities of product or service development, with the goal of generating improved margins on that product or service. Typically, margins reflect financial goals, but a "margin" can also be achieved in efficiency, safety, quality, and satisfaction. The key to successful use of this model is to make the processes within each category as efficient as possible while addressing the relationship between them. Table 2, page 282 identifies each category, some relevant practice processes for each value chain activity, and examples of approaches to addressing some of these processes.

Porter also described four support activities: firm infrastructure, human resource management, technology development and procurement. Examples of activities in these categories are noted in the Table 3, page 283. Examples later in this chapter will illustrate the use of the value chain in health care innovation.

## Key Principles for Innovation

There are three important principles for strategic innovation. The first is to recognize the tendency to go for a quick fix and to avoid this energy-wasting diversion. It is tempting to go after the most irritating and obvious problems first. Typically, the result of such shortsighted efforts is a layering of new processes on top of dysfunctional, old ones without getting at the true source of the problems. It's like pulling out a weed by its leaves rather than digging up the roots. True innovation requires a deep dive, not a swim on the surface.

## Table 2. The Value Chain and Examples of Practice Activities and Innovation

| The Value Chain – Primary Activities | Practice Activity | Practice Innovation |
|---|---|---|
| **Inbound Logistics** | Front desk; telephone intake; scheduling; template-building; reception area work-flow; patient pre-visit education; transportation support; insurance verification; retrieval of prior medical records; patient pre-visit data collection | • Pre-visit completion of patient information database<br>• Pre-visit assessment of clinical concerns, educational needs and potential coordination of care needs<br>• Open access scheduling<br>• Computer-based patient requests<br>• Advanced template development<br>• Group visits<br>• Practice management system upgrade<br>• Scheduled telephone visits |
| **Operations** | Visit process (flow); clinical visit; standardization of clinical processes; allocation of care responsibilities across the health care provider team; generation of office note; use of clinical decision support tools; medical record-retrieval and keeping; in-office clinical procedures; exam room management; patient & family education after assessment of learning preferences; laboratory/test ordering; referral generation; prescription management; disease management/population management; biohazard waste management | • Chronic care model implementation<br>• Appropriate educational materials based on literacy level and needs of population<br>• Group visits<br>• Office-based testing and procedures<br>• Clinical decision support<br>• EHR or registry utilization<br>• Safe-needle technology selection<br>• Electronic prescribing |
| **Outbound Logistics** | Check-out; follow-up activities; patient/family post-visit education; referrals; lab & test result notification; reminder/recall systems; billing/coding; coordination and communication with other post-visit care providers (e.g., Physical Therapy, Rehabilitation Services) | • Computerized referral tracking<br>• Tickler files (paper and computer based)<br>• Coding systems<br>• Referral and test-tracking processes<br>• Patient-initiated phone retrieval of lab and test data |

## Table 2. The Value Chain and Examples of Practice Activities and Innovation (continued)

| The Value Chain – Primary Activities | Practice Activity | Practice Innovation |
|---|---|---|
| **Marketing & Sales** | Promotional activities; community involvement; speaking engagements; unique service offerings | • Prepared condition-specific presentations<br>• Technology-enhanced patient education<br>• Office newsletter highlighting quality innovations<br>• Multi-functional website with patient-oriented content and scheduling/communication features<br>• Automated telephone or secure email reminders |
| **Service** | Enabling services (e.g., social services, translation services, health benefits advice, nurse triage and telephone advice); outreach | • Personal health record<br>• On-line communication<br>• Enhanced in-office laboratory procedures<br>• Email consultation |

## Table 3. Supporting Activities of the Value Chain

| The Value Chain – Support Activities | Practice Activity | Practice Innovation |
|---|---|---|
| **Firm Infrastructure** | Leadership functions; strategic/business planning; quality management; accounting; housekeeping | • Leadership development<br>• Business planning |
| **Human Resources** | Recruitment; training; development; team organization | • On-line training for OSHA requirements<br>• Self-paced learning modules<br>• On-line CME/CEU for clinician/nurse education |
| **Technology Development** | Selection, implementation and improving the use of technology (e.g., electronic health records, registries); implementation of safety reporting and tracking; point-of-care educational resources | • Electronic health record implementation<br>• Registry software<br>• E-prescribing<br>• Secure email communication |
| **Procurement** | Purchase of supplies, medications, educational material | • E-ordering<br>• Group purchasing<br>• Just-in-time supply re-stocking |

The second principle is the alignment of objectives with business priorities. Taking care of a nuisance and crafting a way to eliminate that nuisance can be satisfying. But innovative solutions that also produce reductions in costs or enhanced revenues (or both) can truly be rewarding.

Innovation should also create value – the third principle. Innovation can provide a competitive advantage through value generation. What is value? In this context, it can be described by the value proposition equation noted in Figure 1, below.[5] Value is a function of service attributes, image, and relationships. Do not underestimate the intangible value of improved patient, staff, and clinician satisfaction, or the potential for these intangibles to provide a financial return on investment once others recognize this value.

### Figure 1: Value Equation

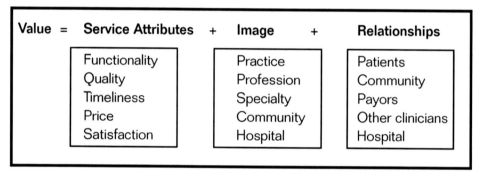

| Value = | Service Attributes | + | Image | + | Relationships |
|---|---|---|---|---|---|
| | Functionality | | Practice | | Patients |
| | Quality | | Profession | | Community |
| | Timeliness | | Specialty | | Payors |
| | Price | | Community | | Other clinicians |
| | Satisfaction | | Hospital | | Hospital |

By assuring that activities for innovation follow the principles above, physicians can be relatively confident that the time and effort expended on these types of projects will provide a return on the investment and be aligned with practice needs.

### Initial Steps: Identifying Areas in Need of Innovative Ideas

It may seem simple, but the first step in undertaking practice innovation involves identifying those potential areas that meet the criteria and principles stated above. This exercise is best accomplished as a team that includes everyone in the practice. Involvement of all staff, especially in small practices, will help avoid creating innovation "killers." In their book, *Sacred Cows Make the Best Burgers*,[6] Robert Kriegel and David Brandt encourage businesses to "...round up sacred cows – outdated beliefs and practices" because they prevent the type of change that is essential to success. They also point out that, "...people are the gatekeepers of change" and, therefore, all stakeholders should be involved whenever possible.

It is at this point that the team should list all the potential issues limiting the practice from operating effectively. The use of structured survey instruments to generate an overall impression or collect ideas can be very useful. Below are two tables from surveys used by the ACP's Center for Practice Innovation (see Table 4, below, and Table 5, page 286). These tables illustrate the collection of clinician and staff concerns about practice processes.

**Table 4: Reported Issues in Practice from American College of Physicians Center for Practice Innovation On-Line Survey of 117 Respondents**

| Issues that Cause Problems in the Office | |
|---|---|
| Have the medical record available at time of visit | 20.5% |
| Unable to stay on office schedule | 40.2% |
| Poor legibility of records | 19.7% |
| Patients unable to access physician when they want/need | 19.7% |
| Patient waits | 34.2% |
| Inefficient use of resources | 41.0% |
| Chart chasing | 35.9% |
| Phone & fax processing | 59.0% |
| Results (e.g., labs, referrals) tracking and follow up | 55.6% |
| Patient satisfaction | 13.7% |
| Medication refills | 42.7% |
| Timely referrals | 18.8% |

Recognize that the perception of operational characteristics of a practice may differ among the personnel even in a small practice. In the table above, 30% of physicians surveyed reported that pre-authorization for a service was a real problem; the corresponding percentage for office administrators and administrative assistants was just 15%. Only 7% of office administrators and their assistants rated phone advice as a real problem, but 20% of the physicians considered it a significant issue. Therefore, it is important to consider the variety of perspectives and priorities among the members of the practice when evaluating potential areas for intervention.

**Table 5:  Representative Survey from American College of Physicians Center for Practice Innovation On-Line Survey. Data represent the responses from 47 physician respondents.  There were a total of 169 respondents including all office staff.**

| | Works Well | Small Problem | Real Problem | Totally Broken | Source of Complaints |
|---|---|---|---|---|---|
| Answering Phones | 41% | 41% | 9% | 0% | 15% |
| Appointment System | 41% | 30% | 13% | 0% | 11% |
| Messaging | 43% | 36% | 9% | 2% | 6% |
| Scheduling Procedures | 37% | 17% | 13% | 0% | 2% |
| Ordering Diagnostic Tests | 36% | 45% | 2% | 0% | 0% |
| Reporting Diagnostic Test Results | 19% | 43% | 23% | 0% | 6% |
| Prescription Renewals | 33% | 42% | 13% | 0% | 4% |
| Making Referrals | 39% | 30% | 24% | 0% | 2% |
| Pre-Authorization for Services | 19% | 28% | 30% | 4% | 0% |
| Billing/Coding | 30% | 43% | 19% | 2% | 4% |
| Phone Advice | 39% | 26% | 20% | 2% | 4% |
| Orientation of Patients to the Practice | 44% | 31% | 4% | 7% | 0% |
| New Patient Work-Ups | 74% | 19% | 0% | 0% | 0% |
| Minor Procedures | 36% | 28% | 0% | 0% | 0% |
| Education for Patients/Families | 49% | 26% | 9% | 4% | 0% |
| Prevention Assessment/Activities | 30% | 38% | 9% | 2% | 0% |
| Chronic Disease Management | 53% | 32% | 4% | 0% | 0% |
| Coordination of Patient Care | 38% | 40% | 15% | 0% | 2% |

## Filtering the Targets of Opportunity

Once a list of potential issues has been identified, the next step is to categorize or group them based on their relationships to common processes. For example, using the value chain framework, issues such as answering phones, appointment-making, messaging, prescription renewals, and phone advice relate to inbound logistics. These processes all depend on communication with the patient, typically by telephone. Chart-chasing, having the medical record available at the time of the visit, legibility of records, and results tracking would be included under the operations component of the value chain.

As ideas are aggregated, additional concerns will be identified; the team should keep track of those. Once the list is generated, it should be matched to the three principles cited above: 1) Avoid quick fixes; 2) Identify issues that align with business priorities; and 3) Select opportunities to create value. An additional consideration at this stage, especially for an initial foray into this type of activity, is to select something that is likely to be achieved within a reasonable period of time, and without a risky financial investment. For example, do not resolve to implement an electronic health record as the one magic solution to the concerns generated by this exercise.

## An Illustrative Example: External Communication

Consider inbound logistics—more specifically, communication with patients and the outside world (physicians, hospitals, pharmacies, etc). External communication is absolutely essential to every practice; and in today's environment, the vast majority is conducted by telephone. This interaction with the external world is the source of others' first impressions of the organization and its operations, and a key element of ongoing patient-physician relationships. Given the importance of managing this element of inbound logistics, why do some practices manage their inbound processes like a gas station with one pump, or a computer help desk that also provides advice on toasters and bicycles?

Does external communication by telephone satisfy the three principles? For most practices, improving these processes does not lend itself to a "quick fix." Therefore, the objective meets the first principle for selecting opportunities for innovation.

In a volume-driven, fee-for-service environment, appointments equate to cash flow. When managed care and capitation prevail, access to care through non-face-to-face care enables practice panels to grow through management of patients at the appropriate level of care. Panel size, therefore, represents cash flow. Responsiveness to other clinicians signals competence, caring, and respect. For a consultant practice, this can easily translate into more referrals. Innovating to solve external communication, therefore, also satisfies the second principle. Addressing this issue aligns with business priorities.

The third principle is also clearly met in that there are considerable opportunities to enhance the perceived value of your practice through improved service attributes, image, and relationships (see Figure 1, page 284).

Once the potential opportunity is identified, filtered, prioritized, and matched against the three principles, the team needs to define the project's parameters. It is important to focus on objectives that are within the influence of the team members, measurable, and have a reasonable expectation of being achieved within an acceptable period of time.  In this example, let's assume that the main source of frustration is patient and physician complaints about getting through to a live person on the telephone.  Most issues relate to long on-hold times, dropped calls, and response time to requests.  The objectives for this project then are to identify the key reasons for long on-hold times, dropped calls, and delayed responsiveness.  The goal is to develop an action plan, test the chosen intervention(s), evaluate the effort and then decide how or if to proceed with further changes.

## Mapping Processes

To improve a process, one must first understand it as it exists.  For this step in the innovation process, flowcharting is essential.  Figure 2, page 289, is an example of a high-level flowchart used to map out the pathway for a patient calling for an appointment.

Once such a map or flowchart is drawn, other techniques need to be used to identify key issues impacting the performance of the processes.  In this example, it is imperative that the team catalog all the functions performed by personnel answering the phones as well as the distractions that keep them from performing their work efficiently.  Table 6, below, was adapted from Outpatient Primary Care Green Book from Dartmouth College.[7]

## Table 6: Tracking Types of Phone Calls by Date/Time

|  | Monday AM  PM | Tuesday AM  PM | Wednesday AM  PM | Thursday AM  PM | Friday AM  PM | Totals for Week |
|---|---|---|---|---|---|---|
| Appt Today |  |  |  |  |  |  |
| Appt Tomorrow |  |  |  |  |  |  |
| Appt Future |  |  |  |  |  |  |
| Test Results |  |  |  |  |  |  |
| Prescription Refill |  |  |  |  |  |  |
| Referral Request |  |  |  |  |  |  |
| Message for Provider |  |  |  |  |  |  |
| Clinical Concern/ Triage |  |  |  |  |  |  |
| Family Member of Patient |  |  |  |  |  |  |
| Hospital |  |  |  |  |  |  |
| Consultant or Referral |  |  |  |  |  |  |
| Totals by Day |  |  |  |  |  |  |

## Figure 2: An example of inbound logistics of a patient calling for an appointment

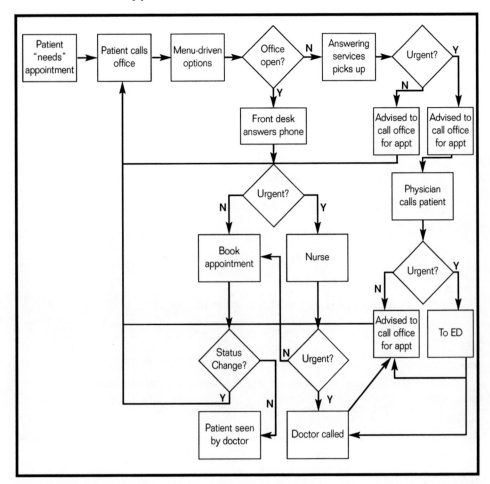

## Identifying Key Concerns with External Communication

Data should be used whenever possible to inform the team. For this example, it would be helpful to have data regarding the volume of phone calls by time of day, dropped calls, average duration of phone calls, and callers' average time on hold. Some telephone service providers can generate these reports upon request (and payment). When combined with staffing levels, telephone utilization data can be used in queuing calculations to model the effect of different staffing complements and numbers of phone lines. One practice used queuing theory[8] to adjust the number of receptionists in a busy practice when it became apparent from the queuing calculations that 85% of patients would wait an average of almost 30 minutes to be registered when only two receptionists staffed the welcome desk—a fact that was confirmed by observational study. The calculation is presented below in Figure 3.

### Figure 3: An Example of Queuing Theory to Calculate Reception Area Waiting Times

## Front Desk Waiting Times

- 7 Clinicians
- Average of 2.25 visits/hour per Clinician
  - — Approximately 16 patients/hour
- 2 Receptionists
- Service Rate = 9 per hour (6.67 minutes each)
- Results of calculations:
  - — Average number in line = **7.67 people**
  - — Average number in line + being served = **9.5**
  - — Average time waiting in line = **29 minutes**
  - — Average time waiting + being served = **36 minutes**
  - — Probability of waiting = **85%**

## Use of QI Tools

It is beyond the scope of this chapter to review quality improvement tools in detail (see Chapter 1). However, useful tools for gaining an understanding of process variation and impediments to successful execution of innovative solutions include the cause and effect diagram (also known as a fishbone diagram or Ishikawa diagram), run charts (for example, to graph the data collected in Table 6, page 288) and Pareto charts to help identify the major drivers of variation in performance.[9,10]

The following charts and tables represent data collected about phone call volumes and reasons for calls.

Figure 4: Volume of Phone Calls by Day and AM/PM

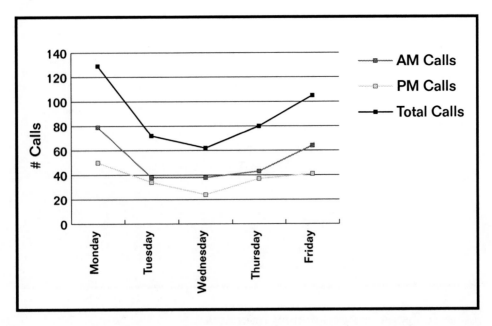

Figure 5: Reasons for Calls

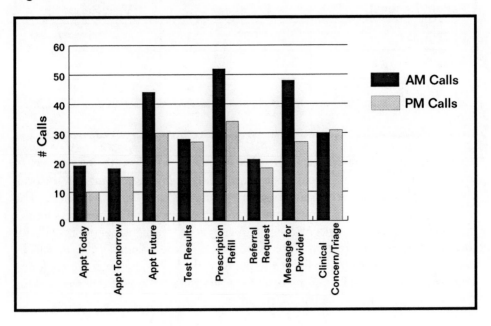

## Figure 6: Volume of Calls by Type of Call and Day of Week

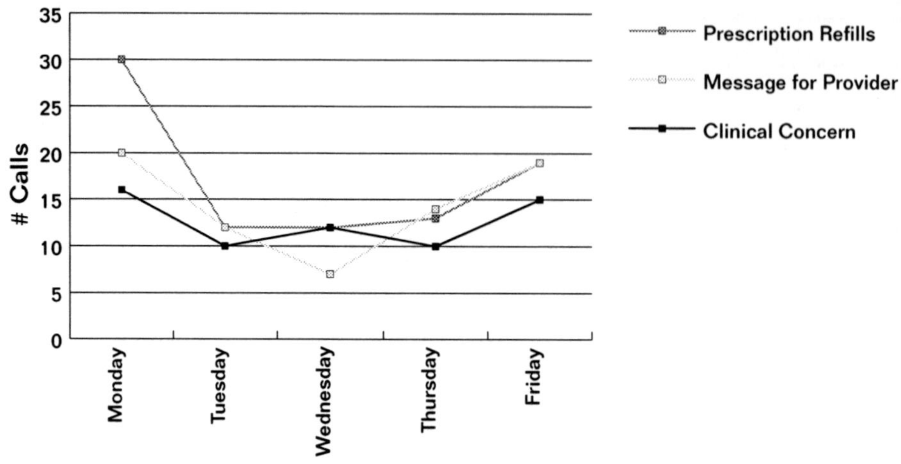

## Table 7:  Types of Appointment Requests

| Patient Request | # Calls/week | % of Total Visit Requests |
|---|---|---|
| Appt Today | 29 | 21% |
| Appt Tomorrow | 33 | 24% |
| Appt Future | 74 | 54% |
| Total | 136 | |

These data suggest some opportunities for innovative solutions to the problem of external communication by telephone.  Figure 4, page 291, points out that the peak volume of phone calls is typically highest on Monday and Friday mornings.  The most frequent types of calls are for future visits, prescription refills, messages for the physician, and clinical concerns.  Figure 6 graphs the frequency of phone calls for three of these popular reasons. Table 7 breaks down the volume of phone calls by type of request.  Note that 54% of the phone calls during the week are for future visits whereas about 45% are requests for visits today or tomorrow, representing some sense of urgency on behalf of the caller.

**Table 8: Percentage of Phone Calls For Future Visits and Prescription Refills by Day**

|  | Monday | | Tuesday | | Wednesday | | Thursday | | Friday | |
|---|---|---|---|---|---|---|---|---|---|---|
|  | AM | PM | AM | PM | AM | PM | AM | PM | AM | PM |
| Rx Refill | 20 | 10 | 6 | 6 | 8 | 4 | 6 | 7 | 12 | 7 |
| Future Visit | 15 | 10 | 5 | 5 | 5 | 4 | 8 | 6 | 11 | 5 |
| Total # Calls | 78 | 51 | 38 | 34 | 35 | 27 | 44 | 36 | 64 | 41 |
| % of Calls | 44.9% | 39.2% | 28.9% | 32.4% | 37.1% | 29.6% | 31.8% | 36.1% | 35.9% | 29.3% |

Further analysis (see Table 8, above) reveals that on Monday prescription refills and non-urgent visit requests (i.e., future visits) accounted for 45% of the phone call volume. If 35% is used as a threshold, these non-urgent visits exceeded that threshold three other times during the week, including Thursday afternoon and Friday morning—the second and third busiest days with respect to total number of phone calls.

If data from the phone service provider were available, the data would probably indicate that the majority of complaints from patients and other callers are directly related to the volume of phone calls at the time the caller tried to access the practice. Therefore, the opportunity for innovation lies in creative ways to manage non-urgent phone calls so that more important and urgent calls can be managed effectively.

## Generating Potential Solutions

What are some potentially innovative solutions? This is where the practice team should generate ideas based on the new understanding of the problem. Brainstorming is a useful technique with which most people are familiar. Searching the Internet and asking colleagues what has been successful are also simple approaches to generating potential solutions. For this example, let's assume the practice has come up with the potential solutions listed in Table 9, page 294, and did some additional research to estimate the cost and impact on operations for each option.

## Table 9:  Potential Ideas, Cost and Impact

| Number | Idea | Potential Cost | Potential Impact |
|---|---|---|---|
| 1 | Do nothing. | No direct cost, but indirect cost of continued inefficiency and poor staff/patient satisfaction. | Continuation of current status would negatively impact practice. |
| 2 | Educate patients not to call during peak times for non-urgent issues. | Minimal cost of materials. | Minimal impact, as changing patient behavior for this issue would be difficult. |
| 3 | More phone lines and phones. | Depending on system, moderate expense both in hardware (phones) and service (lines). | More phones ringing without the personnel to answer them could frustrate patients and staff even more. |
| 4 | Cross-train staff to help with telephones during peak times. | Minimal additional cost; assumes capacity for other staff to supplement telephone receptionists.  There could be an indirect cost of cross-trained staff being distracted from primary responsibilities. | This assumes that the practice has staff that can be temporarily redeployed without negatively affecting primary job responsibilities. |
| 5 | Hire additional staff. | Though more staff would improve the ability to manage calls (assuming there is a workstation available) – there would be considerable additional cost. | Positive impact of additional staff on operations could be offset by additional cost. |

| Number | Idea | Potential Cost | Potential Impact |
|---|---|---|---|
| 6 | Answering service to triage all calls during peak call times. | A pilot to determine the effectiveness of this additional support could be a cost-efficient way of testing both the answering service and to determine how much additional support is needed if contemplating additional staff. | Considerable positive impact if the answering service can do this activity effectively, using structured templates for messages and refill requests. Faxed messages could serve as the record – or secure email to the practice.  Other calls routed directly from the live operator to the practice for immediate response. |
| 7 | Purchase automatic call distribution (ACD) option for phone system (auto-teller). | The cost to purchase automatic call distribution technology can be fairly significant – and if the calls are just distributed to the same limited number of staff, then the effect is to increase call frustration. | ACD technology, if balanced with appropriate staffing levels can significantly improve service levels. However, many people object to the menu-driven, non-human interface. |
| 8 | Introduce secure email messaging for non-urgent communication. | Subscribing to an existing secure email service to communicate with patients is typically done on a monthly basis. The actual costs depend on the types of services selected.  For the basic package of a popular service, the cost is approximately $75/month per doctor. | The impact for this service would be highly variable for the concerns being addressed and would depend on patients' access to email and their willingness to use email to communicate with the office. |

Given the options in Table 9, page 294, it is often useful to then rate the options numerically. In this example, Table 10, below, applies a rating scale (1-10) for feasibility, cost and the potential positive impact of each strategy. Figure 7, below, is a bubble chart presentation of the same data from Table 10 where the size of the bubble reflects the potential impact of the solution. The bubble chart presents these same data in a way that allows better comparisons between options.

## Table 10:  Rating the Options

|  | Feasibility* | Cost** | Impact*** |
|---|---|---|---|
| 1  Do nothing | 9 | 1 | 1 |
| 2  Educate patients | 7 | 2 | 2 |
| 3  More phones & lines | 4 | 6 | 4 |
| 4  Cross train staff | 6 | 3 | 3 |
| 5  More staff | 2 | 5 | 5 |
| 6  Answering service | 6 | 7 | 8 |
| 7  ACD technology | 4 | 9 | 4 |
| 8  Secure email | 8 | 5 | 6 |
| * higher is more feasible    ** higher is more cost    ***higher is potentially larger impact | | | |

## Figure 7: Bubble Chart (numbers in bubbles correspond to numbered options in Tables 9 and 10)

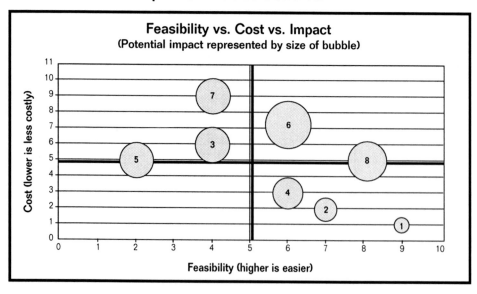

In this example, options 1 (do nothing), 2 (educate patients) and 4 (cross-train staff) are fairly feasible and low cost, but cross-training staff is the only one in this grouping that the team estimated would have a measurable impact (rating of 3 out of a scale of 10) on the problem. Options 3 (more phones and phone lines) and 7 (automatic call distribution technology) wound up in the high cost/relatively low feasibility quadrant and the size of their bubbles reflects an estimate that the potential impact would be relatively modest (4 out of 10). The costs for option 6 (answering service) and option 8 (use of secure email) place them in the upper right quadrant, but their impacts are estimated to be significant compared to most of the other potential choices.

Based on this exercise, this practice could develop a pilot program—perhaps combining a low cost/highly feasible option (educating patients, #2) with a more costly solution on a trial basis (such as engaging the answering service, #6). Ideally, the phone service provider would provide pre- and post-implementation data for the practice to assess the effectiveness of this strategy. At the end of the trial period, the practice would conduct an assessment of the impact of the pilot. Metrics would include call statistics, the cost of the enhanced service, and the satisfaction of the staff and callers. Based on the assessment, the practice would decide whether to adjust, continue or terminate the experiment in lieu of another option.

This relatively simple example, using a common issue in medical practice, highlights the use of the three innovation principles, the use of teams to generate ideas, the filtering of ideas and selection of potential solutions using data and basic graphs to permit easier analysis.

## Conclusion

Innovative ideas can be as simple or complex as the situation demands. Providing health care services is challenging under the best of circumstances. The current environment is placing additional pressure on physicians in all specialties. Many physicians find it difficult to tackle common problems while doing their best to provide quality care to their patients. Responding to the economic imperatives while enhancing quality requires innovation – and appropriate reimbursement to promote and sustain creative solutions.

This chapter focused on one simple example to demonstrate assessment of a common issue and the development of options using a framework for creating value, standard quality improvement tools, and data analyses available to anyone who is able to use a calculator or spreadsheet.

It is important that projects undertaken satisfy the key principles identified and that change efforts include all stakeholders in the process being evaluated. Following the principles and keeping staff involved will help insure that innovation becomes part of the culture and, if done correctly, add value to patients, the practice—and contribute to improving health care in the United States.

## Suggested Readings

American College of Physicians Center for Practice Innovation Annotated Bibliography. www.acponline.org/cfpi/anno_bib.htm.

## References

1. Hing E, Cherry DK, Woodwell DA. *National Ambulatory Medical Care Survey: 2004 Summary*. Advance data from vital and health statistics; no. 374. Hyattsville, MD: National Center for Health Statistics; 2006.

2. American College of Physicians. Center for Practice Innovation. Available at: www.acponline.org/cfpi/. Accessed September 26, 2006.

3. Tzu S. *The Art of War*. Mineola, NY: Dover Publications; 2002.

4. Porter ME. *Competitive Advantage: Creating and Sustaining Superior Performance*. New York, NY: The Free Press; 1985.

5. Kaplan RS, Norton DP. *The Balanced Scorecard: Translating Strategy into Action*. Boston, MA: Harvard Business School Press; 1996, 73-85.

6. Kriegel RJ, Brandt D. *Sacred Cows Make the Best Burgers*. New York, NY: Warner Books; 1996.

7. Accessed at: http://cms.dartmouth.edu/gbook/OPPC/OPPC%20Primary%20Care.doc

8. Chase RB, Aquilano NJ. *Production and Operations Management: Manufacturing and Services, 7th ed.* McGraw-Hill/Irwin, 1995, 130-153.

9. Walton M. *The Deming Management Method*. New York, NY: Putnam; 1986.

10. Brassard M, Ritter D. *The Memory Jogger II: A Pocket Guide of Tools for Continuous Improvement and Effective Planning*. New Hampshire: Goal QPC; 1994.

# Section 5
# Financial Management

# Chapter 18

## *Joining or Starting a Medical Practice*

Geoffrey T. Anders, JD, CPA, CHBC and Anne E. Jorgensen, JD

### Executive Summary

This chapter explores options for the new physician coming out of residency or fellowship. The two main options are establishing a solo practice or joining a group practice. We will compare and contrast these two types of practices, and review the issues you should weigh in making your decision. Finally, we will illustrate the steps to take towards either option.

### Learning Objectives

1. Understand the advantages and disadvantages of solo practice and group practice.

2. Understand the challenges of practice business management.

3. Evaluate your personal strengths and weaknesses.

4. Weigh the factors to consider in making this determination.

### Keywords

business plan; business systems; capital investment; compensation; coverage; group practice; market share; negotiating; risk; solo practice

### Introduction

At least half of the physicians entering practices this year will change practices within 2 years.[1] Many physicians change practices because they did not initially identify what they really wanted from their professional careers. As their goals become clearer, they began to seek practice situations more compatible with those goals. Identifying what is important at the start increases the chance of choosing a practice situation that enables you to develop both personally and professionally.

## Comparing and Contrasting Solo Practices and Group Practices

Physicians are most commonly employed in an institutional setting, solo practice, or group practice. The institutional setting is typically a hospital, health plan, or university setting (academic medical center). A solo practice involves either starting a new practice or purchasing an existing practice. A group practice could be a single or multi-specialty practice that is either a private practice or a practice owned by an HMO or hospital group.

Physicians completing training are generally faced with a choice of beginning a solo practice or joining a group. Those who choose institutional work often do so to pursue specific specializations or research. In exchange, these physicians give up a measure of control over practice finances, workload, and career advancement, as well as future income and equity prospects.

Solo practices and group practices have distinctive features that set them apart from one another. These features include aspects of independence, finance, business acumen, market share, and practice practicalities, to name a few.

### Independence and Control

The most visible difference between solo and group practice is the degree of independence and control exercisable by the physician. Physicians in solo practice work for themselves. In contrast, the group practitioner is an employee subject to the rules and regulations of the employer.

Control issues include patient treatment, work hours, insurance participation, and financial practices. In exchange for a regular paycheck and less financial risk, the group practitioner gives up complete control over billing, collection, work hours, and patient assignments. The group practitioner must work as agreed, and follow the policies and procedures of the practice, which often limits individual physician control and autonomy. By contrast, the solo practitioner is in charge of his or her own work hours, patients, and the procedures he or she performs. The solo practitioner is in control of contracts and billing, but also takes on the financial responsibility and risks involved. Overall, the solo practitioner has full autonomy in decision making for the business; the group practitioner must deal with "partners."

Control varies by degree, dependent on a variety of factors. For example, a hospital group may be under a specific contract, hindering the independence and control of all of the physicians, including its owners. A small group practice may ask the new physician to become an owner quite quickly. This, consequently, allows more input into decisions as others teach you how to manage the practice. A multi-specialty group practice permits varying degrees of control, depending on the specialty and group organizational structure. Though not as independent as the solo practitioner, the group practitioner may have the freedom to exercise a greater or lesser degree of independence and control based on the particular practice situation.

### Capital Investment

Opening a new medical practice requires a significant amount of capital. A new practice requires planning, advisors, equipment, supplies, rent, and payroll—all of which are due and payable before you even see one patient or bill for any services. Furthermore, accounts receivable from services rendered will not be paid immediately. The practice should have enough capital to pay all costs for at least three months, if not more, plus initial equipment costs. How much capital is required varies by specialty—from less than $100,000 to well over $500,000.

Obtaining financing for a new practice may not be easy. A physician must go through many years of training to attain the ultimate goal of practicing medicine, regardless of specialization. Those years of schooling and training come with a high price tag, putting the physician in significant debt. Without some type of collateral or a solid business plan, a bank may be reluctant to loan a physician the funds needed to start a solo practice.

In contrast, the group practitioner will not have a capital investment initially. The capital for the group practice has already been funded by the current members of the practice. In some cases, moving costs or signing bonuses may be available as a recruitment incentive from the group.

### Coverage

Your job as a physician is to treat patients. Patients may need care at any time. Thus, you must either be available to the patient or arrange for coverage during the times you are not available. The continued availability of care must be provided for the patient.

The group practitioner, by definition, should have fellow practice members available to treat patients during periods of absence. The employed physician can take vacation and professional absences without securing coverage because those absences are approved by the practice for times when the practice can provide such coverage. The solo practitioner must make arrangements for vacation and professional absences on his or her own. In some cases, the solo physician may have a reciprocal relationship with another solo physician or group of physicians. However, the solo practitioner must put forth the effort to secure this coverage.

In addition to coverage for vacation and professional absences, a physician must also supply night and weekend call coverage. The group practice will have additional physicians to staff all on-call needs so the group doctor need not be available 24/7. The solo practitioner will once again have to secure such call coverage, or be tied to the beeper every hour of the day.

Perhaps one of the most serious weaknesses of solo practice is the potential for absence due to disability or illness. Should the solo doctor become unable to practice and generate an income, the practice overhead continues; and, very soon, patients will seek other doctors. Some solos have pre-agreed arrangements with their colleague-competitors for practice coverage in the event of sickness or sudden death.

### Business Knowledge and Training

By training, physicians practice medicine, but a medical practice is a business. Entering into private practice requires more than an exceptional knowledge of medicine. In order to have a financially viable practice, one must also learn the skills for running a successful business.

In this regard, the obvious difference between solo practice and group practice is the time the physician has to learn the business aspects of practicing medicine. The group practitioner will initially rely upon others to perform the business functions of the practice. This allows the group practitioner time to learn how to effectively run a practice or, alternatively, compensate another group doctor to do so. The solo practitioner is responsible for performing the business functions of the practice without the luxury of a grace period for learning.

At the most basic level, a physician starting a solo practice must have some accounting and financial knowledge, as well as negotiation and management skills. Chapter 19 offers more information about the key accounting and finance concepts and practices. Every practice requires at least one administrative employee, and usually more. It would be a poor use of physician time to check every patient in and out, file charts, answer the phone, and handle all billing and office management duties. Once an employee is hired, the physician must consider employment laws, fringe benefits, and personnel policies. Additionally, the physician must train, motivate, and monitor this employee, as well as formulate job descriptions, rules, and standards for the office.

Amongst myriad other things, the physician must be aware of all the rules and regulations regarding billing. Billing codes and rules change yearly, and sometimes more frequently. Improper billing and coding carry significant penalties under both federal and state laws. Chapter 20 offers the basics on billing and coding. The physician must also decide with which insurance companies he or she will negotiate, contract, and participate. Overexposure to managed care or a lack of understanding of a managed care environment and systems will potentially cost the physician significant revenue.

With proper training and courses, it is possible for a physician to attain the skills necessary to run a solo practice. Furthermore, it is advisable for the physician to focus on developing these skills since he or she will be ultimately responsible for the business success or failure of the practice.

### Division of Labor

In economics, the division of labor is the specialization of function to increase productivity. If your corn grows better and my wheat is more plentiful, the most economic approach is for each of us to specialize and then trade.

Division of labor applies to the economics of medical practices just as it applies to the rest of the business world. When a business can compartmentalize and specialize, those functions become more efficient and productive because personnel become experts in those particular areas. The same can be said for physicians. In a group practice, the physicians can specialize in different treatments, thereby becoming more efficient. For example, a nephrology group can divide itself into treatment teams for kidney stones, chronic kidney disease, hypertension, and transplant. In this way, the group becomes better equipped to treat patients with specific conditions and more efficient at doing so. However, this division of labor will only work in group practices.

### Business Systems

Every practice should run on business systems—a series of pre-defined steps performed by designated individuals to accomplish a task. These systems include scheduling systems, billing and collection systems, bookkeeping, purchasing and management reporting programs on the technical side, and recruitment, personnel management, and documentation on the human resources side. Few businesses can implement perfect business systems on the first try. Most have trial and error periods as they find what routines best fit their particular business needs. Medical practices are no different. A solo practitioner should expect growing pains and many changes at the outset. But the solo physician should be careful not to adjust systems to meet each individual set of circumstances that arise. If systems are varied daily to meet yesterday's new crises, things will never settle into an efficient routine.

A group practice, presumably, will have already established the business systems that work for that practice. If a group practice grows, it too may experience growing pains and adjustment, but the backbone for the office systems will be in place — which is not to say that already established systems cannot be improved.

### Application to Particular Specialties

Certain medical specialties lend themselves to group practice over solo practice due to the nature of the medicine. Likewise, certain specialties are more viable as solo practices. For example, cardiologists are often found primarily in group practice because of the different subspecialties that have developed within cardiology, and the need for access to these varying specialties. Additionally, cardiologists are on call at hospitals and often have agreements with hospitals to provide all cardiology call services. Providing these services is much easier within a group, as is shouldering the capital expense of the essential imaging devices that cardiologists rely upon. Radiology and anesthesiology are also disciplines that are more difficult to do as a solo practitioner because of coverage issues and hospital contracts.

In contrast, plastic surgeons, dermatologists, allergists, pain medicine physicians, and retinal surgeons often have successful solo practices. Each of these specialties has a limited practice area, which tends to be highly compensated. Because of the income potential, these physicians can absorb the overhead costs of an office and staff more easily than some of their counterparts in other specialties. Furthermore, these physicians' call responsibilities are usually not very burdensome.

Other specialties, particularly in primary care fields, can also be practiced solo. However, the typically poorer reimbursement and financial prospects for primary care physicians tends to suggest that group practice is preferable. In addition to shared overhead, larger groups of primary care physicians may serve sufficiently large patient populations, making a variety of ancillary services—anything from hearing-aid dispensing to prescription dispensing to physical therapy—viable.

Depending on the physician's specialty, solo practice may or may not be a viable option. In determining the viability of a solo practice, the physician should consider the requirements of the specialty and the practical implications of that type of practice.

### Compensation

Compensation is one of the final keys in comparing solo and group practices. A group practice will typically agree to pay the new employee/physician a salary. Despite the work production of the physician, the physician will be paid (at least until employment is terminated). If the physician produces sizable revenues, a bonus or incentive payment may be available. However, most employees are expected to produce a profit for their employer. Not benefiting from the full fruits of one's labor is normally a short-lived situation. After only a few years, private practice group physicians are most often invited into co-ownership. And while that equity opportunity requires a capital investment, it also involves a return on that investment, including the right to benefit fully from the fruits of one's work.

The solo practitioner does not receive a set salary, and only gets paid after all creditors are paid. If production is down, the physician's personal income draw will decline. Of course, the contrary is true in that if the physician has considerable collections and is able to pay all expenses, the physician keeps all the excess money produced.

Over the long term, very few solo practitioners become top earners. Far and away, the bulk of private group practice doctors earn more than do the solo practitioners. Institutional or academic employment tends to start at a slightly higher pay than group practice opportunities, but the increases in salaries are measured and slow. And institutional settings do not offer any equity position or the possibility to benefit from investments in ancillary services.

## Evaluating Your Practice Options

Because of the differences in the solo practice and the group practice, it is easy to conclude that not every physician will thrive in each workplace. There are more considerations in choosing either a solo or group practice over an academic position. Solo practitioners face financial risk, possible professional isolation, and potential long hours in exchange for controlling their own work and building value in their practice. Group practitioners face a lack of practice control and potential personality conflicts in exchange for income predictability, camaraderie, and shared patient responsibility. It is your job as a physician entering the workforce to determine which characteristics you possess that would enable you to flourish in a particular practice setting.

### Initial Assessment

A good starting point might involve consideration of four specific areas: 1) entrepreneurialism, 2) management abilities, 3) social style, and 4) lifestyle choices. In relation to entrepreneurialism, you should consider how aggressive you are and how comfortable you are with taking risks. You need to decide if you want to be a leader and boss, and if you enjoy dealing with myriad non-patient care issues, including finance, personnel, legal, and operational concerns. An affirmative response to these considerations may point you to the solo practice option.

In relation to management, you should consider how well you handle administrative details, hospital and referring doctor politics, and support staff. Are you good at spotting new business opportunities and dealing with people, including providing motivation, direction, feedback, and discipline? If not, you may be better off in a group practice environment where other physicians' talents may shore up management weaknesses.

Socially, consider your ability to develop new referral and business sources. Do you open up to new people, enjoy meeting new people, and enjoy socializing? Finally, what type of lifestyle do you prefer? Are you a workaholic? What are you willing to sacrifice to meet your professional, business, or financial goals? How relatively valuable are money, family time, professional recognition, and recreation time?

Once completed, you should review these initial assessments and expect these traits to remain constant. In all likelihood, your personality and skill set will not change. Personal values may well change, but only over the long term. Note that excess compensation rarely compensates for other significant lifestyle sacrifices.

### Assessment of Risk Tolerance

Some practice arrangements contain significantly more or less financial and clinical risk than others. A solo practitioner will be responsible, solely, for the practice's financial profits and losses. A member of a large practice group will likely not be responsible for individual losses, as an associate, and will not likely benefit exclusively from any profits. However, a member of a smaller group practice may be more directly liable for the financial health of the practice.

For a physician coming out of residency with loans and other financial obligations, financial risk is an important factor in determining the physician's practice choice. Those with strong ideas and support, and a practice specialty conducive to this course of action may opt to establish their own practice, taking on significant financial risk. Others will seek out the highest compensated position in an effort to become financially independent, perhaps planning to launch a solo practice in the years to come. Those primarily interested in lifestyle and avoiding financial risk may see group practice as the best permanent solution. Whichever course is chosen, it is up to you to evaluate the risks, the potential rewards, and the possible pitfalls of any situation before taking action.

### Personal Relationships

In addition to performing the initial assessment, you must also consider the socialization and happiness of those who are affected by your decisions. Your choice to accept a position may affect not only you, but also your family. If you conclude that you are a workaholic, who enjoys being independent and wants to practice on your own, will this decision create a strain on your family life and relations? An unhappy social life due to family or personal issues will undoubtedly have an impact on the physician's ability to flourish in his or her professional life. You must also consider how your decisions will influence those around you.

### Training and Abilities

Every physician has both personal and clinical strengths. Though personal strengths may lead you to the select one form of medical practice setting, your clinical abilities must also play a role in determining the best choice. For example, if you have limited research experience, you may not be quite right for an institutional position. Also, if you seek additional education and guidance with regard to certain procedures, you may not be suited to solo practice.

All prospective employers will want to know what you have to offer and what distinguishes you from your colleagues. They will want to know about your training, personality, and demeanor. Physicians who opt for solo practice may not want to be controlled by others, and their personality and demeanor will reflect that type of work ethic. You must always be aware of your own clinical and personal strengths when deciding a future course for your practice.

### Market Share and Location

The key to a successful practice is patients. Without patients, you cannot provide treatment and bill for services. Thus, market share and location are critically important in considering when, where, and how to practice medicine. Entering a saturated market with plenty of physicians providing similar services may hurt the productivity of all of the physicians. Market share becomes increasingly important when opening a solo practice. Without unique skills, a solo cardiologist new to an area will not be competitive with the 12-member group that has served the community with comprehensive cardiac services for over 20 years. However, if that cardiologist instead joins the 12-member group, he or she would have the benefit of the referrals to the group—a known community entity.

The solo practitioner faces a tougher battle in establishing a practice if he or she does not have ties to an area or built-in referral sources. Conversely, if the area is underserved, the solo practitioner will not need to work as hard to build the practice. In underserved areas, the driven physician opening a solo practice may be in a better position than the group practitioner, particularly if the solo physician provides an "alternative" to a presently existing monopoly.

### Characteristics of Successful Practitioners

Regardless of the path you choose, your ultimate goal is to be successful. A successful solo practitioner is often a person with good organizational skills who is independent and driven. The solo practitioner is comfortable taking risks and exhibits a high degree of self-confidence. Typically, this physician has fewer outside interests, allowing more time to devote to developing the practice.

The group practitioner should enjoy being part of a team and get along well with others. Depending on the size of the practice, the group practitioner will be more willing to conform or compromise with his or her "partners." The group practitioner frequently seeks more of a balance between professional and personal life.

Although these characteristics are important, they are not blueprints to lead a physician to a particular type of practice. They do illustrate, however, the innate differences between preferences for solo practice and group practice, and should be considered as part of any decision-making process.

## Steps to Establishing a Solo Practice

Once you decide that a solo practice is the choice for you, you must take many steps before you can hang your shingle. First and foremost, you must decide where you want to practice and what types of services you would like to provide. However, wanting to practice in a particular area does not automatically mean that it is possible. The area must be in need of the practice.

Once a suitable area has been located for the practice, you must take certain other steps before choosing an office location, purchasing supplies, and hiring personnel. You must choose advisors, create a business plan, and establish financial relationships and lending arrangements. Additionally, before any work can be performed, you must secure licensure, malpractice insurance, privileges, if applicable, and credentialing with third-party payors. Only when these plans are in place can you begin to acquire the tangible items of office space, equipment, supplies, and support staff.

### Evaluating a Location

First and foremost, you must determine the proposed location or area for practice. To determine if a physician with a particular skill set is needed in the area, a feasibility study should be conducted by obtaining demographic information, both current and projected, for the chosen location. For example, an aging population with limited new growth and a low birth rate is likely not suitable for a pediatrician to open a practice. Physician-to-population ratios can help determine whether a need exists, as can informal interviews with hospital personnel, potential referral sources, and even possible competitors.

Furthermore, you should evaluate your physical space requirements, and whether appropriate office space is available in the desired location at the right price. Consider utilizing a "tenant's representative," a real estate agent who will negotiate on your behalf and is paid by the landlord. Don't forget local municipal ordinances and requirements for permits and licenses. Next, you should visit area hospitals to gather information regarding the availability of staff privileges. If privileges are required, what do you have to do to secure these privileges? What assistance can the hospital provide in establishing the practice? For example, some hospitals, where there is a need for your specialty, will provide income guarantees in exchange for your promise to stay in the area for a set period of time. Other hospitals will provide assistance in purchasing furniture and equipment, recruiting staff, and so forth. Is emergency department call available? Is it mandatory? Are "unassigned" patients rotated among all members of the department?

In addition to the hospital, learn what information, advice and assistance pharmaceutical company representatives can offer.

### Choosing Advisors

The next step to starting a practice is choosing advisors. The advisors should have experience working with physicians. Though many different types of advisors exist, the basic advisors that every practice should have are an accountant, an attorney, and a property and casualty insurance broker. A medical practice management consultant is an excellent idea. Depending upon a variety of other factors, the practice might also have a real estate broker (the aforementioned tenant's representative), a banker, a benefits consultant or salesperson, or another type of consultant.

The accountant (or management consultant) and attorney should be able to work together to formulate a plan that works financially and legally for the practice. The management consultant should recommend office layout, business systems, software systems, job descriptions, recruitment efforts, and other practice aids.

### Creating a Business Plan

Before you can go further in establishing your practice, you must create a business plan. This business plan should outline the goals for the practice, the anticipated finances—thus, capital needs—an assessment of competition, and a plan for achieving the goals. The plan should include an analysis of your skills as a physician and how you believe you will be able to structure a financially viable business. Financial relationships are established and revolve around the business plan.

### Establishing Financial Relationships

Once you have a well thought-out and workable business plan, you will need to get your finances in order. You must choose a bank and secure details for loans, checking accounts, savings accounts, and lines of credit for start-up costs. To obtain this funding and financial backing, you will need to provide the pro-forma financial estimate, which is part of the business plan, for the bank.

You may encounter some difficulty obtaining financing, regardless of the solidity of the business plan/pro-forma. Most physicians have significant debt in the form of school loans. Without some type of collateral, a financial institution may not be willing to take on the risk of a new business. This is a time when the advisors, who have experience, may be able to step in and lead you through the process to obtain the financing. Also various medical societies make financing services available through financial "partners."

### Securing All Licenses, Insurance, and Privileges

In order to practice medicine, you will need a state medical license and, usually, a DEA registration. In many states, professional liability insurance is required (and, in any event, advisable). Medical licenses are issued by the state according to each state's particular rules. These licenses can take several months to be approved. During that time, you cannot practice medicine, so if you are leaving the state in which you trained, good advance planning is needed.

Likewise, you need professional liability insurance. While some states permit doctors to practice "bare," i.e., without insurance, that is rarely a good idea. In seeking this insurance, you should review a variety of insurance plans to determine the best program with a financially sound insurer.

Plans can vary from "occurrence" to "claims made," and an entire spectrum in-between. Depending on start-up costs, financial ability, and the professional liability insurance market, you may not have as many options as you would like. Here again, check with the local hospital, which may have an insurance program for its medical staff doctors.

In addition to malpractice insurance, the practice will also need various other insurances. Workers' compensation insurance, overhead insurance, premises liability, health insurance, non-owner's automobile insurance, and employee dishonesty insurance are all of concern. The insurance brokers will review the need and options for each insurance type.

Depending on the specialty involved, the physician may need to obtain hospital or facility privileges.  Depending on the entity, it may take several months to obtain privileges.  Credentials committees rarely meet more than once a month, and as a soon-to-be solo practitioner, you may not have any friends on the committee pushing your application through the review labyrinth.

### Regulatory Compliance

In addition to licensure and privileges, a medical practice needs regulatory procedures and protocols to operate.  Among the plethora of health care regulations are the Health Insurance Portability and Accountability Act (HIPAA) laws[2] and Occupational Health and Safety Administration (OSHA) blood-borne pathogen laws.[3]  Furthermore, you need to be sure that you are not violating any Stark or fraud and abuse laws with arrangements that you may make.[4]  When developing your compliance plans, you should also adopt a personnel policy manual.  Although this is not required for regulatory purposes, it will allow you to officially set office policy—including your regulatory compliance plans.  Your management consultant and attorney should be able to help you with these processes.

### Equipping the Office

After all other steps have been taken, the final task is equipping and staffing the office.  Even when an appropriate space is located, a build-out will most likely be needed to properly fit the office and the clinical areas.  Once all the furniture and hardware are in place, and the pictures and plaques hung, the equipment and supplies for the office must be ordered.  Prices for equipment and supplies can vary significantly, so it is wise to comparison shop.

Obviously, the practice will need personnel, computers, and software.  The management consultant will aid the physician in determining human resource requirements.  The new staff will need training on the computer systems chosen, which should be arranged as part of the purchase of the computer systems and programs.  Office protocols and hours of work all need to be established, and the staff oriented to the practice's procedures and benefits.

Outsourcing billing, transcription, practice management, human resource functions, and other tasks can make great sense.  You can focus the practice's functions on what you do best—treat patients—while other issues are farmed out.  Remember that while outsourcing reduces the need to recruit, train, and manage staff, you must instead manage the outside contractor and the contract.

### Opening the Doors

Opening the practice will require a bushel of other details; notably, office stationery, forms and business cards, signage, office and clinical supplies, telephone numbers and the like. You must also decide whether or not to participate with certain health insurance programs or provide services at different facilities. Billing procedures and a collection agency must be in place. Marketing the new practice through advertising and networking is a must so you have patients to see. While "personal selling" is difficult for many doctors, it brings substantially better results than a mailing and an office open house. Each practice should have one or more unique selling points: clinical procedures not performed by others, e.g., better availability and access (often most easy to provide for a new doctor!), perhaps availability through night, weekend hours, or same-day appointments; new technology; a better customer care attitude; or some other distinguishing feature that not only will bring patients back. All of these will give you talking points for personal selling of patient sources. Chapter 7 offers more options for advertising and communicating about your practice.

## Steps to Joining a Group Practice

If you decide to join a group practice, you must begin to research your options. Group practices come in varying sizes, shapes, orientations, and specialties. For example, an orthopedist would have the choice of a single-specialty group, a musculoskeletal group (orthopedists, rheumatologists, podiatrists, physiatrists and, perhaps, other specialists), or a broad-based, multi-specialty group. Accordingly, the practices will have different and unique attributes that may or may not suit you and competition for desirable positions may be high. You must present yourself well on paper, the phone, and during the personal interview. Hopefully, an offer will be extended, which you will need to evaluate, and then negotiate before signing on.

### Researching Options

Finding a group practice begins with research. Research begins with your own self-analysis. Based upon the initial assessment discussed above, you should begin to streamline your search by eliminating certain practice options. Formulating a list of "ideal characteristics" for a practice may aid in the winnowing process.

In some specialties, the offers may come directly to you. In others, you must seek out the opportunity, especially if you have specific requirements for location. Similar to the solo practitioner, you should evaluate the market in the area. While a group may think it needs a doctor, there may not be that actual need in the community, so a second evaluation is in order. Will the market bear an additional physician? If not, is a doctor in the hiring group preparing to leave practice? If there is not a clear need in the area, the growth potential and potential for co-ownership in the future will be lower.

In researching group practices, several questions should be asked. What is the history of the practice? Have any physicians in the practice been disciplined or excluded from federal programs? What types of cases does this practice handle? Would you be adding new skills or expanding the group's scope of service? What hospitals are affiliated with the practice? These answers can be had without much trouble and can help you in the decision-making process.

Once the research has been completed, or while it is in process, you should begin making connections with target practices. Curriculum vitae (CV) and cover letters should be tailored to the specific groups in which you are interested. For example, you would not want a cover letter indicating a love of the Midwest to go to a Seattle practice. Detail is important, because you must put your best foot forward since, at least at the outset, the practice can only evaluate you based on the quality of the product you provide—your CV and cover letter.

### Interviewing

Interviewing is an art form. Both the interviewer and interviewee want to show themselves in the best possible light. You may be picked up from the airport with a car service and taken out to the best restaurant in town. During the interview, the group practice will likely not volunteer practice negatives, unless a group doctor is looking to sabotage the hiring (not a terribly unusual event). Likewise, you should treat this opportunity as though it were your number one choice, regardless of whether it is or is not. Each side must wade through the fanfare and find the truth about its potential future "partner."

You should be prepared for questions regarding your training, qualifications, and work ethic. Prior to entering the interview, you should rehearse and review your answers to certain pertinent questions:

- Do my qualifications meet or surpass the needs of the situation for which I am interviewing?

- What are my greatest strengths and weaknesses?

- Do I get along well with others; am I a team player and am I flexible?

- Am I a star or superstar?

- What does working "hard" mean to me?

- What interests other than medicine are important to me?
- Do I inspire trust?
- Do I appear too competitive?

Each of these questions answers more about you than the actual question asked. Outside activities could demonstrate other interests, or appear to be too time-consuming for the hiring practice. Strengths and weaknesses are significant not only for the merit of the action, but also for the weakness or strength not mentioned.

Conversely, you must do your own interviewing as well.

- Why does the practice believe it needs another physician?
- How will the practice promote a new doctor?
- Does the group have a strategic business plan?
- On what basis do the partners compensate themselves?
- What will the practice look like in five years?
- What comprises a typical work day?
- What is expected of me as an associate physician?
- How will you communicate with me about whether I am succeeding in the practice?

These thoughtful but pointed questions allow you to gain perspective on the values of the group.

The interview process is rarely a one-day affair, especially if travel is involved. You should take this opportunity to evaluate the practice and surroundings. Visiting schools, driving through neighborhoods, and talking to local community members are important to get a feel for the area. Will your family, if applicable, be happy here? Professionally, you should speak with employees at the hospital and with practices in a position to refer to the group. Does the group treat nurses and support staff well? Do they have a good reputation in the area? Are they in favor with the hospital? What types of cases do they bring in? If possible, the physician may want to ask comparative questions with regard to competing groups in the same specialty.

Once the interview is completed, you should have a good working knowledge of the practice and the members of the practice, as well as knowledge of the expectations of employment and how the group functions.

### Evaluating an Offer

When evaluating an offer, keep the following points in mind: 1) people exaggerate; 2) the better the offer, the more rule number 1 applies; 3) if you weren't there, you don't really know; and 4) you never *really* know what the practice is like until you work there. Additionally, the written contract is *the* contract. Oral agreements, handshake agreements, and other offers are not "the deal." Be wary of promises that are not in writing, or contract terms that are reported to not actually be enforced. A contract is a legally binding recitation of your mutual intent. If it is not in the contract, it does not exist. Best intentions have been known to go awry when circumstances change and memories are faulty, to boot—sometimes conveniently so.

The contract should be in common, easy-to-understand language that is free of ambiguity (easier said than done, especially when lawyers are involved!). The offer will have the standard categories of term, termination, compensation and incentives, business expenses, malpractice insurance, fringe benefits, vacation and sick pay, and restrictive covenants/non-solicitation agreements. The agreement should clearly specify the starting date for employment and ability for either party to terminate (the initial draft of institutional contracts is notorious for allowing the institution to terminate for a host of reasons, but not allowing you to terminate for any reason). Fortunately, this is all negotiable, if you take your time, and have the sense to negotiate. You should be aware of any liability for early contract termination, and whether the start date will affect access to benefits that have waiting periods.

Compensation and bonuses vary by practice, specialty, and geographic area. The structure of compensation may be set or variable in accordance with productivity. Bonuses may or may not be available. You should know the average starting salary for your specialty nationally and, if possible, in the chosen location. Compensation increases for subsequent years should be as specific as possible.

Business expenses and malpractice insurance are generally paid by the practice. Business expenses should include continuing medical education costs, beeper or cell phone, license fees, and hospital fees, as they are necessary for practice. Dues for societies and journal subscriptions are often approved by the practice. Malpractice insurance should be provided, but payment for "tail coverage" for claims-made policies varies, and there is currently no standard.

Fringe benefits should include family basic and major medical health insurance, and retirement plan participation (after a waiting period), and may include disability insurance, life insurance, vision care and dental insurances. Additional perquisites may involve moving expenses and signing bonuses. Each practice will have certain benefits available to physician employees. While these benefits are often non-negotiable, you must have an understanding of what you will receive. Vacations, leaves of absence, call obligations, and sick pay should also be set out in the agreement.

A restrictive covenant is an agreement not to compete with a former employer. The general law regarding these covenants is that they must be reasonable in time, scope, and place, and they may not violate the public interest. The enforceability of restrictive covenants and non-solicitation agreements varies by state. Some states do not allow restrictive covenants (e.g., Alabama, Massachusetts) or place specific guidelines on the scope of the covenant (e.g., Delaware, Colorado, and California).

The non-solicitation agreement prohibits the physician from soliciting patients, contracts, employees, or referral sources upon leaving the practice. The purpose of this clause is to prohibit the taking of patient lists and soliciting those patients to seek treatment at the physician's new office, wherever it may be. While the theft of a practice's patient lists and conversion to a purpose contrary to the practice's interest is illegal in any event, non-solicitation agreements generally make other solicitations improper, i.e., "I want you to be my number one assistant in my new practice!"

In virtually all privately-owned, group practices, you will want to know about potential co-ownership arrangements and what happens if the senior physician in a two-doctor group dies or becomes disabled.

In reviewing the contract, you should always try to clarify the meaning or intent of terms in the agreement. An attorney or consultant familiar with these types of contracts should review the contract to help determine if, in business terms, the contract is fair, reasonable, and complete. An attorney's services may be needed if there are specific legal issues, such as the enforceability of indemnification or restrictive covenant clauses.

Most often, the physician should deal directly with the practice doctors to discuss contract terms rather than using attorneys to represent each side. A physician negotiating with the practice's attorney will be at a disadvantage; lawyers do this for a living and, most often, will work to protect the practice, rather than to reach an equitable resolution to issues.

### Negotiating a Contract

The negotiating power of the physician is a direct function of how much the potential employer believes it needs the new doctor, and the size, type, and location of the group. Larger groups have standard contracts, which are necessary for administration and keeping things fair as among all members. Conversely, small groups of physicians have minimal contracting experience and are more willing to alter terms to attract the right physician. In larger groups, the only real negotiable terms may be salary, bonus, permissible amount of business expenses, and vacation allowance. Before beginning the negotiation, you must be aware of your trade-offs. Regardless of how it is received, the practice only has a certain amount of money to go around. The money spent on each physician either goes to salary, benefits, or expenses.

When negotiating, you should begin with the points of most importance. In order to negotiate from a position of strength you should know what the "going rates" are, so be sure to do your research. Additionally, pay attention to the practice's negotiating style. Presumably when co-ownership comes up in the future, you will have to negotiate again. Does the practice's negotiation style lead you believe that there may be problems reaching consensus?

Above all, you should be open, honest, and fair during the negotiation stage. A negotiation does not have winners or losers. "Winning" the negotiation occurs when both parties have reached a mutually agreeable set of terms, and nobody is left in the dust. If you win a negotiation by beating the other party into the ground, you will lose as the subsequent years unfold; physicians have remarkably long memories for actual and perceived wrongs. A contract with ambiguous language, or one based upon verbal assurances contrary to the stated contract language, should never be signed.

## Conclusion

In today's ever-changing medical climate, you must be able to evaluate and assess your best practice options, keeping an eye towards the future. What do you wish to be doing five years from now? How about ten years from now? To make these determinations, you must plan carefully and well in advance, assess risk, and negotiate well (or delegate that negotiation to an experienced advisor). Most importantly, whether in solo practice or a group, you must be open to change and be willing to adapt. Even with the best planning, many physicians change jobs within the first four years, and for some, more than once during that timeframe. As such, immediately putting down roots with large mortgages and expensive toys may not be the wisest course. During the recruitment period and initial work "honeymoon," everyone's best foot is forward. If that is not the case in long-term practice, you must be able to assess the situation and change positions, if warranted.

## Case Study

Dr. Jay is a dermatologist with a specialization in Mohs surgery. She is currently finishing her training in Los Angeles, but remains an "East Coast" girl at heart. Dr. Jay has two children, and a husband whose job is very mobile. Her children have just started junior high and are very active in their schools. Her son has developed a talent for surfing, and her daughter spends weekends snowboarding in Northern California.

Dr. Jay and her husband have been trying to decide where she will start her practice. Dr. Jay has several offers from different East Coast and West Coast practices to join existing dermatology practices as a Mohs specialist. Dr. Jay has always been very independent, which is one of the reasons she chose dermatology as her specialty. She has had dreams since she was a young girl of having her own medical practice. Dr. Jay's husband has said he will support whatever decision she chooses.

Logistically, Dr. Jay realizes that having her own practice will require a significant portion of her time. Recognizing that family is important, she would prefer to have a family member step in to help her and her husband with the children, if needed. She is wary of the influences on children when they are not properly supervised and looked after. However, her family is located in the Philadelphia area, and her husband's family is located in a retirement community in Florida. Though she would like to return to the East Coast, her own family is quite settled on the West Coast.

What issues should Dr. Jay consider? What facts tend to favor a group practice setting or a solo practice? What other considerations should play a role in her personal decision?

## Study/Discussion Questions

1. Use a matrix to quantify your decision:

    —List your most important points and rank them in order (best–lowest number)

    —List the opposing points and rank them in order (worst–highest number)

    —Be sure to consider your personal relationships and how your points affect them and factor that in the equation

    —Add together each important and opposing point for a total score and rank your final points

2. Does this decision feel right?

3. Are you doing this for the money? If so, is it more important than your happiness?

## Suggested Reading/Websites

### General Knowledge and Advising

| | |
|---|---|
| The Health Care Group, Inc. | www.healthcaregroup.com |
| American College of Physicians | www.acponline.org/counseling |
| Karen Zupko & Associates, Inc. | www.karenzupko.com |
| National Association of Healthcare Consultants | www.healthcon.org |

### Evaluating your Business Options and Practice Options

| | |
|---|---|
| *Medical Economics* Magazine | www.memag.com |
| United States Small Business Association | www.sba.gov |
| Physician Specialty Associations | |

### Physician Starting Salary Information

| | |
|---|---|
| Physician Starting Salary Survey | www.healthcaregroup.com |
| Student Doc | www.studentdoc.com/salaries.html |
| Jackson & Coker Salary Tool | jacksonandharris.com/physicians/salarytool.aspx |

### Assessing a Location, Demographic Data, Compliance

| | |
|---|---|
| Census Bureau Quickfacts | www.census.gov (Quick facts) |
| Department of Labor & Industry | www.dol.gov |
| State and County Medical Societies Websites and Newsletters | |

## References

1. Abdo W, Broxterman MP. Reasons Why Physicians Change Jobs Results from PHG 2nd Annual Survey. 2004. Available at: http://www.phg.com/article_a052.htm. Accessed October 6, 2006.

2. The Health Insurance Portability and Accountability Act of 1996. Available at: http://www.cms.hhs.gov/HIPAAGenInfo/Downloads/HIPAAlawdetail.pdf. Accessed September 26, 2006.

3. Occupational Safety and Health Administration. Available at: http://www.osha.gov/. Accessed September 26, 2006.

4. Self-Referral Law. Available at: http://www.cms.hhs.gov/PhysicianSelfReferral/. Accessed September 26, 2006.

# Chapter 19

## Fundamentals of Health Care Accounting and Finance

Barbara J. Grant, CPA, MST

### Executive Summary

Good financial management is key to the success of a physician practice. As the financial managers of their practices, physician leaders must be able to manage data—to pull together many little pieces of a puzzle and create the big picture that forms the basis for good decisions.

Before they can make good financial decisions, financial managers must first understand how the data are gathered and what they mean. They must also be familiar with certain basic accounting and finance terminology, ratio analysis, and the various types of reports needed to manage a practice. There are several key concepts to grasp:

- The decision regarding which metrics to monitor depends on the practice's profile, and the issues facing the practice at any particular point in time.

- Budgeting is a process that should involve all key personnel, and careful analysis of anticipated revenue and expenses. The budget should be used by management throughout the year to identify variances, control costs, and manage cash flow.

- The "cost" of an asset is the amount of resources given up to acquire that asset. Certain costs "behave" differently and financial managers must understand these behaviors in order to predict and manage costs.

- The lifeblood of any practice is accounts receivable, because of the direct impact on cash flow. The best way to prevent cash flow problems is to be proactive about collecting patient payments at the time of service, and to have a tightly structured process for capturing charges, submitting claims, and following up on open accounts.

- Investment decisions should be made based on sound economic principles, including considerations of the time value of money.

- Every investment decision requires a financing decision. Financing can be obtained from various sources: capital contributions from the owners, retained earnings, third-party lenders, leasing companies, or hospital systems. Regardless of the source of funding, the practice should have a business plan to support any major undertaking.

Financial management of a medical practice is an ongoing and complex process. Physician leaders must work together to ensure that the practice has the reporting tools and information needed to make good financial decisions.

## Learning Objectives

1. Understand the meaning of basic accounting and finance terms and their application to medical practices.

2. Analyze standard month-end reports to elicit operational and benchmarking data for a practice.

3. Discover the benefits of utilizing benchmarks to monitor the financial well-being of a practice.

4. Create and utilize a budget as a management tool.

5. Understand the various cost components of a medical practice, and how each component relates to profitability.

6. Understand what drives cash flow and why accounts receivable should be monitored closely.

7. Understand the process for making long-term investment decisions.

8. Learn the factors to consider when determining how to finance practice operations.

## Keywords

accounting; benchmarks; budgeting; cash flow; finance; financing; return on investments (ROI)

## Introduction

Good financial management is key to the success of a physician practice. As the financial managers of their practices, physician leaders must be able to manage data —to pull together many little pieces of a puzzle and create the big picture that forms the basis for good decisions.

Financial managers are responsible for designing a system for tracking and reporting key data, implementing controls that ensure their integrity so that short-term and long-term decisions can confidently be based on those data. The profile of the practice determines the nature of the data to be tracked and the appropriate reporting format. For example, the size of the practice influences the complexity of its financial decisions, as does the specialty, the ownership structure, and the individual skills, interests, and level of sophistication of the management team.

## Basic Financial Terms and Applications

Before you can make good financial decisions, you must first understand how the data are gathered, and what they mean. The flow of financial data in any practice can be broken down into six general categories, and recorded in separate "journals" as depicted in Appendix A. The six journal types include:

1. The *Patient Revenue Journal* records income generated by patient encounters, surgeries, procedures, diagnostic tests and other medical services.

2. The *Cash Receipts Journal* records payments made by insurance companies and patients for the services rendered.

3. The *Purchase Journal* records the purchase of services and goods, such as medical supplies, rent, and equipment needed for practice operations.

4. The *Cash Disbursements Journal* records the practice's payment of its bills.

5. The *Payroll Journal* records the salaries, bonuses, and other compensation paid to the practice's employees.

6. The *General Journal* records any transactions that were not captured by the other journals.

The totals from the various journals are posted into a central file, called the *General Ledger*, which is then used as the basis for producing the practice's tax returns, financial statements, and management reports.

Financial managers must be familiar with and understand basic accounting and finance terminology. Appendix B is a Glossary of Terms that are used in business generally. Armed with an understanding of the flow of financial data and basic accounting and finance terms, financial managers are prepared to analyze and interpret the data. The primary approach used to make sense of financial data is "ratio analysis," where one piece of data is measured in relationship to another piece. There are four categories of ratios. *Profitability ratios* indicate the net return on sales or assets; *activity ratios* indicate how efficiently the business uses its assets; *leverage ratios* measure a business' debt burden; and *liquidity ratios* measure a business' ability to fulfill short-term financial commitments. Appendix C is a summary of common financial ratios, how they are calculated, and what they mean. Appendix D is a list of ratios commonly used in medical practice management.

## Financial Statements and Management Reports

There are four general categories of reports needed to manage a practice. Most reports are produced routinely each month or quarter. *Accounting system reports* include financial statements and other special reports based on the General Ledger generated by accounting software. *Billing system reports* are generated by practice management software and include details of patient services and collection activity. *Management reports* are prepared using Excel or other spreadsheet software and include key data that management has determined to be relevant to monitoring the financial health of the practice. Finally, *ad hoc reports* are produced only as needed to address a particular financial issue.

There are three primary financial statements.

1. The *Income Statement* (a.k.a. *Statement of Revenue and Expenses or Profit and Loss Statement*) shows details of income, expenses, and the resulting profit for a specific period of time (month, quarter, or year-to-date). It provides critical information necessary to determine key operating indicators, such as overhead percentage or collection ratio.

2. The *Balance Sheet* (a.k.a. *Statement of Assets and Liabilities*) shows details of assets, liabilities, and owners' equity at a given point in time. It reflects the accumulation of transactions since the inception of the business. For example, the owners' equity section of the Balance Sheet represents all the money invested in the practice by the owners plus the profits generated by operations and either retained in the business or distributed to the owners.

3. The *Cash Flow Statement* (a.k.a. *Statement of Sources and Uses of Funds*) provides details of the sources and uses of cash generated by the practice, broken down by the type of activity: operations, investing (e.g., purchase of medical equipment) and financing (e.g., bank loans).

Financial statements can be prepared either on the "accrual basis" or the "cash basis." *Accrual basis* financial statements record income when it is earned and expenses when the liability is incurred. *Cash basis* financial statements do not record income until payment is received and only record expenses once the bills are paid. Most private practices use the cash basis of accounting because: 1) it's better for tax purposes (taxes are paid only on income actually received); and 2) it's easier for physicians to understand "real cash" in and out. For management purposes, however, the accrual method is better because it shows the true financial picture, regardless of the timing of collections and disbursements.

Billing system reports vary with each practice management system. However, standard monthly reports should include a summary of charges, payments, and adjustments by provider; details of mandated adjustments (insurance contractual allowances) and non-mandated adjustments (e.g., bad debts and small balance write-offs); accounts receivable aging by payor; and productivity reports of the charges and frequencies of each CPT code for each provider. In addition, there are numerous reports that can be produced as needed to monitor provider productivity, collection efforts, and patient trends. Most reports can be filtered to "slice and dice" by range of dates, type of service, provider, place of service, payor, or patient type.

When designing management reports, the financial manager should follow these guidelines.

1. Present historical data to compare trends.

2. Add perspective with charts, graphs, ratios or narrative commentary.

3. Keep the reports simple and self-explanatory.

4. Layer the detail by putting an executive summary first, followed by supporting detail in order of importance.

5. Check the reports for mathematical accuracy before issuing.

## Financial Benchmarks and Gauging Performance

The four ratios that every medical practice should monitor are :1) overhead expenses as a percent of revenue; 2) gross collection ratio; 3) adjusted collection ratio; and 4) days (or months) fee-for-service charges in accounts receivable. The decision of which other metrics should be monitored depends on the practice's profile and the issues facing the practice at any particular point in time. Table 1 lists some of the possible indicators to be monitored.

## Table 1. Indicators to be Monitored

| Area of Concern | Indicators to be monitored |
|---|---|
| Patient volume | • Charges by provider<br>• Number of encounters, surgeries, procedures, diagnostic tests, or hospital admissions<br>• New visits as a percentage of total visits<br>• Number of physician shifts worked<br>• Number of no-shows<br>• New visits by referral source<br>• Patients by gender, age or zip code |
| Collections | • Gross collection ratio<br>• Payments by payor<br>• Co-payments collected as a percentage of total collections. |
| Billing office performance | • Adjusted collection ratio<br>• Number of days (or months) of fee-for-service charges in accounts receivable<br>• Accounts receivable balances over 120 days<br>• Number of claims processed |
| Managed care reimbursement | • Payor percentage of total charges compared to payor percentage of total payments<br>• Gross collection ratio by payor |
| Overhead | • Operating costs as a percentage of revenue<br>• Operating costs per FTE physician |
| Staff salaries | • Salaries as a percentage of revenue<br>• Salaries per FTE physician<br>• Number of FTE employees per FTE physician |
| Supplies expense | • Supplies per FTE physician<br>• Supplies as a percentage of revenue |
| Facility costs | • Rent per square foot<br>• Square feet per FTE physician |
| Short-term cash | • Current ratio<br>• Accounts payable over 30 days |
| Long-term debt | • Debt ratio<br>• Long-term debt to fixed assets ratio |

When calculating ratios, determine which "normalization" calculations are most appropriate. Examples include calculations based on dollars per physician (or provider), percent of medical revenue, per square foot, or per patient. Also, per-physician and per-employee calculations should be based on full-time equivalents (FTEs), not pure head counts.

The ratios for the practice should be compared to benchmarks, starting with the practice's own historical data. Then, compare to external benchmarks, such as surveys produced by the Medical Group Management Association (MGMA)[1] and similar professional associations, medical specialty societies, and health care research organizations. But remember: surveys are great, but they can be skewed depending on the number of participants, accuracy of their responses, inconsistent definitions, and different demographics. Therefore, the best benchmark is an internal "target" developed by management based on a combination of the practice's historical data and external surveys.

## The Budgeting Process

Budgets provide management with a tool for making better informed decisions about operations, capital investments, and financing needs. There are two types of budgets, each having a distinct purpose. The *static budget* is prepared annually, before the fiscal period starts. It reflects anticipated revenue and expenses based on facts as they are known at the time. Once adopted, the static budget does not change. Accordingly, management can use the budget throughout the year to identify unanticipated variances.

The *dynamic budget* is periodically or systematically updated throughout the year based on new information. Accordingly, management can use the dynamic budget to plan cash flow. However, once revised, the budget is no longer useful for identifying variances. Therefore, some organizations use both types of budgets.

The budgeting process begins with a meeting of key personnel, who review the strategic plan, discuss anticipated changes, and determine baseline assumptions such as salary increases, capital acquisitions and sources of financing. Then the financial manager gathers historical data to use as a starting point for the budget. Documents such as leases, contracts, and quotes for new equipment are reviewed and considered. The financial manager needs to decide whether to create a single budget for the practice, or to create budgets by location or activity center. A spreadsheet is created with rows reflecting sources and uses of cash and columns reflecting each month during the fiscal year. Amounts are then entered based on the combination of historical data, contractual obligations, and baseline assumptions provided by the key personnel, paying careful attention to items that are seasonal or non-recurring. Projected cash balances are calculated monthly, and any excess cash or shortfall is identified.

The financial manager circulates a draft of the budget among the key personnel, who provide their comments and, ultimately, approval of the final version. The budget is then used by management throughout the year to identify variances, control costs, and manage cash flow.

## Understanding and Controlling Costs

The "cost" of an asset is the amount of resources given up to acquire that asset. Sometimes a cost is hard to quantify. Costs can be classified in different ways depending on the purpose of the analysis: direct and indirect; differential/incremental/marginal; controllable versus non-controllable; discretionary versus sunk (funds have already been expended); opportunity costs; actual versus standard costs. Appendix B lists definitions of each of these costs. When used in the context of operating expenses, costs are categorized according to the accounting system's Chart of Accounts, e.g., salaries, supplies, and rent.

Certain costs "behave" differently. Financial managers must understand these behaviors in order to predict and manage costs. Fixed costs, such as office rent, do not change as patient volume increases. Variable costs, such as medical supplies, do increase with volume. Semi-variable costs are a mixture of fixed and variable costs; for example, the cost of x-ray equipment is fixed but the cost of film is variable. Finally, step-fixed costs remain fixed in total over a wide range of volume and then increase in step fashion when patient volume goes beyond this range; for example, support staff costs. Figures 1-4 depict the behavior of these types of costs.

## Figure 1.  Fixed Cost

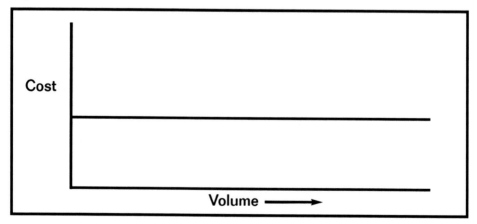

Figure 2. Variable Cost

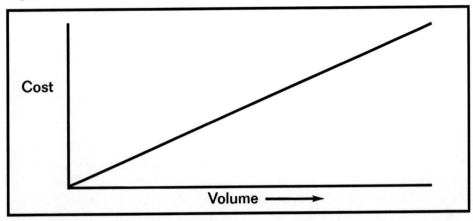

Figure 3. Semi-variable Cost

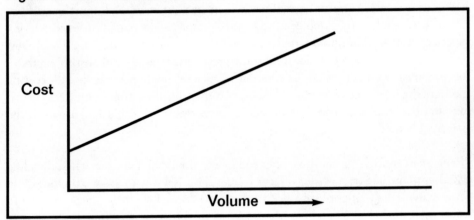

Figure 4. Step-fixed Cost

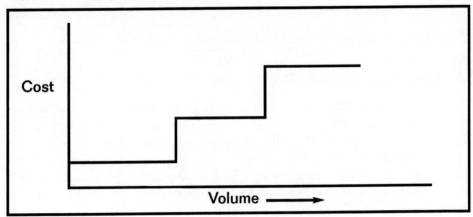

Since the advent of managed care, many practices are using "full cost" methods to measure the cost of their services and, thereby, justify higher reimbursements when negotiating managed care contracts. The process is complicated but, in certain circumstances, well worth the effort. First, identify the "cost centers" in the practice, including administrative departments (medical records, reception, billing and corporate), as well as clinical departments (e.g., providers, lab, x-ray). Next, trace all revenue and expenses to a respective cost center. Then, allocate the expenses of each administrative cost center to each clinical cost center based on assumptions of how those administrative resources are consumed. The sum of the cost center's direct costs and its allocated indirect costs equals its "full cost." To calculate the cost of a particular procedure, divide the "full cost" of each clinical cost center by a relevant metric, such as per-procedure or Relative Value Unit (RVU), which "quantify the work, practice expense, and malpractice costs for specific physician services to appropriately establish payment."[2]

Full costing methods are also useful when management wants to know the profit or loss of a service line (e.g., lab or x-ray), a class of providers (e.g., non-owners), or a practice location. Hospital-owned practices use full costing methods to allocate system-wide costs to each practice, and some group practices use full costing methods for physician compensation calculations. Before implementing a full costing method, financial managers should be certain that the allocation of indirect costs is fair, and that the administrative burden of preparing the calculations is worth the potential benefits.

"Breakeven analysis" is another tool available to financial managers when deciding whether to initiate or continue a service line. This is a way to answer the question: How many units (patient visits, lab tests, x-rays) do we have to produce in order to cover our costs? The formula for determining the breakeven volume is:

Breakeven = Fixed Costs divided by Contribution Margin per Unit
(Where Contribution Margin per Unit = Price per Unit minus Variable Cost per Unit)

Figure 5, page 333, depicts a breakeven analysis.

## Managing Cash Flow and Receivables

The lifeblood of any practice is accounts receivable because of the direct impact on cash flow. Financial managers use various reports to help them monitor cash flow and predict any cash shortfalls. A weekly *Cash Available* report reflects the cash balance at the beginning of the week, plus collections and minus cash disbursements, to reconcile to the ending cash balance. It also lists a total of payroll and accounts payable that need to be paid within the next week. Another

**Figure 5. Breakeven under fee-for-service**

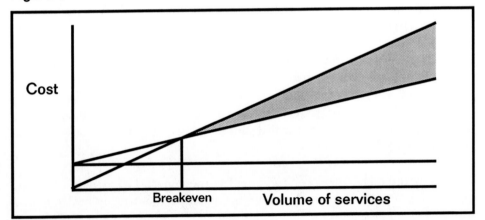

method is to compare the actual cash balance to the budgeted cash balance and investigate any major variances.

The best tool for monitoring accounts receivable is the monthly Accounts Receivable Aging report. When each aging "bucket" is listed beside the previous months, the financial manager can quickly identify trends and investigate any unexpected increases in the older aging categories. This report can be presented in either dollars, percentages of total, or both. To pinpoint problem areas, the Accounts Receivable Aging report can be filtered to represent only amounts due from patients, primary insurance, or secondary insurance. Since insurance accounts are typically easier to collect, collection efforts can be redirected accordingly.

Most medical billing professionals agree that the best way to prevent cash flow problems is to be proactive about collecting patient payments at the time of service and to have a tightly structured process for capturing charges, submitting claims, and following up on open accounts.

## Measuring Return on Investments

From the first day that they hang out a shingle, physicians make investment decisions. Whether purchasing equipment, opening a satellite office, offering a new service line, or hiring a new associate, decisions should be made based on sound economic principles.

A simplified approach to measuring return on investment (ROI) is to compare the projected profit (revenue minus expenses) generated over the life of the investment to the original cost of the investment, and hope that the former exceeds the latter. The better analyses also consider the "time value of money." A dollar received today is worth more than a dollar expected tomorrow. Why? Because inflation will eat away at tomorrow's dollar, and there's always some risk that the dollar will never be collected. When we quantify the time value of money, we use "compound interest" theory to determine the *future value* (the amount to which a given amount of cash invested will grow at the end of a given period of time when compounded by a given rate of interest) or the *present value* (the amount that, if invested today at a designated rate of return for a specified period of time in the future, would accumulate to a specified amount).

The "Look-up Table" in Appendix E depicts the concepts of present value and future value. As you can see, there are three variables that need to be determined when using either approach.

- *Amount:* the best possible estimate of future cash flows (revenue, expenses and original cost) to be derived from the project. This is often the hardest variable to determine because it involves assumptions about patient volume, reimbursement rates, and fixed and variable costs. Be sure to consider all incremental operating costs and all acquisition costs, such as delivery, installation, and training.

- *Time:* the estimated length of time involved in the project; for example, the expected useful life of a proposed piece of equipment.

- *Rate:* the rate of return that your investors will require to compensate them for the risk involved in the project; the higher the risk, the higher the expected rate of return.

There are many models for evaluating ROI. Following is a description of four such models. The first two are preferred methods that consider the time value of money. The second two are simplified approaches, which are presented because they are popular, "quick and dirty" approaches.

**Net Present Value:** Using a financial calculator or computer software, calculate the present value of the net cash inflows (projected annual revenue minus expenses) over the life of the project. If the present value of the net cash inflows is less than the initial cash outlay, then No Go.

**Internal Rate of Return (IRR):** Using a financial calculator or computer software, calculate the rate of return that equates the initial cash outflow and the stream of cash inflows. If the calculated rate of return is less than the required rate of return, then No Go.

**Payback Period:** Divide the required initial cash outlay by the annual cash inflows to determine the number of years over which the initial outlay will be received. If the payback period is more than, equal to, or slightly less than the economic life of the project, then No Go.

**Average or Unadjusted Rate of Return:** Divide the average annual income from the project (net of depreciation) by the required initial cash outlay to get the average rate of return. If the average rate of return is less than the required rate of return, then No Go.

No one method should be considered in isolation. Instead, these models should be considered, and only then selected in the context of other non-economic factors, such as the impact on patient care and the overall strategic plan of the practice.

## Financing Considerations

The need for capital arises throughout the life cycle of a medical practice. Every investment decision requires a financing decision. Financing can be obtained from internal sources by capital contributions from the owners and retained earnings, or from external sources such as third-party lenders, leasing companies, or hospital systems.

The most common source of third-party financing is *commercial lenders*. When selecting a financial institution, interest rates alone should not be the determining factor. The financial manager should also look for a bank whose service representatives understand the health care industry, are stable, service-oriented, and can make local decisions.

Loan underwriting criteria will usually require the practice to offer its accounts receivable and fixed assets as collateral for the loan. Depending on the credit history of the practice, the lender may require personal guarantees. There may be other financial and reporting covenants, such as the requirement to maintain all banking relationships with the lender, to submit regular financial reports, or to maintain minimum debt coverage or equity ratios.

The specific terms of the loan will depend on the type of loan. *Short-term loans* are typically used for temporary swings in working capital, due in 3 to 12 months, and require interest-only payments. *Intermediate-term loans* are typically used for the acquisition of tangible personal property, the term is tied to the life of the asset (usually 1 to 8 years), and require fixed principal and interest payments. *Long-term loans* are typically used for purchasing real estate, and require fixed principal and interest payments over 15 to 30 years.

Another source of financing is *leasing companies*. Leases can be true (operating) leases or capital (finance) leases. The term of an operating lease is often shorter than the useful life of the asset. The lessor retains the title to the asset at the end of the lease, or the lessee has the right to purchase the asset at its then-fair market value. Neither the asset nor the liability is shown on the lessee's balance sheet. Most operating leases are for office space, automobiles, or office equipment.

The term of a capital lease usually approximates the useful life of the asset and the lessee has the option to purchase the asset at the end of the lease for a nominal amount. Because a capital lease is similar to a commercial loan, the lessee does show the asset (and liability) on its balance sheet.

The advantages of leasing rather than purchasing fixed assets are that: 1) leases do not require a large down payment; 2) it's easier to get credit for a lease since the lessor retains the title; 3) a lease limits the lessee's risk of obsolescence, if the asset is one that involves rapidly changing technology; and 4) the liability is not reflected in the lessee's balance sheet, which otherwise could impact the lessee's credit rating. The disadvantage of leasing is that leases usually have higher interest rates compared to commercial lenders.

There are also tax issues involved in the decision whether to lease or purchase, which are outside the scope of this textbook. Since tax laws change frequently, the practice should consult its tax advisor before making a final decision.

Hospitals or other health care organizations can be sources of financing for physician practices, but only within the constraints of self-referral, anti-inurement, and other fraud and abuse legislation that generally require that transactions between hospitals and physicians must be done at fair market value. However, in limited circumstances and subject to specific rules and regulations, hospitals can subsidize physician practices when there is a demonstrated need in the community for physicians in the particular specialty.

Regardless of the source of funding, the practice should have a business plan to support any major undertaking. A business plan should contain a statement of the goals and objectives of the venture, a description of the planned services, an action plan, a description of the practice's organization and management team, a survey of market data for the service area, and financial projections.

## Conclusion

Financial management of a medical practice is an ongoing and complex process. Physician leaders must work together to ensure that the practice has the reporting tools and information needed to make good financial decisions.

## Case Study

Review the Accrual Basis Balance Sheet and Income Statement below.

**Anytown Medical Group**
**Accrual Basis Balance Sheet**
**December 31, 20x1**

**ASSETS**

Current Assets

| | |
|---|---:|
| Cash – unrestricted | $ 50,000 |
| Cash – certificate of deposit | 100,000 |
| Accounts receivable | 500,000 |
| Less: provision for allowances | (200,000) |
| Supplies | 30,000 |
| Prepaid insurance | 20,000 |
| Total current assets | 500,000 |

Fixed Assets

| | |
|---|---:|
| Medical equipment | 25,000 |
| Office furniture & equipment | 15,000 |
| Software | 10,000 |
| Less: accumulated depreciation | (20,000) |
| Net fixed assets | 30,000 |

Other Assets

| | |
|---|---:|
| Security deposits | 5,000 |
| Investment in Surgery Center | 2,000 |
| Total other assets | 7,000 |
| Total Assets | $ 537,000 |

**LIABILITIES AND STOCKHOLDERS' EQUITY**

Current Liabilities

| | |
|---|---:|
| Accounts payable | $ 20,000 |
| Line of credit | 30,000 |
| Payroll withholdings | 25,000 |
| Accrued payroll liabilities | 15,000 |
| Total current liabilities | 90,000 |
| Notes Payable | 25,000 |

Stockholders' Equity

| | |
|---|---:|
| Common stock | 1,000 |
| Additional paid in cpaital | 20,000 |
| Retained earnings | 401,000 |
| Total stockholders' equity | 422,000 |
| Total liabilities and stockholders' equity | $ 537,000 |

## Anytown Medical Group
## Accrual Basis Income Statement
## December 31, 20x1

**Revenue**

| | |
|---|---:|
| Gross charges | $ 2,200,000 |
| Less: contractual allowances | (1,150,000) |
| Less: bad debts | (50,000) |
| Net revenue | 1,000,000 |

**Operating Expenses**

**Support staff salaries and fringe benefits**

| | |
|---|---:|
| Administrative staff salaries | 105,000 |
| Clinical staff salaries | 50,000 |
| Ancillary staff salaries | 40,000 |
| Total salaries | 195,000 |
| Support staff benefits | 50,000 |
| Total support staff salaries and fringe benefits | 245,000 |

**Other operating expenses**

| | |
|---|---:|
| Information technology | 15,000 |
| Medical and surgical supplies | 14,000 |
| Building and occupancy | 46,000 |
| Furniture & equipment | 12,000 |
| Administrative supplies and services | 15,000 |
| Professional liability insurance | 20,000 |
| Other insurance premiums | 2,000 |
| Outside professional fees | 7,000 |
| Promotion and marketing | 3,000 |
| Clinical laboratory | 4,000 |
| Radiology and imaging | 50,000 |
| Other ancillary services | 7,000 |
| Total other operating expenses | 195,000 |

| | |
|---|---:|
| **Total Operating Expenses** | 440,000 |
| **Income Available for Providers** | 560,000 |

**Provider salaries and benefits**

| | |
|---|---:|
| Physician salaries | 400,000 |
| Nonphysician provider salaries | 100,000 |
| Employee benefits | 50,000 |
| Total provider salaries and fringe benefits | 550,000 |

| | |
|---|---:|
| **Net Income** | $    10,000 |

1. How would these financial statements be different if the organization's accounting practices were on a cash basis?

2. How can you tell whether this practice is "profitable"? What if I told you that net revenue last year was $800,000? What if income available for providers last year was $650,000?

## Study/Discussion Questions (Answers are in italics.)

1. Patient revenue, cash receipts, purchase, cash payment and payroll represent: (a) balance sheet items, (b) income statement items, (c) *accounting journals*.

2. Ratios should be broken down into categories (profit, leverage, activity and liquidity) and compared to (a) external standards, (b) revenue, (c) internal trends, (d) assets, (e) *a and c*.

3. View costs from various perspectives: categorical (e.g., salaries, supplies, rent, utilities) and behavioral. Examples of how costs "behave" include _____, _____, _____ and _____. (*fixed, variable, semi-variable, and step-fixed*).

4. Four key evaluation models include: *net present value, internal rate of return*, payback period and average rate of return. The two models that consider the "time value of money" are _____ and _____.

5. Which type of financing includes the following advantages: no large down payment, ease of obtaining credit, limited risk of obsolescence, and the liability is not reflected on balance sheet? (a) bank loan, (b) *operating lease*, (c) both.

## Suggested Readings

*Financial Management for Medical Groups*, Ernest J. Pavlock, Ph.D., CPA, Medical Group Management Association, Second Edition, 2000.

*Medical Practice Management Handbook*, Reed Tinsley, CCH, Incorporated, Eighth Edition, 2002.

*Physician Compensation and Production Survey: 2005 Report Based on 2004 Data*, Medical Group Management Association, August 2005.

*Cost Survey for Single Specialty Practices: 2005 Report Based on 2004 Data*, Medical Group Management Association, October 2005.

*Cost Survey for Multispecialty Practices: 2005 Report Based on 2004 Data*, Medical Group Management Association, October 2005.

*Chart of Accounts for Health Care Organizations*, Neill Piland, Dr. P.H. and Kathryn P. Glass, MBA, MSHA, Center for Research in Ambulatory Health Care Administration.

*Medical Practice Business Plan Workbook, Second Edition*, Peter D. Lucash, Digital CPE Press/MGMA, November 2003.

## References

1. Medical Group Management Association. MGMA Practice Data and Surveys. Available at: http://www.mgma.com/surveys/. Accessed August 18, 2006.

2. Johnson SE, Newton WP. Resource-based relative value units: A primer for academic family physicians. *Fam Med.* 2002;34:172-176.

## Appendix A

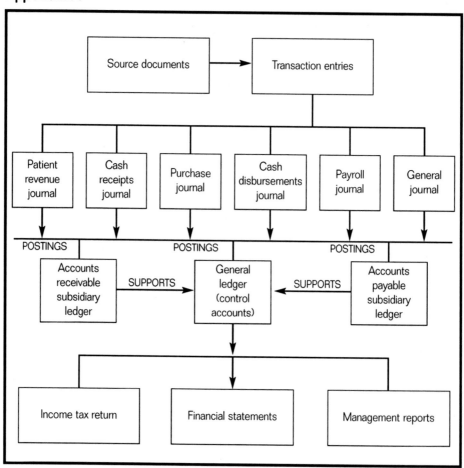

## Appendix B

### Glossary of Accounting and Finance Terms

**Accelerated depreciation** – Any method of depreciating an asset that produces higher depreciation in earlier years than in later years.

**Accounting (average) rate of return** – The rate of return on an investment computed as accounting profit divided by some measure of investment; e.g., average profit per year divided by initial investment.

**Acid-test ratio** – Ratio of cash and other current monetary assets to current liabilities.

**Activity ratio** – A financial ratio that indicates how efficiently a firm uses its assets: inventory turnover, average collection period, fixed-asset turnover, and total asset turnover are activity ratios.

**Administrative costs** – The costs of the different activities or functions included under the broad heading of administration; includes the activities associated with such officials as the president, administrative vice-presidents, the controller, the treasurer, the personnel director, the director of purchasing, the legal counsel, and the director of information systems.

**Annuity** – A series of equal periodic payments or receipts.

**Asset turnover** – Ratio of sales to total assets; average total assets preferred.

**Balance sheet** – A financial statement summarizing the assets, liabilities, and net worth (equity) of an individual or business as of a given date.

**Balance sheet method** – Forecasts of future financing requirements and available cash based on forecast income statements and balance sheets.

**Benefit-cost ratio** – For an investment, the ratio of the present value of its future cash flows to its initial cost. The benefit-cost ratio method uses the ratio to evaluate investment opportunities.

**Book value** – The original cost of an asset minus total depreciation deductions made to date; this is the value indicated by the firm's financial statements.

**Break-even sales; break-even point** – The volume of sales at which the sales revenue equals total costs.

**Budgeted balance sheet** – Balance sheet based on planned activities; part of the master profit plan.

**Budgeted income statement** – Income statement based on planned activities; part of the master profit plan.

**Capital asset** – A physical asset (plant and equipment) used by a firm in producing goods or services.

**Capital budget** – A statement of the firm's planned investments, generally based upon estimates of future sales, production needs, and availability of capital.

**Capital budgeting** – Planning of long-term capital investments; often refers to the process of evaluating the costs and benefits of long-range projects.

**Capital gains (losses)** – The difference between the original cost of an asset and its selling price. Capital gains (losses) are *realized* when the asset is sold.

**Capital income** – Income produced from investing money, such as dividends and interest.

**Capital structure** – The composition of a firm's financing; often refers to the proportion of long-term debt, preferred stock, and common equity on the firm's balance sheet.

**Cash budget** – Statement that shows expected cash receipts and expected cash disbursements; part of master profit plan.

**Cash flow forecasts** – Forecasts of cash receipts and payments for one or more periods.

**Cash flow from an investment** – The dollars coming to the firm (cash inflow) or paid out by the firm (cash outflow) as a result of adopting the investment.

**Cash flows** – Cash receipts and cash disbursements expected over the life of a capital investment.

**Collateral** – Property pledged by a borrower as security on the loan.

**Collection period** – The time period from the date of sale of the firm's product to the date of collection of cash from the customer.

**Committed cost** – A fixed cost arising from past decisions to provide for a certain production capacity; also capacity cost.

**Common stock** – A document that represents the ownership of a corporation.

**Compensating balance** – Money that must be on deposit at a bank to compensate the bank for services; may be a requirement of a loan.

**Compound interest** – Interest that is paid or received on interest accumulated from prior periods.

**Consumer price index** – The average price (in a certain period) of a typical package of consumer goods and services expressed as a percentage of the average price of the same package in a base period.

**Contribution margin** – Sales revenue less variable costs.

**Controllable cost** – A cost that can be influenced by a manager's decisions and actions; contrast with noncontrollable cost, which is outside a manager's influence.

**Controllable profit** – A measure of profit center profit that excludes those expenses that cannot be controlled by the profit center manager.

**Corporation** – A business that has been chartered by a state and whose owners are not personally responsible for the business' debts.

# Chapter 19: *Fundamentals of Health Care Accounting and Finance* 343

**Cost** – A sacrifice incurred in economic activity.

**Cost of capital** – The average cost of long-term financing expressed as an interest rate.

**Covenant** – A promise by the firm, included in the debt contract, to perform a certain act (e.g., to pay interest on the debt); a *restrictive covenant* is one that imposes constraints upon the firm in order to protect the debt-holders' interest (e.g., a requirement that the firm maintain a particular current ratio).

**Current ratio** – Current assets divided by current liabilities; a measure of a firm's liquidity.

**Debt capacity** – The maximum amount of debt that can feasibly be outstanding for a firm at a given point in time.

**Debt financing** – Acquisition of assets with the use of borrowed money.

**Debt ratio** – Total firm debt divided by total assets; a measure of a firm's debt burden.

**Depreciation** – A deduction of part of the cost of an asset from income in each year of the asset's life.

**Differential costs** – Costs that change as a result of a decision; same as incremental costs.

**Differential revenue** – Change in revenue as a result of a particular decision.

**Direct costs** – Costs that can be traced unequivocally to a cost objective.

**Direct labor** – Labor applied directly to a product.

**Direct materials** – Cost of materials that enter into, and become a constituent part of the product.

**Discretionary cost** – A cost (usually fixed) that results from a management decision to carry out a specific program or undertake a specific policy; same as programmed cost.

**Earned income** – Income produced by an individual's personal services.

**EBIT** – Earnings before debt interest and income taxes are deducted.

**Equity financing** – Acquisition of assets with the use of money received from stockholders from the issuance of stock.

**Equity investment** – That portion of firm investment financed from retained earnings or from the sale of equity securities such as common stock or warrants.

**Expenditure** – The payment of money or the incurrence of a liability as a result of acquiring resources; for example, the purchase of materials or the payment of salaries.

**External financing** – Raising money by issuing new securities or by borrowing.

**Financial lease** – A lease that is noncancellable (except by mutual consent of both lessor and lessee) and that generally has a duration equal to most of the economic life of the asset.

**Financial ratio** – A ratio of dollar magnitudes, obtained from a firm's financial statements, that reflects some aspect of the firm's performance.

**Financial risk** – The uncertainty as to the future returns to a firm's owners resulting from the use of debt or preferred stock.

**Fixed cost** – A cost that does not change as output changes.

**Flexible budget** – A production cost budget or expense budget that can be adjusted to different levels of volume.

**Funds** – A term that normally refers either to cash or to working capital (current assets minus current liabilities).

**Funds flow** – The flow of funds through the firm; this flow is described by a sources and uses statement.

**Future value** – Amount to which a given amount of cash invested will grow at the end of a given period of time when compounded by a given rate of interest.

**General partnership** – A business in which each partner is personally responsible for any debts of the business.

**Historical cost** – Cost measured by the past actual sacrifice.

**Incremental costs** – Costs that will change as a result of a decision; same as differential costs, relevant costs.

**Incremental internal rate of return method** – A method for comparing two or more mutually exclusive investments using the IRR approach. This method examines the IRR on the additional (or "incremental") cash flow produced by one investment relative to any mutually exclusive alternative in order to determine which is more profitable.

**Incremental investment** – In an asset replacement decision, the difference between the investment required for the new asset and the investment in the old asset; usually means the investment in the new asset less the sales value of the old asset.

**Incremental profit (income)** – Difference between incremental revenue and incremental costs; the change in income arising because of a decision.

**Incremental revenues** – The change in revenues as a result of a decision.

**Indirect costs** – Costs incurred for more than one cost objective.

**Inflation** – Increase in the general price level.

**Interim financing** – Short-term loans to be repaid from long-term debt or other financing in the future.

**Internal financing** – Financing with money earned and retained in the business.

**Internal investment** – A firm's investment that involves the direct acquisition of productive assets rather than the acquisition of another firm or the productive assets of another firm (**external investment**).

**Internal rate of return** – The interest rate that makes the present value of the cash flows of an investment equal to the investment.

**Lessee** – The user of a leased asset who pays the lessor for the usage right.

**Lessor** – The owner of a leased asset.

**Letter of credit** – A written statement by a bank that money will be loaned provided that conditions specified in the letter are met.

**Leverage** – The degree of firm borrowing.

**Leverage ratio** – A financial ratio that measures a firm's debt burden; the debt, times interest earned, and fixed-charges coverage ratios are leverage ratios.

**Leveraged lease (or "third-party lease")** – An arrangement under which the lessor borrows funds to cover part or all of the purchase price of the asset.

**Limited liability** – A legal term that means that the owner of a business is not personally responsible for its debts; only his investment in the business is available to its creditors.

**Limited liability company** – An unincorporated business in which the partners (members) are not personally liable for any debts.

**Limited partnership** – A business in which some partners (the general partners) are personally responsible for any debts, but the other partners (the limited partners) are not.

**Limiting factors** – Physical or economic conditions that restrict production; in most cases, the demand for a product will restrict the production of that product; in some cases, production capacity will restrict production below the limit set by market demand for a product.

**Line of credit** – An agreement by a bank to loan money to a customer, as needed, up to a stated maximum amount.

**Line-item budget** – A budget expressed in objects of expenditure; a budget that shows the planned expenditures for the different resources such as materials, personal services, and purchased services.

**Liquidation** – The sale of a firm's assets when the company is dissolved.

**Liquidity ratio** – A financial ratio that measures a firm's ability to fulfill short-run financial commitments; the current and quick ratios are liquidity ratios.

**Market value (or market price)** – The value that an asset (e.g., a security such as a share of stock or a physical asset such as a machine) is bought and sold for in the market.

**Marketing costs** – The costs of the different activities associated with selling and promoting a company's products, warehousing merchandise or finished goods, shipping goods to customers, advertising, and market research.

**Master profit plan; master budget** – The financial statements that are based on the operating plans for the period; includes the planned income statement, the planned cash receipts and disbursements, and the planned balance sheet.

**Matching principle** – A principle that holds that the firm should finance short-term needs with short-term sources and long-term needs with long-term sources.

**Merger** – The combination of two or more firms with one of them surviving (e.g., firm A merging with firm B with firm A surviving).

**Minimum acceptable rate of return** – The lowest rate of return that an investment can be expected to earn and still be acceptable; same as the investment's **cost of capital, required rate of return, hurdle rate,** or **capitalization rate.**

**Mortgage** – A pledge of specific property given by a borrower as security on a loan.

**Net lease** – A lease under which the lessee pays all maintenance and upkeep of the asset.

**Net present value** – The difference between the present value of the cash flows of an investment (when cash flows are discounted by a specified interest rate) and the amount of the investment.

**Net profit** – After-tax net income to stockholders; sometimes also used to refer to the annual annuity that is equivalent to a given net present value.

**Noncontrollable costs** – Costs that an individual manager cannot influence by his or her decisions.

**Operating lease** – A lease that is cancelable by the lessee at any time upon due notice to the lessor; also called a **service lease.**

**Opportunity costs** – the sacrifice associated with a specific alternative.

**Payback period** – The amount of time required for an asset to generate enough cash flow to just cover the initial outlay for that asset; an asset costing $1,500 and generating an after-tax cash flow of $500 per year has a payback period of three years ($1,500/$500).

**Payback period method** – A capital budgeting technique that specifies that an investment is acceptable only if it has a payback period less than or equal to some specified time period, e.g., three years.

**Percentage analysis** – Constructing the income statement to show sales as equal to 100% and each item as a percent of sales.

**Period costs** – Costs not assigned to products but charged as expenses of the period.

**Personal property** – All property other than **real property.**

**Present value** – Amount that, if invested today at a designated rate of return for a specified time in the future, would accumulate to a specified amount.

**Present value index** – The ratio of the present value of the cash flows of an investment to the investment.

**Prime rate** – Interest rate charged by banks on short-term loans to large, low-risk businesses.

**Principal** – The amount on which interest is paid by a borrower or the amount on which interest is received by a lender.

**Product costs** – Manufacturing costs incurred to produce products; the costs of direct materials, direct labor, and factory overhead that constitute the cost of manufactured products.

**Profit center** – A division or segment of the business that is responsible for revenues and expenses.

**Profit objectives** – A company's goal for income; may be expressed as the rate of net income on sales, rate of net income on owners' equity, or percentage of operating income to assets.

**Profit performance report** – Income statement that compares actual revenue and expenses with budgeted revenue and expense.

**Profitability index** – A measure of the profitability of an investment computed by dividing the net present value (or simply present value of future cash flows) by the initial cost of the investment.

**Profitability ratio** – A financial ratio that indicates the net returns on sales or assets; net operating margin, profit margin on sales, return on total assets, and return on net worth are profitability ratios.

**Proprietorship** – A business owned by an individual who is personally responsible for all its debts.

**Quantity or usage variance** – A variance from standard arising because the actual quantity or hours differed from the standard quantity or hours.

**Quick ratio (or acid test ratio)** – A measure of the firm's liquidity equal to [(current assets – inventory) ÷ current liabilities].

**Rate of return** – The interest rate earned on an investment; may be an actual or expected rate.

**Rate of return on sales** – Ratio of net income to sales.

**Real property** – Land and buildings.

**Replacement costs** – The cost today to replace an asset.

**Responsibility accounting** – A system of accounting that collects revenues and expenses by areas of managerial responsibility.

**Retained earnings** – The earnings in a given period that have been retained by the firm rather than paid out as dividends; also refers to the balance sheet account that is the sum of all earnings retained to date.

**Return on investment** – Ratio of income to investment; may be operating income to total assets or net income to owner's equity

**Return on total assets** – Ratio of operating income to total assets; average total assets preferred to either beginning or ending total assets.

**Revolving credit** – Legal commitment by a bank to loan money to a customer, as needed, up to a stated maximum amount. The time period covered by the agreement may extend for several years.

**Sales budget** – Planned sales for each product or product group; expressed in units of product for individual products and in dollars for product groups.

**Sales forecast** – A prediction of sales based on economic conditions and other environmental factors that are expected to affect sales.

**Semi-fixed cost** – A cost that remains fixed in total over a wide range of volume and that increases in step fashion when volume goes beyond this range.

**Semi-variable cost** – A cost that is a mixture of variable and fixed costs.

**Sensitivity analysis** – Analysis of the effect on a project's cash flows or profitability of possible changes in factors that affect the project (e.g., sales, various costs, etc.).

**Simple rate of return** – Net income on investment divided by the average investment.

**Spending variance** – A variance from standard overhead cost arising because the amount actually incurred for overhead differed from the amount of overhead budgeted; thus, if overhead is budgeted on the basis of direct labor hours, the spending variance would be the difference between actual overhead and the overhead budgeted for the actual direct labor hours.

**Standard cost** – The direct materials, direct labor, and overhead cost of a product that should be incurred under reasonably efficient conditions of production.

**Statement analysis** – Development of ratios and percentages from information taken form the financial statements.

**Sunk costs** – Those cost that do not change as a result of a decision; sunk costs are past costs and are irrelevant to decisions.

**Time value of money** – Value of money expressed as a function of time; value of money decreases as the length of time increases; illustrated by the fact that a dollar received today is worth more than a dollar to be received in the future.

**Time-adjusted rate of return** – The rate of return on an investment that recognizes the time value of money; the rate reflects the fact that a dollar of cash flow in the future is worth less than a dollar of cash flow to be received now.

**Trend analysis** – Percentage analysis of income statements for several years; may include other important ratios and percentages.

**Variable cost** – A cost that changes as output changes.

**Variable rate loan** – A loan with an interest rate that varies according to the general level of interest rates. The interest rate is not fixed over the period of the loan.

**Variance analysis** – The analysis of the difference between actual manufacturing costs and standard manufacturing costs to derive price, rate, efficiency, spending, and volume variances.

**Volume variance** – The variance from standard cost arising because actual volume of production differed for the standard or normal volume.

**Working capital** – Current assets *minus* current liabilities (sometimes referred to as **net working capital**).

**Working capital budget** – Budget that shows the components of working capital that the company expects to have at the end of the planning period.

**Zero-base budgeting** – An approach to budgeting that considers whether an activity is really necessary; for necessary activities, budgeting begins at a minimum, bare existence level of expenditure and adds increments of expenditure in a decreasing order of priority.

## Appendix C

### Summary of Common Financial Ratios

| RATIO | FORMULA | INDICATION |
|---|---|---|
| *Profitability ratios:* | | |
| Profit as a percent of sales | $\dfrac{\text{Profit after taxes}}{\text{Sales}}$ | Profit margin on sales |
| Return on total assets | $\dfrac{\text{Earnings before interest + Taxes}}{\text{Total assets}}$ | Return on total investment |
| Return on net worth | $\dfrac{\text{Profit after taxes}}{\text{Owners' equity}}$ | Return on owners' investment |
| *Activity ratios:* | | |
| Fixed assets ratio | $\dfrac{\text{Sales}}{\text{Fixed Assets}}$ | Turnover on plant and equipment |
| Total assets turnover | $\dfrac{\text{Sales}}{\text{Total assets}}$ | Turnover on all assets |
| Inventory turnover | $\dfrac{\text{Costs of goods sold}}{\text{Inventories}}$ | Level of inventory |
| Average collection period | $\dfrac{\text{Accounts receivable}}{\text{Sales per day}}$ | Length of time between making a sale and receiving cash for it |
| *Leverage ratios:* | | |
| Debt ratio | $\dfrac{\text{Total debt}}{\text{Total assets}}$ | Level of funds collected by creditors |
| Times interest earned | $\dfrac{\text{Earnings before interest + Taxes}}{\text{Interest charges}}$ | Ability to meet current debt obligation |
| Fixed charge coverage | $\dfrac{\text{Earnings before taxes + Interest charges + Lease obligation}}{\text{Interest charge + Lease obligations}}$ | Ability to meet current debt and lease obligation |
| Days payable | $\dfrac{\text{Accounts payable}}{\text{Purchases per day}}$ | Level of financing by suppliers |
| *Liquidity ratios:* | | |
| Current ratio | $\dfrac{\text{Current assets}}{\text{Current liabilities}}$ | Short-term solvency |
| Quick ratio | $\dfrac{\text{Current assets - Inventories}}{\text{Current liabilities}}$ | Very short-term solvency |

## Appendix D

### Ratios Commonly Used in Medical Practices

| Formulas for Ratios | Data Normalization Calculations |
|---|---|
| Adjusted fee-for-service collection percentage = <br><br> $\dfrac{\text{(Net FFS revenue)}}{\text{(Adjusted FFS charges)}}$ | Per FTE physician = <br><br> $\dfrac{\text{<performance measure>}}{\text{(Total physician FTE)}}$ |
| Current ratio = <br><br> $\dfrac{\text{(Current assets)}}{\text{(Current liabilities)}}$ | As a percent of total medical revenue = <br><br> $\dfrac{\text{<performance measure>}}{\text{(Total medical revenue)}}$ |
| Days of gross fee-for-service charges in accounts receivable = <br><br> $\dfrac{\text{(Total accounts receivable)}}{\text{(Gross FFS charges) x (1/365)}}$ | Per FTE provider = <br><br> $\dfrac{\text{<performance measure>}}{\text{(Total provider FTE)}}$ |
| Debt ratio = <br><br> $\dfrac{\text{(Total liabilities)}}{\text{(Total assets)}}$ | Per square foot = <br><br> $\dfrac{\text{<performance measure>}}{\text{(Square feet)}}$ |
| Debt to equity ratio = <br><br> $\dfrac{\text{(Total liabilities)}}{\text{(Total net worth)}}$ | Per total RVU = <br><br> $\dfrac{\text{<performance measure>}}{\text{(Total RVUs)}}$ |
| Gross fee-for-service collection percentage = <br><br> $\dfrac{\text{(Net FFS revenue)}}{\text{(Gross FFS charges)}}$ | Per work RVU = <br><br> $\dfrac{\text{<performance measure>}}{\text{(Physician work RVUs)}}$ |
| Months of gross-fee-for-service charges in accounts receivable = <br><br> $\dfrac{\text{(Total accounts receivable)}}{\text{(Gross FFS charges) x (1/12)}}$ | Per patient = <br><br> $\dfrac{\text{<performance measure>}}{\text{(Number of patients)}}$ |
| | Per encounter = <br> $\dfrac{\text{<performance measure>}}{\text{(Patient encounters)}}$ |

# Appendix E

## Look Up Table for TVM Problems

**Present Value Factors: Present Value of $1 to be Received after T Periods = 1/(1 + r)T**

Interest Rate

| Period | 1% | 2% | 3% | 4% | 5% | 6% | 7% | 8% | 9% | 10% | 12% | 14% |
|---|---|---|---|---|---|---|---|---|---|---|---|---|
| 1 | 0.9901 | 0.9804 | 0.9709 | 0.9615 | 0.9524 | 0.9434 | 0.9346 | 0.9259 | 0.9174 | 0.9091 | 0.8929 | 0.8772 |
| 2 | 0.9803 | 0.9612 | 0.9426 | 0.9246 | 0.9070 | 0.8900 | 0.8734 | 0.8573 | 0.8417 | 0.8264 | 0.7972 | 0.7695 |
| 3 | 0.9706 | 0.9423 | 0.9151 | 0.8890 | 0.8638 | 0.8396 | 0.8163 | 0.7938 | 0.7722 | 0.7513 | 0.7118 | 0.6750 |
| 4 | 0.9610 | 0.9238 | 0.8885 | 0.8548 | 0.8227 | 0.7921 | 0.7629 | 0.7350 | 0.7084 | 0.6830 | 0.6355 | 0.5921 |
| 5 | 0.9515 | 0.9057 | 0.8626 | 0.8219 | 0.7835 | 0.7473 | 0.7130 | 0.6806 | 0.6499 | 0.6209 | 0.5674 | 0.5194 |
| 6 | 0.9420 | 0.8880 | 0.8375 | 0.7903 | 0.7462 | 0.7050 | 0.6663 | 0.6302 | 0.5963 | 0.5645 | 0.5066 | 0.4556 |
| 7 | 0.9327 | 0.8706 | 0.8131 | 0.7599 | 0.7107 | 0.6651 | 0.6227 | 0.5835 | 0.5470 | 0.5132 | 0.4523 | 0.3996 |
| 8 | 0.9235 | 0.8535 | 0.7894 | 0.7307 | 0.6768 | 0.6274 | 0.5820 | 0.5403 | 0.5019 | 0.4665 | 0.4039 | 0.3506 |
| 9 | 0.9143 | 0.8368 | 0.7664 | 0.7026 | 0.6446 | 0.5919 | 0.5439 | 0.5002 | 0.4604 | 0.4241 | 0.3606 | 0.3075 |
| 10 | 0.9053 | 0.8203 | 0.7441 | 0.6756 | 0.6139 | 0.5584 | 0.5083 | 0.4632 | 0.4224 | 0.3855 | 0.3220 | 0.2697 |

**Future Value Factors: Future Value of $1 to be Received after T Periods = (1 = r)T**

Interest Rate

| Period | 1% | 2% | 3% | 4% | 5% | 6% | 7% | 8% | 9% | 10% | 12% | 14% |
|---|---|---|---|---|---|---|---|---|---|---|---|---|
| 1 | 1.0100 | 1.0200 | 1.0300 | 1.0400 | 1.0500 | 1.0600 | 1.0700 | 1.0800 | 1.0900 | 1.1000 | 1.1200 | 1.1400 |
| 2 | 1.0201 | 1.0404 | 1.0609 | 1.0816 | 1.1025 | 1.1236 | 1.1449 | 1.1664 | 1.1881 | 1.2100 | 1.2544 | 1.2996 |
| 3 | 1.0303 | 1.0621 | 1.0927 | 1.1249 | 1.1576 | 1.1910 | 1.2250 | 1.2597 | 1.2950 | 1.3310 | 1.4049 | 1.4815 |
| 4 | 1.0406 | 1.0824 | 1.1255 | 1.1699 | 1.2155 | 1.2625 | 1.3108 | 1.3605 | 1.4116 | 1.4641 | 1.5735 | 1.6890 |
| 5 | 1.0510 | 1.1041 | 1.1593 | 1.2167 | 1.2763 | 1.3382 | 1.4026 | 1.4693 | 1.5386 | 1.6105 | 1.7623 | 1.9254 |
| 6 | 1.0615 | 1.1262 | 1.1941 | 1.2653 | 1.3401 | 1.4185 | 1.5007 | 1.5869 | 1.6771 | 1.7716 | 1.9738 | 2.1950 |
| 7 | 1.0721 | 1.1487 | 1.2299 | 1.3159 | 1.4071 | 1.5036 | 1.6058 | 1.7138 | 1.8280 | 1.9487 | 2.2107 | 2.5023 |
| 8 | 1.0829 | 1.1717 | 1.2668 | 1.3686 | 1.4775 | 1.5938 | 1.7182 | 1.8509 | 1.9926 | 2.1436 | 2.4760 | 2.8526 |
| 9 | 1.0937 | 1.1951 | 1.3048 | 1.4233 | 1.5513 | 1.6895 | 1.8385 | 1.9990 | 2.1719 | 2.3579 | 2.7731 | 3.2519 |
| 10 | 1.1046 | 1.2190 | 1.3439 | 1.4802 | 1.6289 | 1.7908 | 1.9672 | 2.1589 | 2.3674 | 2.5937 | 3.1058 | 3.7072 |

# Chapter 20

## Documenting, Coding, and Billing: Getting it Right the First Time

Brian M. Aboff, MD, FACP and Rosemary Bell, RN, CPC

### Executive Summary

Proper documentation and coding are essential to providing quality patient care and to ensuring that physicians are appropriately reimbursed for services rendered. Good documentation improves communication among health care providers, allowing them to go back in time to better understand what happened to a patient and to assess progress. It also affords "proof" that care was given and standards were followed. The record helps to support accurate and timely claims review and, for the inpatient setting, appropriate utilization and quality of care reviews.

The standards for coding non-operative physician-patient interactions, known as evaluation and management (E/M) services, were established by the American Medical Association and the Centers for Medicare and Medicaid services in 1992, with subsequent revisions in 1995 and 1997. The E/M codes are predicated on three factors: location of care (e.g., inpatient, outpatient, emergency room), relationship of the patient to the physician (e.g., new patient, established patient, or consultation), and the complexity of the service provided. This last item, in turn, is determined by the completeness of the history, physical examination, and the intricacy of the medical decision making. The nature of the presenting problem, time spent on the coordination of care and counseling are contributory factors to the E/M code. While the rules are complex, mastering the criteria for accurate coding is important to providers to help ensure compliance with Medicare and other insurance carrier guidelines and for proper remuneration.

### Learning Objectives

1. Value the importance of proper documentation and coding.
2. Identify the key elements used to determine the proper E/M service.
3. Accurately assign E/M codes to sample physician notes.

### Keywords

evaluation and management services; history; medical documentation

## Introduction

Proper documentation and coding are essential to providing quality patient care and to ensuring that physicians are appropriately reimbursed for services rendered. There are many reasons health care providers should maintain quality medical documentation. First, good documentation improves communication across all health care providers. It allows the physician or other individuals to go back in time to better understand what happened to a patient in the past and assess progress. Secondly, documentation affords "proof" that care was given and that standards were followed, which in turn can lead to accurate and timely claims review and, for the inpatient setting, appropriate utilization, and quality of care reviews.

Getting into the habit of writing quality notes will pay long-term dividends. All medical records should be complete and legible. At a minimum, notes should include the reason for the encounter, a relevant history, pertinent physical examination, assessment, and management plan. If the patient is being followed over time, notes should comment on the patient's progress and include any response and/or changes to therapy. All notes should be dated and signed legibly. While documentation skills are refined during medical school and residency, what most perplexes the newly practicing physician is proper coding.

In the past, physicians' charges to insurance carriers for evaluation and management (E/M) services had the potential to be arbitrary. Insurance carriers expect to be billed similarly for an outpatient treated with an uncomplicated urinary tract infection, whether they were seen in California or New Jersey. In order to standardize the process, the American Medical Association and the Centers for Medicare and Medicaid Services (CMS) developed documentation guidelines for E/M services in 1992, with revisions in 1995 and 1997.[1,2] The guidelines and billing codes remove some of the ambiguity by providing a common language for physicians and insurance carriers. If you want to get paid what you deserve and avoid being fined by CMS, it is worth your while to gain an understanding of E/M services documentation guidelines.

This chapter will review the method for establishing an E/M service billing code. These services cover almost all non-operative interactions with patients in both the inpatient and outpatient setting. Discussion of billing codes for operative procedures is beyond the scope of this chapter; the reader is referred to the American Medical Association Current Procedural Terminology (CPT) manual for further information.[3]

All insurance carriers require the submission of the proper billing codes. While insurance plans vary in terms of reimbursement of each E/M service level and covered services, the billing code numbers are the same. The code numbers are predicated on three factors: location of care, relationship of the patient to the physician, and the complexity level of the E/M service. The first key factor, location of care, includes: outpatient services, hospital-based visits, nursing home visits, and home visits. The second key component to the billing code describes the relationship of patient to provider, i.e., new patient, established patient, or consultation.

As you can see from the billing code numbers (Table 1), there is a range of numbers within each type of visit service (e.g., new outpatient visit codes are from 99201-99205). Most visit types consist of three to five code numbers. The range of numbers reflects the complexity of the case and, subsequently, the level of reimbursement. A simple new outpatient visit (coded 99201) takes less time and is paid less than a more complex case (coded 99205).

## Table 1. Common Evaluation and Management Codes

| Category/Subcategory | Code Numbers |
|---|---|
| Outpatient services<br>    New patient<br>    Established patient<br>    Consultation | <br>99201- 99205<br>99211- 99215<br>99241- 99245 |
| Hospital services<br>    Initial care (first visit)<br>    Subsequent care<br>    Discharge services | <br>99221- 99223<br>99231- 99233<br>99238- 99239 |
| Other hospital-based services<br>    Emergency dept. visits<br>    Critical care – adult<br>    Critical care – pediatric<br>    Critical care – neonatal | <br>99281- 99288<br>99291- 99292<br>99293- 99294<br>99295- 99296 |
| Other outpatient services<br>    Preventive medicine<br>    New patient<br>    Established patient | <br><br>99381- 99387<br>99391- 99397 |
| Nursing facility services<br>    Initial (first visit) care<br>    Subsequent care | <br>99304 - 99306<br>99307 - 99310 |
| Home services<br>    New patient<br>    Established patient | <br>99341 - 99345<br>99347 - 99350 |

How does one determine the level of code for a particular type of visit? The level of the complexity of the case, and hence the level of the E/M service, is determined by three key components:

- History
- Examination
- Medical Decision Making

While these three key components are the principal drivers for coding billing levels, other contributory factors such as counseling, coordination of care, the nature of the presenting problem, and visit length may influence the level of the E/M coding. We'll discuss this in more detail later in the chapter.

For coding purposes, the history, examination, and medical decision making can each be categorized in terms of completeness and complexity. Assessing all of the key components together leads to the determination of E/M service level.

## History

The history is gleaned from the patient and, as appropriate, from family members, caregivers, and other medical records. From the E/M service-level perspective, there are four components to the history:

- Chief complaint (CC)
- History of present illness (HPI)
- Review of systems (ROS) (Table 2, page 357)
- Past medical history, family history, and social history (PFSH)

With the exception of the chief complaint, each of these components can vary in complexity. The chief complaint is a brief statement, usually in the patient's own words, that describes the primary reason for the encounter. All histories must include a chief complaint.

**History of Present Illness (HPI).** The history of present illness can vary in complexity and detail. For coding purposes, the HPI can be a single problem addressed in some detail or multiple chronic problems assessed individually. For a single problem, the eight HPI elements are:

- Location — for example, chest pain;
- Quality — pressure or vice-like;
- Severity — 7 on a scale of 1 – 10;

- Duration — lasts 5-10 minutes at a time;

- Timing — started about a month ago;

- Context — comes on whenever the patient climbs a hill or runs;

- Modifying factors — gets better with rest; and

- Associated signs and symptoms — is associated with left arm heaviness, shortness of breath, and diaphoresis.

The E/M service level for the HPI of a single problem is determined by the number of elements documented. For most inpatient issues, it will focus on a single issue and the aforementioned HPI elements. In the outpatient setting, the number of different chronic problems addressed in the HPI may also determine the E/M service level. There are two E/M service categories for the HPI: Brief and Extended.

- A *brief HPI* includes the chief complaint and one to three elements. For example:

    CC: Burning when urinating

    HPI: Patient complains of a 3-day history of dysuria

- An *extended HPI* includes the chief complaint and at least four elements, or the discussion of the status of three or more chronic conditions. A single problem, extended HPI may look like this:

    CC: Burning when urinating

    HPI: Patient complains of a 3-day history of dysuria. For the past 24 hours, she has also been experiencing 4 out of 10 pain in the left costovertebral area of the back, along with fever and chills. The symptoms transiently improve with acetaminophen, but overall she has been feeling progressively worse.

## Table 2.  Review of Systems (ROS)

| The review of systems section of the HPI consists of 14 organ systems: | |
| --- | --- |
| • Constitutional symptoms (e.g., fever, weight loss) | • Integumentary (skin and/or breast) |
| • Eyes | • Musculoskeletal |
| • Ears, nose, mouth, throat | • Neurological |
| • Cardiovascular | • Psychiatric |
| • Respiratory | • Endocrine |
| • Gastrointestinal | • Hematologic/Lymphatic |
| • Genitourinary | • Allergic/Immunologic |

When documenting the review of systems section, it is important to comment on the signs or symptoms for each ROS category. For example, instead of "respiratory ROS negative," one should document "no shortness of breath, coughing, or wheezing." From the E/M service level perspective, there are three types of ROS:

- **Problem-pertinent ROS:** focuses on the positive and negative responses to the system directly related to the presenting problem in the HPI.

- **Extended ROS:** focuses on the positive and negative responses to the system directly related to the presenting problem in the HPI plus a limited number (2-9) of pertinent additional systems.

- **Complete ROS:** inquires about a minimum number of 10 systems, including the positive and negative responses to the system directly related to the presenting problem in the HPI.

**Past history, family history, and/or social history (PFSH).** The past, family, and/or social history (PFSH) section represents the final component of the history. The past history can include prior major illnesses and injuries, prior surgeries, current medications, allergies, age-appropriate immunization status, and age-appropriate feeding/dietary status. The family history is a review of medical events, diseases, and hereditary conditions of biologic relatives that may place the patient at risk for health problems. With regards to family history, avoid the term "non-contributory" as this is insufficient detail to "count" for coding.[4] The social history represents an appropriate review of past and current activities such as living conditions, marital status, employment, occupational history, drug, alcohol, tobacco use, education level, and sexual history. The E/M service coding guidelines identifies two types of PSFH: pertinent and complete.

- Pertinent: at least one specific item from PFSH that directly relates to the HPI

- Complete: two or all three items of the PFSH are reviewed

Now it's time to put the pieces together. The history is classified into one of four levels of detail: problem-focused, expanded problem-focused, detailed, and comprehensive (Table 3, page 359).

## Examination

The same labels are used for the physical examination levels: problem-focused, expanded problem-focused, detailed, and comprehensive. The examination may be of body areas or organ systems. Per 1995 E/M Documentation Guidelines, the Body Areas and Organ Systems recognized are (Table 4, page 359):

## Table 3. Elements Required for Each Level of History

| Type of History | Definition |
|---|---|
| Problem-focused | CC + Brief HPI (1-3 elements) |
| Expanded Problem-focused | CC + Brief HPI (1-3 elements) + Problem pertinent ROS (1) |
| Detailed | CC + Extended HPI (4+ elements or in the outpatient setting may also be a discussion of 3 or more chronic problems) + Extended ROS (2-9) + Pertinent PFSH (1) |
| Comprehensive | CC + Extended HPI (4+ elements or in the outpatient setting may also be a discussion of 3 or more chronic problems ) + Complete ROS (10+) + Complete PFSH (2-3) |

## Table 4. Body Areas and Organ Systems

| Body Areas | Organ Systems |
|---|---|
| Head | Eyes |
| Neck | Ears, nose, mouth, and throat |
| Chest, including breasts and axilla | Cardiovascular |
| Abdomen | Respiratory |
| Genitalia, groin, buttocks | Genitourinary (male) |
| Back | Genitourinary (female) |
| Each extremity | Musculoskeletal |
| | Skin |
| | Neurologic |
| | Hematologic/lymphatic/immunologic |
| | Psychiatric |

A problem-focused examination is limited to the affected body area or organ system. An expanded problem-focused physical examination is limited to the affected body area or organ system and any other symptomatic or related body area or organ system. A detailed exam represents an extended examination of the affected body area(s) or organ system(s) and any other symptomatic or related body area(s) or organ system(s). A comprehensive exam is a multi-system examination or complete examination of a single organ system and other symptomatic or related body area(s) or organ system(s).

The E/M level for the physical exam relates to the number of body areas or organ systems examined and/or the level of detail examined of a specific organ system. The 1995 and subsequent 1997 guidelines permit the coding level of the physical examination to be determined by either a multi-system exam or by an in-depth examination of one organ system/body area. The following are the content and documentation requirements for the 1997 multi-system examination (Table 5):

## Table 5.  Content and Documentation Requirements of a Multi-System Examination

| System/Body Area | Elements of Examination |
|---|---|
| Constitutional | • Measurement of any three of the following vital signs: 1) sitting or standing blood pressure;  2) supine blood pressure; 3) pulse rate and regularity; 4) respiratory rate; 5) temperature; 6) height; 7) weight<br>• General appearance of the patient |
| Eyes | • Inspection of conjunctivae and lids<br>• Examination of pupils and irises<br>• Ophthalmoloscopic examination of optic discs |
| Ears, Nose, Mouth, and Throat | • External inspection of ears and nose<br>• Otoscopic examination of external auditory canals and tympanic membranes<br>• Assessment of hearing<br>• Inspection of nasal mucosa, septum, and turbinates<br>• Inspection of lips, teeth, and gums<br>• Examination of oropharynx, oral mucosa, palates, tongue, posterior pharynx |
| Neck | • Examination of neck<br>• Examination of thyroid |

| System/Body Area | Elements of Examination |
|---|---|
| Respiratory | • Assessment of respiratory effort<br>• Percussion of chest<br>• Palpation of chest<br>• Auscultation of lungs |
| Cardiovascular | • Palpation of heart<br>• Auscultation of heart<br>• Examination of:<br>— Carotid arteries (pulse, amplitude, bruits)<br>— Abdominal aorta<br>— Femoral arteries<br>— Pedal pulses<br>— Extremities for edema and/or varicosities |
| Chest (Breasts) | • Inspection of breasts<br>• Palpation of breasts and axillae |
| Gastrointestinal (Abdomen) | • Inspection of abdomen with notation of masses or tenderness<br>• Examination of liver and spleen<br>• Examination for presence or absence of hernia<br>• Examination of anus, perineum and rectum<br>• Obtain stool sample for occult blood |
| Genitourinary | Male<br>• Examination of scrotum and contents<br>• Examination of penis<br>• Digital rectal examination of prostate<br><br>Female (pelvic examination)<br>• Examination of external genitalia<br>• Examination of urethra<br>• Examination of bladder<br>• Cervix<br>• Uterus<br>• Adnexa |
| Lymphatic | Palpation of lymph nodes in two or more areas:<br>• Neck<br>• Axilla<br>• Groin<br>• Other |

| System/Body Area | Elements of Examination |
|---|---|
| Musculoskeletal | • Examination of gait and station<br>• Examination of digits and nails<br>• Examination of joints, bones and muscles of one or more of the following six areas: 1) head and neck, 2) spine, ribs, pelvis; 3) right upper extremity; 4) left upper extremity; 5) right lower extremity; 6) left lower extremity.<br>• The examination of a given area includes<br>— Inspection and palpation<br>— Assessment of range of motion<br>— Assessment of stability<br>— Assessment of strength and tone |
| Skin | • Inspection<br>• Palpation |
| Neurologic | • Cranial nerves<br>• Deep tendon reflexes<br>• Examination of sensation |
| Psychiatric | • Description of patient's judgment and insight<br>• Assessment of mental status (including orientation to time, place and person, recent and remote memory, and mood and affect) |

Like the history, the physical examination is classified into one of four levels of detail: problem-focused, expanded problem-focused, detailed, and comprehensive (Table 6, below).

## Table 6.  Elements Required for Each Level of the Physical Examination Based on a Multi-System Examination

| Level of Exam | Perform and Document (refer to Table 5 for bulleted elements) |
|---|---|
| Problem-focused | Affected body area with one to five elements identified by a bullet |
| Expanded problem-focused | Affected body area + other symptomatic/related organ systems for a total of at least six elements identified by a bullet |
| Detailed | At least two elements identified by a bullet from each of 6 areas/systems, OR  At least 12 elements identified by a bullet in two or more areas/systems |
| Comprehensive | Perform and document the exam for at least two elements identified by a bullet from each of nine areas/systems (for a total of at least 18 bulleted elements examined) |

The aforementioned physical examination levels are based on the multi-system examination. However, there will be times when very detailed, in-depth examination of single organ system and related systems are in order. The 1997 E/M Documentation Guidelines list in great detail what is required for the following single organ system examinations:

- Eyes
- Cardiovascular
- Genitourinary
- Skin
- Hematologic/lymphatic/immunologic
- Ears, nose, mouth, and throat
- Respiratory
- Musculoskeletal
- Neurologic
- Psychiatric

It is beyond the scope of this text to highlight all of the elements listed for each of these individual organ system examinations. As an example, the following are the components of a single organ eye examination:

Eyes:
- Visual acuity
- Gross visual fields by confrontation
- Test ocular motility
- Examination of ocular adnexae including lids
- Examination of pupils and irises
- Slit lamp examination of the corneas
- Slit lamp examination of the anterior chambers
- Slit lamp examination of the lenses
- Measurement of intraocular pressures

Ophthalmoscopic examination through dilated pupils
- Optic discs
- Posterior segments including retina and vessels

Neurological/psychiatric
- Orientation to time, place, person
- Mood and affect

Similar to the multi-system examination, a single organ system exam can be categorized as problem-focused, expanded problem-focused, detailed, or comprehensive (Table 7, below).

### Table 7.  Content and Documentation Requirements for a Single Organ System Examination

| Type of Examination | Description |
| --- | --- |
| Problem-focused | 1-5 elements identified by a bullet |
| Expanded problem-focused | At least 6 elements identified by a bullet |
| Detailed | Examinations other than the eye and psychiatric examinations should include at least 12 elements identified by a bullet<br><br>Eye and psychiatric examinations include at least 9 elements identified by a bullet |
| Comprehensive | Include performance of all elements identified by a bullet |

## Medical Decision Making

The third and final key component to determining an E/M service level is medical decision making. Medical decision making refers to the complexity of the determining a diagnosis or selecting a management plan. Factors affecting the level of medical decision making include:

• The number of possible diagnoses and/or the number of management options that must be considered. The different levels in this category are:

— Minimal

— Limited

— Multiple

— Extensive

• The amount or complexity of the data to be reviewed, such as: medical records, diagnostic tests and/or other information that needs to be obtained, reviewed, and analyzed. The different levels in this category are:

— Minimal

— Limited

— Multiple

— Extensive

• The risk of complications, morbidity, and mortality associated with the underlying problem and/or the management options. The different levels in this category are:

— Minimal

— Low

— Moderate

— High

The documentation guidelines are intricate when it comes to determining what constitutes the various levels of complexity in the first two categories mentioned: the number of diagnosis and management options, and the amount and/or complexity of the data to be reviewed. While not articulated in the 1995 or 1997 guidelines, most auditors commonly use a scoring system to determine the extent of these first two factors.[5] The guidelines emphasize the importance of documenting the factors that go into the coding decision. Every note should contain an assessment, which, as appropriate, includes the differential diagnosis and management options considered along with documentation of what data was reviewed and their results. The level coded should reflect the complexity of the problem(s) addressed. Risk of morbidity or mortality from the underlying disease or treatment is the last of the categories which determine the level of medical decision making. Below is a table of risk that can provide guidance in selecting the appropriate level (Table 8).

## Table 8. Table of Risk

| Degree of Risk | Presenting Problem | Diagnostic Procedure(s) Ordered | Management Options Selected |
|---|---|---|---|
| Minimal | One self-limited or minor problem, e.g., viral URI, tinea corporis. | Laboratory test requiring venipuncture<br>Chest X-ray<br>ECG<br>Urinalysis | Rest<br>Elastic bandage<br>Superficial dressing |

| Degree of Risk | Presenting Problem | Diagnostic Procedure(s) Ordered | Management Options Selected |
|---|---|---|---|
| Low | Two or more self-limited or minor problems. One stable chronic illness (e.g., well-controlled hypertension, cataract, benign prostatic hypertrophy, type 2 diabetes mellitus). Acute uncomplicated illness (e.g., cystitis, allergic rhinitis, simple sprain). | Superficial needle biopsy. Clinical laboratory tests. requiring arterial puncture. Physiologic tests not under stress (e.g., PFTs). Non-cardiovascular imaging studies with contrast (e.g., barium enema). | Over-the-counter drugs. Minor surgery with no identified risk factors. Physical therapy. Occupational therapy. Intravenous fluids without additives. |
| Moderate | One or more chronic illnesses with mild exacerbation, progression, or side effects to treatment. Two or more stable chronic illnesses. Undiagnosed new problem with uncertain prognosis (e.g., breast lump). Acute illness with systemic symptoms (e.g., pyelonephritis, pneumonia). Acute complicated injury (e.g., head injury with brief loss of consciousness). | Physiologic tests under stress (e.g., cardiac stress test, fetal contraction test). Diagnostic endoscopies with no identified risk factors. Deep needle or incisional biopsy. Cardiac catheterization. Lumbar puncture. Thoracentesis. Culdocentesis. | Minor surgery with identified risk factors. Elective major surgery with no identified risk factors. Intravenous fluids with additives. Closed treatment of fracture or dislocation without manipulation. |
| High | One or more chronic illnesses with severe exacerbation, progression, or side effects of treatment. Acute or chronic illnesses or injuries that pose a threat to life or bodily function (e.g., multiple trauma, acute MI, pulmonary embolus, severe respiratory distress, progressive severe rheumatoid arthritis, peritonitis, acute renal failure, seizure, stroke, psychiatric illness with potential threat to self or others). | Cardiovascular imaging studies with contrast with identified risk factors. Cardiac electrophysiologic tests. Diagnostic endoscopies with identified risk factors. Discography. | Elective major surgery with identified risk factors. Emergency major surgery. Parenteral controlled substances. Drug therapy requiring intensive monitoring for toxicity. Decision not to resuscitate or to de-escalate care because of poor prognosis. |

Four types of medical decision making are recognized: straightforward, low complexity, moderate complexity, and high complexity. In order to determine the level of medical decision making, the factors of diagnostic or management options, amount or complexity of the data to be reviewed, and the risk for morbidity and mortality must be taken into account. Two of the three elements must either be met or exceeded (Table 9, below).

## Table 9. Elements of Medical Decision Making

| Type of Decision Making | Number of Diagnosis or Management Options | Amount and/or Complexity of Data to be Reviewed | Risk of Significant Complications, Morbidity, and/or Mortality |
|---|---|---|---|
| Straightforward | Minimal | Minimal or None | Minimal |
| Low complexity | Limited | Limited | Low |
| Moderate complexity | Multiple | Moderate | Moderate |
| High complexity | Extensive | Extensive | High |

## Putting it All Together

When determining the final E/M code, one must consider the level of the history, physical, and medical decision making involved in the case. For initial patient visits, all three key components are required for calculating the proper E/M code; for subsequent/established visits, only two of three components are required. While visit length is not explicitly used to determine the level of the E/M code, there are general guidelines of how much time each code level should take. In the outpatient setting, this refers to face-to-face time with the patient. For the inpatient setting, the time includes face-to-face time with the patient and time spent with the patient's chart on the floor or nursing unit.

## Office Visits

Office Visit, New Patient (3 of 3 components required)

| E/M Code | History | Exam | Medical Decision Making | Avg. Time (min) |
|---|---|---|---|---|
| 99201 | Focused | Focused | Straightforward | 10 |
| 99202 | Exp. problem focused | Exp. problem focused | Straightforward | 20 |
| 99203 | Detailed | Detailed | Low | 30 |
| 99204 | Comprehensive | Comprehensive | Moderate | 45 |
| 99205 | Comprehensive | Comprehensive | High | 60 |

Office Visit, Established Patient (2 of 3 components required)

| E/M Code | History | Exam | Medical Decision Making | Avg. Time (min) |
|---|---|---|---|---|
| 99211 | N/A | N/A | Straightforward | 5 |
| 99212 | Focused | Focused | Straightforward | 10 |
| 99213 | Exp. problem focused | Exp. problem focused | Low | 15 |
| 99214 | Detailed | Detailed | Moderate | 25 |
| 99215 | Comprehensive | Comprehensive | High | 40 |

Office Consultations, New or Established Patient (3 of 3 components required)

| E/M Code | History | Exam | Medical Decision Making | Avg. Time (min) |
|---|---|---|---|---|
| 99241 | Focused | Focused | Straightforward | 15 |
| 99242 | Exp. problem focused | Exp. problem focused | Straightforward | 30 |
| 99243 | Detailed | Detailed | Low | 40 |
| 99244 | Comprehensive | Comprehensive | Moderate | 60 |
| 99245 | Comprehensive | Comprehensive | High | 80 |

## Inpatient Care

Initial Inpatient Care (3 of 3 components required)

| E/M Code | History | Exam | Medical Decision Making | Avg. Time (min) |
|---|---|---|---|---|
| 99221 | Detailed or Comprehensive | Detailed or Comprehensive | Straightforward or Low | 30 |
| 99222 | Comprehensive | Comprehensive | Moderate | 50 |
| 99223 | Comprehensive | Comprehensive | High | 70 |

Subsequent Hospital Care (2 of 3 components required)

| E/M Code | History | Exam | Medical Decision Making | Avg. Time (min) |
|---|---|---|---|---|
| 99231 | Focused | Focused | Straightforward or Low | 15 |
| 99232 | Exp. problem focused | Exp. problem focused | Moderate | 25 |
| 99233 | Detailed | Detailed | High | 35 |

Discharge Day Management

| E/M Code | Time |
|----------|------|
| 99238 | 30 minutes or less |
| 99239 | More than 30 minutes |

Initial Inpatient Consultations (3 of 3 components required)

| E/M Code | History | Exam | Medical Decision Making | Avg. Time (min) |
|----------|---------|------|-------------------------|-----------------|
| 99251 | Focused | Focused | Straightforward | 20 |
| 99252 | Exp. problem focused | Exp. problem focused | Straightforward | 40 |
| 99253 | Detailed | Detailed | Low | 55 |
| 99254 | Comprehensive | Comprehensive | Moderate | 80 |
| 99255 | Comprehensive | Comprehensive | High | 110 |

Follow-up Inpatient Consult (2 of 3 required elements)

| E/M Code | History | Exam | Medical Decision Making | Avg. Time (min) |
|----------|---------|------|-------------------------|-----------------|
| 99261 | Focused | Focused | Straightforward or Low | 10 |
| 99262 | Exp. problem focused | Exp. problem focused | Moderate | 20 |
| 99263 | Detailed | Detailed | High | 30 |

Emergency Department Services

| E/M Code | History | Exam | Medical Decision Making |
|----------|---------|------|-------------------------|
| 99281 | Focused | Focused | Straightforward |
| 99282 | Exp. problem focused | Exp. problem focused | Low |
| 99283 | Exp. problem focused | Exp. problem focused | Moderate |
| 99284 | Detailed | Detailed | Moderate |
| 99285 | Comprehensive | Comprehensive | High |

Visit length is usually not a key component to determining an E/M code, but there are exceptions. As noted above, inpatient discharge day codes are time-dependent. So, too, are critical care codes. In addition, when counseling or coordination of care dominates an office or hospital visit (i.e., > 50% of the visit), then time may be used as the determining factor. When using this option, it is critical to document the amount of time spent face-to-face with the patient, and the extent and details of the counseling and/or coordination of care. For example: "20/30 minutes spent discussing…" would indicate that the physician spent 20 minutes out of a 30-minute visit discussing specific counseling issues.

There are a number of other E/M coding situations that are not mentioned above. These include preventive medicine visits, nursing facility care, home visits, domiciliary or custodial care services, and prolonged services with face-to-face patient contact. The reader is referred to the Evaluation and Management Services Guidelines for further details.

## Coding Made Easy

Here are some suggestions for making the coding easier for outpatient visits.

Please note that what we are about to explain is not the traditional method of determining medical documentation for coding purposes, as per the Evaluation and Management guidelines. In the experience of the authors, it is challenging for a busy clinician to go through each of the aforementioned steps to code during a demanding session of seeing patients. Since clinicians tend to think in terms of problem lists and how many issues or concerns are being addressed, we will offer an alternative method for coding. Each problem, its evaluation, and management options are associated with risk. We can use Medicare's Table of Risk of Complications and/or Morbidity or Mortality to approximate a billing code (Table 10, page 372). Remember, you only need one bullet from the table to determine the level of risk.

- Consider that the "Minimal" level = 99201, 99202, or 99212; the "Low" risk level = 99203 or 99213; "Moderate" risk level = 99204 or 99214; and "High" risk level = 99205 or 99215. (Table 8)

- Choose the level that best fits the patient you have just seen.

  —If the patient's illness is such that a simple over-the-counter drug is recommended, the visit <u>may</u> qualify as a "Low" level of risk (99203 if a new patient, or 99213 for an established patient).

  —If the patient has "two or more stable chronic illnesses", the patient <u>may</u> qualify as a "Moderate" level of risk (99204 if a new patient, or 99214 for an established patient).

- These assumptions presume that an adequate history and physical examination are performed. You must document in the patient record the chief complaint (CC), history of present illness (HPI), review of systems (ROS), and past history (PFSH), as well as the physical exam and medical decision making, to support the code you selected based on the Table of Risk of Complications and/or Morbidity or Mortality, to meet the level requirements. Refer to the coding guidelines outlined earlier in this chapter for those requirements. Remember that medical necessity also drives your code selection. If a patient presents with a straightforward, uncomplicated viral upper respiratory tract infection, no matter how much you document, you cannot code for a high level of care. If a patient presents with two or more chronic problems, you can only "count" it toward your coding level as potentially moderate risk if you are taking an active role in the evaluation, assessment, or management of the problem.

The risk table (Table 10, page 372) is useful to determine the appropriate level; however the documentation in the progress note must also meet the level requirements, including HPI, physical exam and medical decision making. Medical necessity must also be considered.

## Medical Necessity

According to the Medicare Carrier Manual, Chapter 12, Section 15501:

- Medical necessity is the overarching criterion for payment, in addition to meeting individual requirements of a CPT code.

- It <u>would</u> <u>not</u> be medically necessary or appropriate to bill a higher level evaluation/management service when a lower level of service is warranted.

- The volume of documentation <u>should not</u> be the primary influence upon which a specific level of service is billed.

- Documentation should support the level of service reported.

## Other Tips:

- After you have interviewed and examined your patient, document your findings in the patient record as soon as possible. Be sure you are recording all the important information, as well as ensuring timely, correct code submission to the payers.

- <u>Always</u> consider "medical necessity." Ask yourself if it is medically necessary to remove that lesion; or to do a complete review of systems on the patient with a URI. If you believe it is medically necessary, you must document your rationale.

## Table 10.  Using Medicare's Table of Risk of Complications and/or Morbidity or Mortality to Approximate a Billing Code

| Level of Risk and Possible E/M Coding level (assumes adequate documentation) | Presenting Problem | Diagnostic Procedure(s) Ordered | Management Options Selected |
|---|---|---|---|
| **Minimal** New patient visit 99201 or 99202 Established patient visit 99212 | One self-limited or minor problem, e.g. viral URI, tinea corporis. | Laboratory test requiring venipuncture Chest X-ray ECG Urinalysis | Rest Elastic bandage Superficial dressing |
| **Low** New patient visit 99203 Established patient visit 99213 | Two or more self-limited or minor problems. One stable chronic illness (e.g., well-controlled hypertension, cataract, benign prostatic hypertrophy, type 2 diabetes mellitus). Acute uncomplicated illness (e.g., cystitis, allergic rhinitis, simple sprain). | Superficial needle biopsy Clinical laboratory tests requiring arterial puncture Physiologic tests not under stress (e.g., PFTs) Non-cardiovascular imaging studies with contrast (e.g., barium enema) | Over-the-counter drugs Minor surgery with no identified risk factors Physical therapy Occupational therapy Intravenous fluids without additives |
| **Moderate** New patient visit 99204 Established patient visit 99214 | One or more chronic illnesses with mild exacerbation, progression, or side effects to treatment. Two or more stable chronic illnesses. Undiagnosed new problem with uncertain prognosis (e.g., breast lump). Acute illness with systemic symptoms (e.g., pyelonephritis, pneumonia). Acute complicated injury (e.g., head injury with brief loss of consciousness. | Physiologic tests under stress (e.g., cardiac stress test, fetal contraction test). Diagnostic endoscopies with no identified risk factors. Deep needle or incisional biopsy. Cardiac catheterization Lumbar puncture Thoracentesis Culdocentesis | Minor surgery with identified risk factors. Elective major surgery with no identified risk factors. Intravenous fluids with additives. Closed treatment of fracture or dislocation without manipulation. |
| **High** New patient visit 99205 Established patient visit 99215 | One or more chronic illnesses with severe exacerbation, progression, or side effects of treatment. Acute or chronic illnesses or injuries that pose a threat to life or bodily function (e.g., multiple trauma, acute MI, pulmonary embolus, severe respiratory distress, progressive severe rheumatoid arthritis, peritonitis, acute renal failure, seizure, stroke, psychiatric illness with potential threat to self or others). | Cardiovascular imaging studies with contrast with identified risk factors. Cardiac electrophysiologic tests. Diagnostic endoscopies with identified risk factors. Discography. | Elective major surgery with identified risk factors. Emergency major surgery. Parenteral controlled substances. Drug therapy requiring intensive monitoring for toxicity. Decision not to resuscitate or to de-escalate care because of poor prognosis |

It is far easier to do it at the time of the visit, than having to write a letter to the medical director of the insurance company to appeal a denial. The medical record should stand for itself.

- Consider, <u>and record</u>, the differential diagnoses. Co-morbidities, underlying diseases or other factors (e.g., the number and type of medications) that increase the complexity of medical decision making by increasing the risk of complications, morbidity, and/or mortality should be documented.

- One of the important things to remember is:  DOCUMENT, DOCUMENT, DOCUMENT!

## Conclusion

Proper documentation improves communication among health care providers, documents a patient's progress, provides "proof" that care was given and standards were followed, and allows physicians and other reviewers to go back in time and understand what happened to a patient in the past.  Chapters 8, 12, and 16, touch on importance of coding and documentation as it relates to Risk Management, Medical Malpractice, and the Referral Process, respectively. Coding and billing is based on the AMA/CMS Evaluation and Management Services Guidelines. While the rules are complex, mastering the criteria for accurate E/M coding helps to ensure that physicians are appropriately reimbursed for services rendered.

## Case Study

The case study below will serve as an example to demonstrate proper coding.  As you read through the case, think about how you would code the visit.  The answer is provided below in the office visit note.

Patient:  Missy Waters          Record #: 654321

Date of Service:   03/04/06
Type of patient:  Established

Chief Complaint:  pain on urination

HPI: 27-year-old woman complains of pain and burning on urination x 2 days. Has tried drinking a lot of fluids and cranberry juice without relief. Denies fever.

ROS:  No nausea, vomiting, or diarrhea

Past medical history:  Previous UTI once three years ago
Allergies:  No known allergies

Exam:
T. 99.0, BP 118/72, Wt. 124 lbs.
WNWD, NAD
Lungs:  CTA, no respiratory distress
Heart:   regular rate and rhythm
Abdomen:  normal bowel sounds, without tenderness or guarding

Labs:  Urinalysis → + blood and + leukocyte esterase

Impression & Plan:
Urinary tract infection.  Treat with trimethoprim/sulfamethoxazole (Bactrim DS® ) 1 tab orally every 12 hours for 3 days.

James Kildare, MD

## Answer:

HPI = location, quality, duration, modifying factor = Extended history (four or more elements)
ROS = constitutional, gastrointestinal = Extended ROS (2-9 ROS)
PFSH = past medical history (one element)

What type of history has Dr. Kildare taken? Taking a chief complaint, an extended history, an extended ROS, along with one component of the PFSH, is equivalent to "Detailed History." The physical examination contains seven bulleted elements (vital signs, general appearance, two components of the respiratory exam, cardiovascular, and abdominal examination), which is an extended problem-focused examination. Regarding the final key component of the E/M code, medical decision making, the patient has a new problem, but no additional workup or evaluation is needed.  One test result was reviewed, and an acute uncomplicated illness such as a urinary tract infection represents a low risk for complications. Thus, the final medical decision making is considered low complexity.

Putting this all together:
Detailed history + Extended problem-focused examination + low complexity medical decision making  = 99213

## Suggested Readings/Websites

American Medical Association CPT® Resources:
http://www.ama-assn.org/ama/pub/category/3113.html

Centers for Medicare and Medicaid Services Evaluation and Management Services Guide:
http://www.cms.hhs.gov/MLNProducts/downloads/reference1.pdf.

## References

1.  Centers for Medicare and Medicaid Services. 1995 Guidelines for Evaluation and Management Services in Medicare Physician Guide: A Resource for Residents, Practicing Physicians, and Other Health Care Professionals. Available at: http://www.cms.hhs.gov/MLNProducts/downloads/reference1.pdf. Accessed July 9, 2006.

2.  Centers for Medicare and Medicaid Services. 1997 Guidelines for Evaluation and Management Services. Available at: http://www.cms.hhs.gov/mlnproducts/downloads/master1.pdf. Accessed July 9, 2006.

3.  *American Medical Association CPT Professional Edition — 2006* (CPT / Current Procedural Terminology (Professional Edition)). Clifton Park, NY: Thomson Delmar Learning; 2006.

4.  Trailblazer Health Enterprises. Tips for Preventing Most Common E/M Service Coding Errors. Available at: http://www.trailblazerhealth.com/partb/downloads/emcommonerrors.pdf. Accessed July 9, 2006.

5.  Trailblazer Health Enterprises. Evaluation and Management: Coding and Documentation Pocket Reference. Available at: http://www.trailblazerhealth.com/partb/downloads/empocketref.pdf. Accessed July 9, 2006.

# Chapter 21

## Physician Compensation Trends, Models, and Approaches

David Edward Marcinko, DPM, MBA, CFP, CMP
and Hope Rachel Hetico, RN, MHA, CMP, CPHQ

**Executive Summary**

Anyone who has paid a doctor's bill lately knows that health care costs are out of control. It should come as no surprise that the golden era of medicine for physician compensation is over, and that health care is the latest industry to tighten its payment belt.

Physician compensation is also a contentious issue in medical group practice, and fodder for public scrutiny. Few situations produce the same level of emotion as doctors fighting over how a seemingly collegial employment contract should be interpreted. This situation often springs from a failure of both sides to understand mutual compensation terms of art when the deal was negotiated.

This chapter will help you to avoid this contentiously polarizing human and economic polemic. It begins with the basic principles of student-debt avoidance, the intangible concept of goodwill, and the compensation versus value paradox of medical practice worth. Employer-employee deferred compensation arrangements are also visited as important fringe benefits. Compensation benchmarks for medical and allied health care specialties are then presented. Finally, newer health delivery models, such as consumer-directed health plans, cash-based compensation extenders, and concierge medicine, are mentioned.

This physician salary and compensation information is offered to serve as a reference point for further individual investigation.

## Learning Objectives

1. Define mutual terms-of-art in order to reduce compensation discord among all health care professionals.

2. Understand old and new models of independent and employed medical practice as they affect physician compensation.

3. Review average medical and allied health care provider salaries.

4. Understand the basics of Qualified and Non-Qualified Deferred Compensation Plans in the context of physician fringe benefits.

5. Speculate on future trends of physician compensation and encourage change-management and lifelong learning.

## Keywords

cash-based compensation (CBC); compensation versus value paradox; concierge medicine (CM); consumer-directed health plans (CDHP); goodwill conundrum; independent contractor (IC); locum tenens practitioner (LTP); nonqualified deferred compensation plans (NQDCP); physician practice management companies (PPMCs); qualified deferred compensation plan (QDCP); rabbi and secular trust; value-based health insurance (VBHI)

## Introduction

Several years ago, *Fortune* magazine carried the headline "When Six Figured Incomes Aren't Enough. Now Doctors Want a Union."[1] To the man in the street, it was just a matter of the rich getting richer. The sentiment was quantified by Russ Alan Prince, who reported that 50,000 physicians, with a net worth of $5 million or more, control assets worth $375 billion.[2] Physicians were not complaining under the traditional fee-for-service system; the imbroglio began when managed care adversely impacted incomes. Rightly or wrongly, the public has little sympathy for affluent doctors.

Today, the situation is vastly different as medical professionals struggle to maintain adequate income levels. While a few specialties flourish, others, such as primary care, barely move. In the words of Atul Gawande, MD, a surgical resident at Brigham and Women's Hospital in Boston, "Doctors quickly learn that how much they make has little to do with how good they are. It largely depends on how they handle the business side of practice."[3]

In order to become a compensation-maximizing practitioner, it is critical to understand contemporary thoughts on physician compensation trends, models and approaches.

## Physician Compensation Trends

In 2006, the Medicare Trustees Report projected a 4.7% reduction in physician reimbursement for 2007, and 37% in cumulative cuts over the next nine years. It noted that each year in the next decade will feature a 5% cut in doctors' pay, while physician costs will increase 2% annually. The Bush administration also called for $36 billion in Medicare reductions over five years and advocated pay for performance reimbursement metered against predetermined quality standards. The direct results on physician compensation are predictable, but other trends are more alarming.[4]

- **Medical Student Debt Burden and Loan Defaults:** Medical student debt burdens (averaging $100,000-$250,000) are economically devastating. In FY 2000, the federal Health Education Assistance Loan (HEAL) program squeezed significant repayment settlements from its Top 3 deadbeat doctor debtors, and excluded 303 practitioners from Medicare and other federal/state programs.[5]

- **The Goodwill Conundrum:** In the context of long-term compensation for a lifetime of work, mature practitioners erroneously focus on the intangible of goodwill upon retirement. Goodwill is defined as "The ability of a business to generate income in excess of a normal rate on assets due to superior managerial skills, market position, new product technology, etc. In the purchase of a business, goodwill represents the difference between the purchase price and the value of the net assets."[6] Yet, there are two types of goodwill, with one far more compensable than the other.

  — **Physician Goodwill:** Personal goodwill results from the charisma and reputation of a specific doctor. Its attributes accrue solely to the individual, are not transferable, and can't be sold. They have no economic value. Nevertheless, young uninformed physicians may overcompensate retiring doctors for this non-existent "asset."[7]

  — **Business Goodwill:** Medical practice goodwill, on the other hand, may be transferred and is defined as the unidentified residual attributes that contribute to the propensity of patients and managed care contracts (and their revenue streams) to return in the future.[8] However, one must appreciate the: 1) impact of a changing environment; 2) practice transfer activity in a local market, which can augment or blunt goodwill value; and 3) determination of whether patients or HMOs return because of goodwill, or are mandated by contractual obligations. A good medical practice is not necessarily a good business, and retiring group practice doctors can no longer extract excess compensation for this intangible asset.

## Self-employed Physician Compensation Models

According to medical benefits consultant Eric Galtress, physicians can still select from traditional self-employment compensation models.[9]

- **Independent Physicians:** A self-employed physician has greater freedom, but less security, because relationships with an employer are defined in return for a set compensation. Typically, this option is ideal for those who desire control, don't work well in structured environments, and are committed to maximizing personal compensation.

- **Same-specialty Group Partnerships:** A same-specialty partnership is more restrictive than independent practice, and must balance control with the security that comes from working with colleagues along a continuum-of-care. Internal competition may be fierce, but partners maintain some autonomy while reaping rewards from economies of scale. More personal time is available too, but compensation is based on individual and group performance.

- **Multi-specialty Group Partnerships:** The partners of a multi-specialty group have even more restrictions, but harvest power from an expanded group of physicians and the presence of a vertically integrated referral chain. Because more disciplines are within the group, a partner might be well-positioned to capture additional prospective payment contracts.

- **The Compensation versus Value Paradox:** Regardless of the model, physician compensation is inversely related to practice value. In other words, the more a doctor takes home in compensation, the less the practice is worth and vice versa. This is the difference between a short-term and long-term compensation strategy.

- **Insourced Entrepreneurs:** The classic example is an inpatient specialist or hospitalist. The National Association of Inpatient Physicians (NAIP) estimated the model encompassed 40,000 hospitalists in 2005, with an average salary of $171,001.[10]

- **Outsourced Entrepreneurs:** Some physicians are risk-tolerant and utility-neutral when seeking other compensation opportunities. For example, Vanderbilt University-trained neurologist Michel Burry, MD, is a hedge fund manager at Scion Capital, LLC; Dimitri Sokoloff, MD, MBA, is a venture capitalist on Wall Street; and Harvard-trained emergency room physician Gigi Hirsch, MD, is the founder of a pharmaceutical industry physician executive search firm.

Regardless of the independent physician compensation model, degree or specialty, a review of the Deferred Compensation Plan (DCP) concept is vital for long-term success.

**Qualified Deferred Compensation Plans:** Gary J. Gunnett, Esq., of the Pittsburgh law firm of Houston-Harbaugh, PC, opines that most physicians participate in a Qualified Deferred Compensation Plan (QDCP) as a self-employed benefit.[11] An IRS-qualified plan mandates minimum coverage and nondiscrimination requirements prohibiting benefits to the exclusion of other employees. In exchange, favorable tax treatment is received, such as tax deductions for contributions, tax-deferred growth, and the lack of taxation until benefits are paid. Distributions are generally eligible for transfer or IRA rollover, permitting further tax deferral. Moreover, federal laws governing qualified plans require that all contributions be set aside in trust, beyond the reach of creditors. Therefore, a vested physician in a qualified plan can assume that benefits will eventually be available.

## Salary Ranges for Independent Physicians According to Medical Specialty *+^

| Specialty | All Physicians | Starting | East | West | South | North |
|---|---|---|---|---|---|---|
| Allergy and Immunology | $207,278 | $154,080 | $193,480 | $210,802 | $204,870 | $206,241 |
| Anesthesiology | $315,300 | $250,000 | $275,000 | $298,000 | $334,200 | $334,033 |
| Cardiac & Thoracic Surgery | $421,620 | $310,000 | $387,298 | $343,050 | $421,240 | $469,860 |
| Cardiology | $336,000 | $280,000 | $264,900 | $343,646 | $386,957 | $369,566 |
| Colon & Rectal Surgery | $327,927 | **** | $300,000 | **** | **** | $350,798 |
| Critical Care Medicine | $228,740 | **** | $220,235 | **** | $227,242 | $228,740 |
| Dermatology | $274,014 | $200,000 | $225,000 | $289,409 | $322,138 | $263,201 |
| Diagnostic Radiology – Interventional | $410,250 | $320,000 | $345,860 | $410,000 | $537,942 | $410,250 |
| Diagnostic Radiology – Non-Interventional | $364,899 | $257,367 | $330,000 | $350,224 | $383,319 | $383,256 |
| Emergency Care | $230,930 | $175,500 | $200,327 | $228,814 | $225,905 | $239,984 |
| Endocrinology | $185,000 | $140,000 | $166,675 | $185,000 | $177,665 | $201,241 |
| Family Medicine | $164,209 | $120,000 | $141,225 | $166,750 | $163,417 | $168,488 |
| Family Medicine - with Obstetrics | $163,334 | $125,000 | $140,643 | $162,352 | $161,421 | $167,222 |
| Gastroenterology | $308,246 | $250,000 | $263,594 | $325,698 | $325,033 | $306,994 |
| General Surgery | $294,000 | $200,000 | $250,028 | $275,336 | $301,761 | $330,903 |
| Geriatrics | $159,492 | **** | $150,000 | **** | $158,400 | $170,278 |
| Gynecological Oncology | $334,009 | **** | $290,795 | $345,355 | **** | $347,005 |
| Gynecology | $217,283 | **** | $220,794 | **** | $224,420 | $217,256 |
| Gynecology & Obstetrics | $250,196 | $180,000 | $232,276 | $240,118 | $258,756 | $275,419 |
| Hematology & Medical Oncology | $255,007 | $200,000 | $207,300 | $261,004 | $293,043 | $255,007 |
| Hospitalist | $171,991 | $150,000 | $153,515 | $175,084 | $183,775 | $171,913 |
| Hypertension & Nephrology | $214,751 | $165,000 | $186,683 | $238,750 | $253,228 | $214,751 |
| Infectious Disease | $185,920 | $140,111 | $161,206 | $179,402 | $175,000 | $203,640 |
| Intensivist | $231,111 | **** | **** | $230,391 | **** | **** |
| Internal Medicine | $169,569 | $120,000 | $158,824 | $171,246 | $167,740 | $170,511 |
| Neonatology | $229,486 | $165,000 | $242,492 | $222,750 | $223,312 | $232,738 |
| Neurological Surgery | $465,006 | $400,000 | $352,352 | $495,266 | $553,500 | $465,006 |
| Neurology | $201,241 | $151,960 | $180,882 | $199,614 | $204,000 | $201,241 |
| Nuclear Medicine (MD only) | $268,450 | **** | **** | $277,193 | **** | $267,500 |

| Specialty | All Physicians | Starting | East | West | South | North |
|---|---|---|---|---|---|---|
| Obstetrics | $240,165 | **** | **** | $228,813 | $280,145 | $232,180 |
| Occupational/Environmental Medicine | $181,716 | $140,000 | $157,611 | $182,159 | $173,541 | $187,470 |
| Ophthalmology | $264,422 | $177,500 | $232,863 | $254,743 | $276,280 | $304,994 |
| Oral Surgery | $308,320 | **** | **** | **** | $283,476 | $320,007 |
| Orthopedic Surgery | $381,429 | $250,000 | $336,163 | $374,942 | $390,270 | $393,249 |
| Orthopedic-Medical | $252,803 | **** | $326,938 | $250,650 | **** | $219,502 |
| Orthopedic Surgery - Joint Replacement | $450,000 | **** | **** | $456,912 | **** | $449,839 |
| Orthopedic Surgery – Hand | $389,997 | **** | $335,000 | 378,000 | **** | $393,497 |
| Orthopedic Surg.-Pediatrics | $389,997 | **** | **** | **** | **** | $389,999 |
| Orthopedic Surgery – Spine | $518,937 | **** | **** | $574,345 | **** | $433,658 |
| Otolaryngology | $303,000 | $210,000 | $250,390 | $282,966 | $303,011 | $320,007 |
| Pathology (MD only) | $250,000 | **** | $245,422 | $247,764 | $252,000 | $268,500 |
| Pediatric Allergy | $186,523 | **** | **** | **** | **** | $186,523 |
| Pediatric Cardiology | $219,992 | **** | **** | **** | **** | $221,492 |
| Pediatric Endocrinology | $169,958 | **** | **** | **** | **** | $168,000 |
| Pediatric Gastroenterology | $193,193 | **** | **** | **** | **** | $190,345 |
| Pediatric Hematology/Oncology | $195,249 | **** | **** | $193,387 | $198,940 | $196,897 |
| Pediatric Intensive Care | $200,000 | **** | **** | **** | $200,000 | $200,000 |
| Pediatric Nephrology | **** | **** | **** | **** | **** | **** |
| Pediatric Neurology | $185,212 | **** | **** | **** | **** | $192,528 |
| Pediatric Pulmonary Disease | $158,429 | **** | **** | **** | **** | **** |
| Pediatric Surgery | $326,399 | **** | **** | **** | **** | $354,871 |
| Pediatrics & Adolescent | $169,267 | $115,000 | $155,916 | $168,301 | $191,511 | $168,609 |
| Pediatric Infectious Disease | $173,993 | **** | **** | **** | **** | $173,993 |
| Perinatology | $341,922 | **** | $246,597 | $336,537 | **** | $399,360 |
| Physical Medicine & Rehabilitation | $193,468 | $145,000 | **** | $183,362 | $204,775 | $201,993 |
| Plastic & Reconstruction | $328,764 | $220,020 | $273,000 | $344,059 | $344,998 | $353,983 |
| Psychiatry | $177,000 | $135,000 | $155,673 | $197,021 | $168,160 | $177,000 |
| Psychiatry – Child | $192,416 | **** | **** | $220,055 | **** | $183,621 |
| Pulmonary Disease | $222,000 | $163,626 | $199,831 | $249,865 | $225,400 | $228,359 |
| Radiation Therapy (MD only) | $334,171 | **** | $285,940 | $343,844 | $328,350 | $368,240 |
| Reproductive Endocrinology | $263,568 | **** | **** | **** | **** | **** |
| Rheumatologic Disease | $188,260 | $150,000 | $153,000 | $192,026 | $181,525 | $193,301 |
| Sports Medicine | $193,573 | **** | **** | **** | **** | **** |
| Surgical Pathology (MD only) | $ | $ | **** | **** | **** | **** |
| Surgical Sports Medicine | $391,497 | **** | $485,670 | $459,592 | **** | $389,997 |
| Transplant Surgery – Kidney | $345,000 | **** | **** | **** | **** | $379,995 |
| Transplant Surgery – Liver | $349,788 | **** | **** | **** | **** | $379,995 |
| Trauma Surgery | $312,272 | **** | $265,457 | **** | $310,385 | $352,352 |
| Urgent Care | $176,353 | $125,500 | $179,300 | $179,357 | $180,395 | $173,683 |
| Urology | $324,690 | $219,229 | $270,493 | $302,600 | $351,585 | $358,008 |
| Vascular Surgery | $335,642 | $221,500 | $297,636 | $318,388 | $337,762 | $350,000 |
| Phlebology^ | $170,000 | **** | **** | **** | **** | $170,000 |
| Podiatry+ | $111,130 | **** | **** | **** | **** | **** |

Sources:   * 2003 AMGA Physician Compensation Survey
+ 2005 Podiatry Management Compensation Report
^ 2006 iMBA Inc., Proprietary Compensation Statistics

## Other Professionals

- **Dentists are Different:**   The 2003 Survey of Dental Practice reported net income from dentistry-related sources. Dentists differ from physicians in that 90% are in private practice. In 2003, the average practitioner's net income was $177,340. The average specialist's net was $300,200.[12] These figures represent a 1.7% and a 3.0% increase over 2002, respectively. Net income has risen steadily since 1986, when general dentists made an average of $69,920, and specialists an average of $97,920.

- **So are Chiropractors:** According to Salary.com,[13] the median salary for chiropractors was $78,994 in 2005; while on Collegegrad.com,[14] the median annual earnings of a salaried chiropractor was $65,330 in 2002; with the middle 50% earning between $44,140 and $102,400. The U.S. Bureau of Labor Statistics estimated chiropractors earned an average salary of $82,060 in 2005.[15] A Chiropractic Economics survey in 2005 suggested mean salary at $104,363.[16]

- **Primary Care Doctors Making a Comeback:** Recruitment of primary care physicians soared over the past year. According to a report released by Merritt, Hawkins & Associates,[17] the request for family doctors jumped 55% from March 2005 to April 1, 2006, while the Associated Press reported demand for internists rose 46%. The average overture to a family doctor was $145,000. Salaries offered to internists in the last few months of 2005 were up about 10%-15%.[18]

## Employed Physician Compensation Models

According to corporate medical recruiter Kris Barlow, physicians can select from various employment models that may include fringe benefit packages (i.e., life, health, dental, disability insurance; medical society and hospital dues, journals, vacations, auto, CEUs, etc.) equal to 25%-40% of their salary.[19]

- **Independent Contractor or Employee?** A payor has the right to control or direct only the result of the work done by an independent contractor, and not the means or methods of accomplishing the result. By contrast, anyone who performs services for another is an employee if he or she can control what will be done and how it will be done. Thus, employed physicians are usually not compensated as independent contractors.

- **New Practitioner Salaries:** Published annually for new practitioners by The Health Care Group®, the *Physician Starting Salary Survey* collects and collates nationwide data on new physician employment compensation.[20] The guide reports first, second and third year of starting physicians' salary and incentives, but with large high-low spreads. It also includes information about co-ownership provisions, benefits, and restrictive covenants. The survey is categorized by specialty and results are based on information provided by medical practices, health care advisors, physicians, and health care consultants across the country. The figures represent basic elements of the bid/ask process for establishing optimal salary and benefit amounts for new physicians entering private practice. Available at no charge from the Health Care Group (800.473.0030 or www.HealthCareGroup.com).

- **Public Equity Relationships:** The public equity roll-up model of medical partnerships in the late 1990s offered employed physicians experience within a large group whose decisions were made by managers. Compensation was controlled and replaced with the stress of investor expectations, as physician practice management companies (PPMCs) needed to grow revenues by 10%-15% annually to maintain price-to-earnings ratios. If stock was held in a growing PPMC, physician employees shared in both practice and corporate compensation. A recent survey of the Cain Brothers Physician Practice Management Corporation Index of publicly traded PPMCs, revealed a market capitalization loss of more than 95% since inception.

Regardless of compensation model, a review of the nonqualified deferred compensation plan (NQDCP) concept is vital for the economic success of any physician employee.

- **Nonqualified deferred compensation plans.** More employed physicians than ever are eligible for NQDCPs as a fringe benefit. But, NQDCPs are subject to rules, and those faced with this opportunity should have a basic understanding of the tension between the benefits of taxation and the security of those benefits.

  i. **Federal Income Taxation:** An NQDCP plan is not subject to the minimum coverage and nondiscrimination requirements of a qualified deferred compensation plan (QDCP), and can be designed to cover "highly compensated" physician employees. But, the tax treatment of a NQDCP is not favorable; for example, employers are not entitled to tax deductions until benefits are paid to the physician. And, under the doctrine of "constructive receipt," benefits are taxable when the employee has the right to receive them without regard to when actually paid, unless the employer's obligation remains an "unfunded and unsecured" promise to pay.

  ii. **Tax-Exempt Employers:** Generally, NQDCP benefits are limited by the relationship between payments and timing of an employer's tax deduction. However, since tax-exempt employers (like some hospitals) are not concerned with tax deductions, the Internal Revenue Code imposes taxes when paid (as opposed to the time of deferral) only if the plan meets IRC Section 457 requirements, including annual contribution limits indexed for inflation.

In 2003, employee contributions to a 457(b) plan were limited to 100% of compensation not to exceed $12,000 and increased through 2006. Benefits providing deferred compensation in excess of indexed limitations become taxable when they are not subject to a "substantial risk of forfeiture" (i.e., requiring a physician to remain an employee for a fixed number of years).

iii. **Social Security Taxes:** Employees also experience special timing rules for Social Security (FICA) taxes. Although an amount deferred under a non-qualified plan may not be subject to income tax until paid, the amount is subject to FICA tax when it is no longer subject to a substantial risk of forfeiture. The old-age portion of the FICA tax (6.2% employer plus 6.2% employee) was subject to a taxable wage base of $94,200 in 2006. Therefore, if compensation exceeds that amount, the accrual of a deferred compensation benefit does not increase the 6.2% tax. On the other hand, the Medicare portion of the FICA tax (1.45% employer plus 1.45% employee) is not subject to a wage base. Therefore, the full deferred compensation obligation can be subject to Medicare tax prior to actual payment of the benefit.

iv. **Security of Benefits:** NQDCPs must remain "unfunded and unsecured" and remain assets of the employer, subject to claims of creditors. Thus, there is a possibility that benefits may not be received. There are two situations in which this becomes an issue: 1) bankruptcy and 2) non-bankruptcy. One non-bankruptcy situation is control-change, as new management may not honor obligations adopted by prior management. Another is a cash flow crisis, as management may pay vendors more vital to business continuation at the expense of physician participants.

v. **The Rabbi Trust:** Under this trust, funds used for plan compensation are transferred to a third-party trustee, who is required to pay benefits as they become due without regard to the employer, thus protecting physicians in the event of non-bankruptcy events.

vi. **Bankruptcy of Employer:** Since funds deferred under a NQDCP remain subject to general creditor claims, secured creditors are paid in full first and physician participants are among the unsecured creditors waiting for residual amounts. Thus, a rabbi trust offers no security to participants in the event of bankruptcy.

vii. **Secular Trust:** A secular trust protects the employed physician in bankruptcy, but the price is current taxation on deferred amounts. Occasionally, a hybrid, the "rabbicular trust," may be used, under which a rabbi trust converts to a secular trust (taxable) upon the occurrence of an event signaling employer cash flow difficulty.

## Newer Health Care Delivery and Physician Compensation Models

Today, whether independent or employed, physicians can pursue several creative compensation models not available a decade ago:

- **Management Service Organization (MSO) Contracting:** According to Jeffrey Peters, physicians maintain private practice in this model, but contract with a management services organization to relieve administrative burdens. Physicians maintain control with less stress, but, as MSO contracts are expensive (20%-50% revenue), compensation diminishes, and rests on MSO competence.[21]

- **Locum Tenens Practitioner:** Locum Tenens (LT) is an alternative to full-time employment for most specialties, allowing physicians to work temporarily as a substitute for another provider from a similar speciality. Some younger physicians enjoy the travel associated with this model, while mature physicians like the ability to practice as they desire. Employment factors to consider include: firm reputation, malpractice insurance, credentialing, travel, and relocation expenses (which are negotiable). However, a LT firm typically will not cover taxes.

### Locum Tenens Specialty Compensation per 8-Hour Shift

| | |
|---|---|
| CRNA | $720 to $880 |
| Family Practice | $400 to $450 |
| Internal Medicine | $400 to $450 |
| Pediatrics | $400 to $430 |
| OB/GYN | $600 to $800 |
| Hospitalist | $520 to $760 |
| General Surgeon | $650 to $750 |
| Orthopedic Surgeon | $800 to $900 |
| Neurosurgeon | $1,300 to $1,400 |
| Anesthesiologist | $1,000 to $1,500 |
| Psychiatrist | $500 to $600 |
| Radiologist | $1,200 to $1,500 |
| Cardiologist | $600 to $750 |

Source: LocumTenens.com

- **Cash-based Compensation:** A cash-based compensation (CBC) model attracts patients who pay cash for desirable services, such as surgeons who dispense scar reducers, or in areas such as pain relief, weight loss, aesthetic procedures, and natural health. According to Michael Walerstein, any well-rounded CBC program should include: patient demand; low entry cost; little marketing costs; existing employees to administer the program; and an operational plan. With time and effort, profit for physician compensation may increase 10%-20% annually.[22]

- **Concierge Medicine:** Retainer or boutique medicine first emerged in the mid-1990s. For an annual fee, primary care physicians offer patients top-drawer treatment and amenities like same-day and extended appointments, house calls, enhanced referral coordination and 24-hour access. Patients pay annual out-of-pocket fees, but use traditional health insurance to cover allowed expenses. Annual fees range from $1,000 to $5,000 per patient, to family fees that top $20,000 a year. For these physicians, the opportunity to practice unhurried medicine is priceless compensation.[23]

- **Consumer-Directed Health Plans (CDHPs):** Although patient cost-sharing may be ill-advised in some circumstances, it is unrealistic to completely ignore the need to constrain cost growth. Critics contend that patients and doctors will not negotiate fees, and that CDHPs are harmful as they attract a younger, healthier population.[24] Yet, the sickest 1% of policyholders can constitute up to 40% or more of group health care claims.[25] Nevertheless, when appropriately used, they can cut costs for patients while enhancing the cashflow needs and compensation wants of providers, as presented in these two compensation models:

  — **Medical and Health Savings Account Model (MSAs and HSAs):** MSAs and HSAs allow tax-deferred savings for costs not covered by health insurance plans, based on the concept of high deductibles and low premiums. Incumbent in the model is fee transparency and negotiated private-pay cash payments up to deductible amounts. According to the Government Accountability Office (GAO), the number of patients using these plans jumped from 3 million in January 2005 to 6 million by January 2006.[26] Physician fee information becomes more transparent through search tools such as www.HowMuchDoc.com and www.CashCare.us that enable those with CDHPs to find a doctor or health care facility and offers discounts for drugs, durable medical equipment, and to patients who pay at the time of service.[27,28] The American Hospital Association has acquiesced to market pressures regarding facility price transparency, which fits with the Bush administration's strategy of moving patients into CDHPs in the hope that cost increases will slow as people seek best deals. The Centers for Medicare and Medicaid Services (CMS) are also releasing cost data, broken down to the county level, regarding such procedures as heart operations, back and neck operations, and hip and knee replacement.[29]

  — **Value-Based Health Insurance Model:** According to A. Mark Fendrick, MD, and Michael E. Chernew, PhD, instead of the one size fits all approach of traditional health insurance, a "clinically-sensitive" cost-sharing system that supports co-payments related to evidence-based value for targeted patients seems plausible. In this model, out-of-pocket costs are based on price and a cost/quality tradeoff in clinical circumstances: low co-payments for interventions of highest value, and higher co-payments for interventions with little proven health benefit. Smarter benefit packages are designed to combine disease management with cost sharing to address spending growth.[30]

— **Global Health Care Model:** American businesses are extending their cost-cutting initiatives to include offshore employee medical benefits, and facilities like the Bumrungrad Hospital in Bangkok, Thailand (cosmetic surgery), the Apollo Hospital in New Delhi, India (cardiac and orthopedic surgery) are premier examples for surgical care. Both are internationally-recognized institutions that resemble 5-star hotels equipped with the latest medical technology. Countries such as Finland, England and Canada are also catering to the English-speaking crowd, while dentistry is especially popular in Mexico and Costa Rica. Although this is still considered "medical tourism," Mercer Health and Benefits was recently retained by three Fortune 500 companies interested in contracting with offshore hospitals and Joint Commission on Accreditation of Healthcare Organizations (JCAHO) has accredited 88 foreign hospitals through a joint international commission. To be sure, when India can discount costs up to 80%, the effects on domestic hospital reimbursement and physician compensation may be assumed to increase downward compensation pressures.[31]

Regardless of model, CDHPs are not a panacea to the health care crisis. Novel benefit models that include cost-sharing may allow for more efficient management of resources, although the effects on physician compensation have yet to be discerned.

## Assessment

Money, received as salary in the present, can earn money over a period of time (making the amount ultimately larger than if the same initial sum were received later). Therefore, both the amount of investment return and the length of time it takes to receive that return affect the rate of return (i.e., the value of the return). This principle, known as the time value of money (TVM), is a vital compensation issue regarding ultimate wealth accumulation.

For example, according to the March 31, 2005 issue of *Physician's Money Digest*, a 47-year-old doctor with $184,000 in annual income would need about $5.5 million dollars for retirement at age 65.[32] This should serve as a wake-up call that physicians may need to cut personal consumption and professional expenses, and save more aggressively to harvest the TVM to finance the retirement they're working toward. Remember, compensation is not the sole arbiter of success. To run your own numbers, visit: www3.troweprice.com/ric/RIC.

Therefore, according to Eugene Schmuckler, PhD, it is not too difficult to imagine the following rules for those doctors wishing to maximize compensation:[33]

**Rule No. 1:**  A great idea or competitive advantage can earn generous compensation while still serving the public. It's a *unit-of-one* health care economy, where "Me Inc." is the standard and physicians must maneuver for advantages that boost credibility among patients and payors.  You must also realize the power of networking, vertical integration, and the establishment of PRN "medical practices," which physically or virtually come together to treat a patient or cohort, and then disband when a successful outcome is achieved.

**Rule No. 2:** Differentiate yourself among your peers. Do or learn something new and unknown by your competitors. Market your accomplishments and let the world know. Be a non-conformist. Doctors should create and innovate; do not blindly follow leaders into oblivion.

**Rule No. 3:** Challenge conventional wisdom, think outside the box, recapture your dreams and ambitions, and work harder than you have ever worked before. Remember the old saying, "if everyone is thinking alike, then nobody is thinking."

**Rule No 4:** Realize that the present is not necessarily the future. Attempt to see the future and discern your place in it. Master the art of the quick change, and fast but informed decision making. Do what you love, disregard what you don't, and let the fates have their way with you. Then, decide for yourself if you should be an employer or employee, or adhere to any of the above compensation models.

## Conclusion

Dr. Regina E. Herzlinger, the Nancy R. McPherson professor of business administration and chair at Harvard Business School, and mother of a physician-daughter, opines that there is little wonder that some physicians become depressed and want to give up their careers entirely when pondering the future of medicine, managed care and related compensation issues.

In her book, *Market Driven Healthcare*, Herzlinger implores phsycisians, "don't give up practice, yet." Pragmatically, the future is bright and offers great opportunity to early adaptors who have the foresight to change medicine for the better and be handsomely compensated, too! But, physicians' inability to deal with competitive market forces is well known and many are loath to deal with them.[34]

One way is to seek additional education through a traditional Master's Degree in Business/Health Administration (MBA/MHA), or use an online distance-education resource. Tuition, textbooks and fees may be tax deductible.[35] In this way, doctors may maintain their place as salary and compensation leaders in the U.S. labor force.

## Case Study

*[The New Recruit]*

**Internal Medicine Physician**
**Candidate: Dr. Joe Perez, DO**

New Dr. Joe was being considered by Dr. Mature to join his solo medical practice.

*Personal History*
Dr. Joe grew up in New Jersey and has lived in many locations throughout his medical school and training. He and his wife currently lived in San Diego, CA, where he was completing his residency. They wanted to settle in Massachusetts, as his wife was from the area.

*Education/Training*
See CV. Dr. Joe is licensed in MA and completes his residency in June 2007.

*Professional Goals*
Dr. Joe is seeking a general internal medicine position. He would like an office-based practice with the opportunity to treat hospital and nursing home patients. He has special interest in diabetes care and extensive critical care experience.

*First Impressions*
Dr. Mature's on-site visit and conversation with new Dr. Joe was open, honest and relaxed. He was eager to share his ideas and goals for his first private medical practice. Of course, compensation was an issue too, although new Dr. Joe was just beginning to understand the declining reimbursement environment.

**Key Interpretive Issues**

Improving financial compensation as an employed physician of Dr. Mature was a balancing act for Dr. Joe, between pragmatism and performance. Whether that strategy called for expanding the practice, moving into a key market, or recruiting the right physician, Dr. Mature's plan was important for them both. Simply put, finding and hiring the right physician, at the correct compensation level, was their prescription for mutual economic success.

Additionally, both mature physicians and new residents fresh out of training have become more discerning and skillful in managing the compensation process. Candidates have learned to be selective based on how they're treated on the phone, in-person during site onsite visits; or how smoothly or unique the compensation negotiations proceed. Yet, in truth, some mature physicians like Dr. Mature, look to rule out doctor-hires based only on salary, not in.

### Compensation Levels and Contracts

Dr. Joe wanted a proper compensation package and Dr. Mature needed to offer an employment contract with future performance potential. Putting the financial pieces together began by researching and reviewing all available data about market opportunities. Dr. Mature and Dr. Joe used the American Board of Medical Specialties, the AMA database, and other private resources to learn about numbers and locations of physicians in key specialty areas. They also gathered statistics about the target market nationally and regionally. This helped them determine the financial and competitive nature of the employment process.

### Additional Considerations for Dr. Mature
- Who is the ideal candidate?
- What does the practice need in terms of professional experience?
- Does the candidate need to be proficient in any particular patient skills?
- What about personality?
- Is the candidate seen as a future equity partner?

### Additional Considerations for Dr. Joe
- What do you like or dislike about your current role as a resident physician?
- What factors do you feel make up a satisfying medical practice?
- What type of practice arrangements are you seeking?
- What is your cultural fit with the community?
- Why do you wish to join the practice, or affiliate with the clinic or local hospital, etc?
- What are your future goals?
- Do you wish to become an equity partner?

**More Due Diligence**

Dr. Joe used all available information about the physician compensation process that he could find. Additionally he sought the assistance of a health economist, negotiation consultant and other collegial input. Together, they determined median compensation, per physician work RVU by specialty.

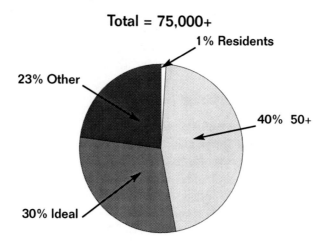

**Research Challenges**

- To obtain a sufficient sample size for medical specialty and sub-specialty.
- To obtain data divided by urban versus rural practitioner information, which may be a greater differential than various geographic regions in most surveys.
- To match survey focus populations with physician specialty.

**Assessment**

A growing number of surveys measure physician compensation, encompassing a varying depth of analysis. And, physician compensation data, divided by specialty and subspecialty, are central to a range of consulting activities like practice assessments and medical entity valuation comparisons between entity and practitioner earnings with national and local averages. The Medical Group Management Association's annual "Physician Compensation and Production Correlations Survey" is a particularly well-known source of these data. One should, however, endeavor to seek out as much information as possible and consider all available data in order to come to a compensation amount that may be reasonable for a comparable entity or practitioner.

### The Outcome

The health economist that Dr. Joe consulted noted that inasmuch as most physicians are not members of the AMA, any salary statistics might be suspect; and private surveys usually project overly optimistic figures, as well. She also suggested that most numbers were for physicians with 3-5 years experience, rather than newbie's.

Additionally, she outlined the following compensation schemes for Dr. Joe to appreciate:

- Physician collections and shared overhead
- Fixed compensation, plus bonus
- Bonus based on percentage of collections
- Bonus based on percentage of net production
- Equal compensation for both doctors
- Fixed compensation, plus percentage of net production
- Percentage of net production

On the other hand, Dr. Joe's Spanish language skills were considered a plus by Dr. Mature, and his wife had strong ties to the local growing community. After several weeks of negotiations, an acceptable compensation package was produced at a 10% salary discount to the norm, since the area had a very reasonable cost-of-living percentage. A health law attorney reviewed the fixed compensation, plus bonus-contract, before final signature.

However, because of Dr. Joe's Spanish fluency and his critical care experience, Dr. Joe's production soon exceeded even Dr. Matures' expectations, and three years later, discussions were underway regarding partnership arrangements.

## Study / Discussion Questions

1. Is physician compensation undergoing salary expansion or compression in the current managed care environment? Can one make any accurate future projections?

2. Which specific medical specialty salaries are benefiting or lagging due to competitive market pressures? How does the aging demographic affect this scenario?

3. How do the goodwill conundrum and valuation paradox affect medical practice value relative to mature physician over-compensation for practice worth? How do the paradox and conundrum differ for buyers and sellers?

4. What is the impact of CDHP fee-transparency on physician compensation? On health care entity profitability?

5. What is the future of the independent medical practitioner model? How about the employed physician model?

## References

1. Marcinko DE. Status of Doctor and Medical Unions. In: Marcinko DE, ed. *Financial Planning for Physicians and Healthcare Professionals*, 2nd edition. New York, NY: Aspen Publishers; 2002.

2. Prince RA. *Wealth Preservation for Physicians*. New York, NY: Primedia, Inc.; 2006.

3. Gawande A. *Complications: A Surgeon's Notes on an Imperfect Science*. New York, NY: Picador USA; 2003.

4. The 2006 Annual Reports, Social Security and Medicare Board of Trustees. Available at: http://www.cms.hhs.gov/ReportsTrustFunds/downloads/tr2006.pdf. Accessed July 27, 2006.

5. The Health Resources and Services Administration. About the Health Education Assistance Loan (HEAL) Program. Available at: http://bhpr.hrsa.gov/DSA/healsite/about.htm. Accessed July 27, 2006.

6. Garner BA, Black HC, eds. *Black's Law Dictionary, 7th ed*. St. Paul, MN: West Publishing Co.; 1999.

7. Cimasi RJ, Alexander T. Valuation of Hospitals in a Changing Regulatory Environment. In: Marcinko DE, ed. *Healthcare Organizations: Financial Management Strategies*. Blaine, WA: Specialty Technical Publishers; 2007.

8. Schilbach v. Commissioner, T.C. Memo 1991-556.

9. Galtress E. Human Resource Options for the Harried Physician. In: Marcinko DE, ed. *The Business of Medical Practice*, 1st ed. New York, NY: Springer Publishing; 2000.

10. Moon S. Big demand, bigger paydays; physician compensation survey shows how far primary-care docs lag behind their specialist colleagues in pay rate, growth. *Mod Health*. July 19, 2004.

11. Gunnett GJ. Nonqualified deferred compensation plans. *Physician's News Digest*, October 2000. Available at www.physiciansnews.com/business/1000gunnett.htm. Accessed July 27, 2006.

12. American Dental Association. 2004 Survey of Dental Practice—Income from the Private Practice of Dentistry, January 2006.

13. www.Salary.com.

14. www.Collegegrad.com.

15. Bureau of Labor Statistics. 2005 Chiropractic Statistics. Available at: http://www.bls.gov/oes/current/oes291011.htm. Accessed July 26, 2006.

16. Segall L. What our 9th Annual Salary and Expense Survey discloses. *Chiropractic Economics Magazine.* 2006: 6:22-52. Available at: http://www.chiroeco.com/article/2006/Issue6/9thSalarySurvey.pdf.

17. Walerstein M. Consider cash based subspecialties, *Physician's News Digest.* April 1998.

18. Agovino T. Demand for primary care physicians rises. Associated Press: New York. May 24, 2006.

19. Barlow K. Establishing Healthy Medical Partner Relations. In: Marcinko DE, ed. *The Advanced Business of Medical Practice,* 2nd ed. New York, NY: Springer Publishing; 2004.

20. The Health Care Group. Physician Starting Salary Survey. Available at: http://www.healthcaregroup.com/servlet/catalog.ProductDetails?pid=2. Access August 4, 2006.

21. Peters J. Alternatives to becoming an employee. *Physician's News Digest.* August 1997. Available at: http://www.physiciansnews.com/business/897peters.html. Accessed October 4, 2006.

22. Walerstein M. Cash based anti-aging medical specialties. *Physician's News Digest.* April 2000.

23. McCarthy A. The Case for Concierge Medicine In: Marcinko DE, ed. *The Advanced Business of Medical Practice,* 2nd edition. New York, NY: Springer Publishing; 2004.

24. Fowles JB, Kind EA, Braun BL, Bertko J. Early experience with employee choice of consumer-directed health plans and satisfaction with enrollment. *Health Serv Res.* 2004; 39:1141-1158.

25. Vrana D. Prozac: Hazardous to your Health Insurance. Available at: http://articles.moneycentral.msn.com/Insurance/InsureYourHealth/ProzacHazardToYourHealthInsurance.aspx?page=all. Accessed July 27, 2006.

26. Government Accountability Office, "Consumer-Directed Health Plans: Early Enrollee Experiences with Health Savings Accounts and Eligible Health Plans," GAO-06-798, August 8, 2006.

27. www.HowMuchDoc.com.

28. www.CashCareUSA.com.

29. Centers for Medicare and Medicaid Services. Healthcare Consumer Initiatives Overview. Available at: http://www.cms.hhs.gov/HealthCareConInit/01_Overview.asp. Accessed October 10, 2006.

30. Fendrick AM, Chernew ME. Value-based insurance design: a "clinically sensitive" approach to preserve quality of care and contain costs. *Am J Manag Care.* 2006;12:18-20.

31. Walker T. Consumers go abroad in pursuit of cost-effective healthcare. *Managed Healthcare Executive*. July 2006. Available at: http://www.managedhealthcareexecutive.com/mhe/article/articleDetail.jsp?id=357668. Accessed July 26, 2006.

32. Kelly GJ. Are You on Your Way to $5.5 Million? *Physician's Money Digest*. March 31, 2005.

33. Schmuckler E. Relinquishing the Role of Physician Leadership. In: Marcinko DE, ed. *The Business of Medical Practice*, 1st ed. New York, NY: Springer Publishing; 2000.

34. Herzlinger R. *Market Driven Healthcare: Who Wins, Who Loses in the Transformation of America's Largest Service Industry*. New York, NY: Perseus Books Group; 1999.

35. Internal Revenue Service. Itemized Deductions. IRS Publication 17.

## Suggested Readings

1. Cimasi RJ, Alexander T. Valuation of Hospitals in a Changing Regulatory Environment. In: Marcinko DE, ed. *Healthcare Organizations: Financial Management Strategies*. Blaine, WA: Specialty Technical Publishers; 2007.

2. Fenton CF. Risk Management in Modern Medical Practice. In: Marcinko DE, ed. *Insurance and Risk Management Strategies for Physicians and Advisors*. Sudbury, MA: Jones and Bartlett Publishers; 2005.

3. Hetico R. Selecting Your Advisory Team. In: Marcinko DE, ed. *Financial Planning for Physicians and Healthcare Professionals*. New York, NY: Aspen Publishers; 2003.

4. Marcinko DE, Hetico HR. *Dictionary of Health Economics and Finance*. New York, NY: Springer Publishers; 2007.

5. McCarthy, A: Physician Recruiting. In: Marcinko DE, ed. *The Advanced Business of Medical Practice*, 2nd ed. New York, NY: Springer Publishers; 2004.

6. Schmuckler E, Shubin-Stein K, Wagner R: Bridging Financial Planning and Human Psychology. In: Marcinko DE, ed. *Financial Planning for Physicians and Advisors*. Sudbury, MA: Jones and Bartlett Publishers; 2005.

## Websites

American Medical Group Association: www.AMGA.org

U.S. Bureau of Labor Statistics: www.BLS.gov

Certified Medical Planners: www.CertifiedMedicalPlanner.com

Health Capital Consultants: www.HealthCapital.com

How Much Doc: www.HowMuchDoc.com

MD Intellinet: www.MDIntellinet.com

## Additional Resources

Related Medical Information Resources
SIC 8043 / NAICS 621391
Physicians

**Bureau of Labor Statistics, U.S. Department of Labor**
*Occupational Outlook Handbook – Physicians*
http://www.google.com/search?hl=en&q=occupational+outlook+handbook
This site describes the nature of the industry, working conditions, employment, occupations in the industry, training and advancement, earnings and benefits, employment outlook, and lists of organizations that provide additional information.

**American Medical Group Association**
*Medical Group Financial Operations Survey*
http://www.amga.org/ Select "Departments – Publications – Data/Statistical Publications"
The financial operations survey provides critical benchmark data on support staff salaries and benefits, staffing profiles, and other key management costs. The data are presented on a per physician basis as well as on a per square foot basis. The summary information pages include financial profiles based on varied managed care revenue percentages and are further broken down by group type, geographic region, and group size, as well as a staffing profile by specialty.

**The Health Care Group**
*Physician Starting Salary Survey*
http://www.healthcaregroup.com   Select "Products – Annual Surveys"
The physician starting salary survey collects nationwide data on new-doctor compensation. The survey reports three initial years of salary and incentive information and includes co-ownership provisions, benefits, and restrictive covenants.

**The Sherlock Company**
*Physician Executive Compensation Analysis*
http://www.sherlockco.com   Select "Analyses"
Douglas B. Sherlock, CFA, is President of Sherlock Company which assists health plans, their business partners and their investors in the treasury, control and compensation functions of healthcare finance.

## Acknowledgements

The authors acknowledge the assistance of Gregory O. Ginn, PhD, MBA, CPA, M.Ed, Assistant Professor, University of Nevada, Department Healthcare Administration, Las Vegas, Nevada.

# Future Trends

# Future Trends

Sara L. Thier, MPH

The goal of this book is to provide you with insight into key issues in health care that will shape how you will practice medicine in the 21st century. The aim of this chapter is to raise some of the questions and concerns that the system and its practitioners face, and to discuss the prominent trends that will ultimately influence the potential resolutions to these concerns.

Will the shift from managed care to consumer-driven health be successful? How will it change the physician-patient relationship? Will the majority of patients actually have an electronic health record by 2014? Will the number of uninsured and underinsured Americans decrease as a result of various local and national efforts? Will pay for performance become the standard, or will another model for reimbursement be implemented? Will reimbursements for Medicare continue to be cut, even as the number of beneficiaries rises in the coming years? Will government-sponsored health care cease, or will it blossom into a universal coverage system?

These and other questions will influence the myriad decisions you will make about how you will practice as this century progresses. You may decide to work in an academic health center or large integrated delivery system. Or, you may select a private group or solo practice. In whichever setting you choose to practice, demographics, socioeconomic conditions, government decisions on coverage, and advancement in treatments and technology will all affect how you practice and how you will be compensated.

## Demographics

Now that the 300 millionth U.S. resident has arrived, either via birth or immigration, the question of demographic changes, and their effects on health care delivery and costs, is a key concern of policy makers and practitioners. Creating solutions for health disparities continues to be problematic and remains a heated topic of political discussion. Differences in the services received, medications prescribed, and health outcomes across races and ethnic populations can be wide and troubling. The lack of reliable solutions to these problems results in delays in receiving care, disruptions in access and other service delivery issues and, for many, creates a faulty safety net at best.

As Chapter 4 suggests, physicians must become more patient-centered in their practices, which includes enhancing their cultural competency and sensitivity to patients from diverse populations. The ensuing debate surrounding immigration and border control is also a factor, as uncompensated services provided for illegal immigrants contribute to the rising cost of health care. Will the United States make a strong statement by refusing to treat illegal immigrants?

Finally, with more Americans entering the older age bracket (60+), the strain upon an already challenged healthcare system is increasing, compounding the issues facing our aging population, such as access to care, coverage, and end-of-life concerns. Will Medicare, and in particular Medicare Part D, be able to provide appropriate and quality care to a population that is expected to be plagued with multiple chronic conditions, complications, and medications? Even with Congress' efforts to eliminate the prescription coverage's "doughnut hole," will Medicare's design and benefits continue to spur disparities in care? Will increasing the eligibility age reduce the threat of depleted funds, or will younger Americans face even more issues if the system is not reformed?

## Information Technology

Is the aim of a nationwide network of electronic health records (EHRs) by 2014 a pipedream or a feasible goal? While larger organizations are embracing the integration of health information technology (HIT), the majority of providers (i.e., small medical groups and practices) are troubled with the acquisition costs, workflow impediments, and uncertainty of return on investment. Yet, the growing use of outcome measurement to inform quality improvement initiatives, payor and consumer choice, and reimbursement ultimately may become the tipping point for widespread adoption of HIT across facilities and practices.

HIT will continue to affect quality of care in general, and how you deliver this care. In the July 2006 report *Preventing Medication Errors: Quality Chasm Series*, the Institute of Medicine recommends that by 2010 all prescriptions should be written and processed electronically (e-prescribing).[1] This and other similar recommendations, along with integration of evidence-based guidelines and decision-making tools, make HIT essential for achieving the IOM's six aims of quality care, (safer, more efficient, patient-centered, timely, effective, and equitable).[2] Many are waiting for earlier adopters of HIT to demonstrate that these technologies can improve workflow and, ultimately, health outcomes. In conjunction with site-specific demonstrations, national work on data standards and interoperability must continue in order to quell resistance to the adoption of technology and to ensure that information sharing across facilities is achieved.

Along with standards and overarching interoperability issues, information-sharing concerns and strategies must be refined. The numerous regional health information organizations (RHIOs) across the country are working hard, albeit differently, to cultivate information-sharing programs that can benefit both individual patients and public health in general. Coordination is lacking, even across individual states, and raises the questions about the government and the country's readiness and ability to adopt the standards and procedures necessary to implement a nationwide health information network (NHIN). Studies across various stakeholders show support and expectations of implementing a NHIN within the next 5-10 years.[3] Without the involvement and feedback of all of the key stakeholders, the NHIN has the potential to become yet another dysfunctional federal program.

## Government and Government Programs

In 2004, the Institute of Medicine's Committee on the Consequences of Uninsurance called upon the federal government to establish universal coverage by 2010.[4] Individual mandates, employer mandates, tax breaks for obtaining coverage, or coverage under a single payor are among the universal coverage models that have been proposed national and locally. As mounting health care costs and consumer-related concerns create pressure for system overhaul, it is unclear what model or combination of models will prevail in the end. The federal government has failed to successfully overhaul Medicare, taking incremental steps (often backwards) in ensuring coverage. The Department of Defense (DOD) and the Veterans Administration (VA) health system, on the other hand, have leveraged their funding and results from health services research to create relatively effective and efficient systems that stand as models for implementing new strategies ranging from care teams to technology. Beyond these two microcosms, the federal government continues to sort through our tattered health care system, trying to piece together a new design from remnants.

Currently, state governments are taking the lead in creating change. Since 1994, the Oregon Health Plan[5] has stood as an example of how cost-benefit analysis can play an important role in creating an essential coverage package for Medicaid recipients. Though not ideal, it uses planning techniques similar to those of certain countries with universal coverage, by recognizing an allotted dollar amount available for care and then creating a utilitarian coverage. Is this the model the country should adopt to rein in costs while providing at least a basic level of care for all?

Massachusetts has already set the pace for refurbishing the way health care services are covered and delivered. The state's individual mandate puts health coverage squarely in the hands of the consumers, while ensuring that their safety net programs are intact and functioning. How this model will play out is yet to be seen, but it promises to offer numerous lessons for other states and perhaps even the federal government. Others states, including Vermont and Rhode Island, are setting additional precedents by pushing for single payor systems.[6,7]

## Reimbursement

Payment models vary depending on the type of organization in which you choose to practice. Each model—fee-for-service, capitation, pay for performance—has its positive and negative effects on containing costs, providing quality of care, and satisfying consumers. The most recent model to enter the fray is the pay for performance design. Though it is still being piloted in several organizations across the country, some are seeing positive returns.[8] This model requires physicians, in group and small practices as well as large health care systems, to document and submit service data, based on a variety of quality indicators. These submissions beg for the widespread use of electronic health/medical records.

Medicare cuts in reimbursement are predicted to continue, and will put additional strain on hospital and physician care. Can providers afford to give up Medicare reimbursements? Can they afford not to? Will patient care and access to care suffer? How much further can payments be cut before care for Medicare patients breaks everyone's bank?[9,10]

## Disease Management and Consumerism

The recent push for consumer activation and accountability around health care costs and choices has created two prominent cost containment strategies: disease management and consumer-driven health care. The impetus for reform comes not only over concern for substandard care for chronic illness, but also from the desire of insurers and payors to shift responsibility for care management (and costs) onto consumers. Physicians have the goal of monitoring and promoting self-management, including encouraging healthy behaviors, medication adherence, and seeking care in a timely manner. Many do an adequate job. However, by enlisting more structured disease management programs, payors have the ability to target those in need of support, especially those who overutilize health services and expend the greatest percentage health care dollars. While disease management programs appear to improve health outcomes, their effects on health care costs are less clear.[11] The potential of this program design to save money must be more clearly documented before there will be full confidence in this strategy. As a result of various mergers and acquisitions, there are fewer numbers of disease management companies, creating a stronger set of competitors. As these companies progress from an individual disease management focus to a more holistic approach, there may be a shift from the current "disease" management vernacular to "care" management.

In order to achieve the goal of creating a more traditional consumer market model in health care, thorough, user-friendly and relevant information is needed. Use of the Internet and other personal technologies, such as PDAs and cell phones, will be essential to meeting this need. Health care consumers will need education on what information is available, how to interpret it, and how to act on it. As a trusted provider, your input and guidance will be sought and you should be prepared to assist. Consumer demand for quality is beginning to grow and physicians must learn how to work within this new patient-activation paradigm rather than be threatened by it. One current strategy for empowering consumers is the roll-out of consumer-driven health plans, which usually include a high deductible health plan supplemented with savings or reimbursement accounts, and appear to have a foothold in the insurance arena. Lower premium costs and availability of portable, tax-sheltered savings accounts make these models attractive to some (primarily younger, healthier, and wealthier) individuals. The greater out-of-pocket risk is making many shy away. It is still unclear if and how these newer models will affect health and health care costs. Yet, regardless of the success or failure of consumer-driven health plans, the accompanying quality and cost data needed to guide consumer choices will be this model's legacy.

## Conclusion

You are entering a rewarding and exciting field, yet the challenges and changes that you may face could seem like an impediment to your work. Your dedication to your patients, and to the professional field of medicine, will allow you to work within the evolving health care parameters.

## References

1. Institute of Medicine Committee on Identifying and Preventing Medication Errors. Aspden P, Wolcott J, Bootman JL, Cronenwett LR, eds. *Preventing Medication Errors: Quality Chasm Series*. Washington, DC: The National Academies Press; 2006.

2. Institute of Medicine. *Crossing the Quality Chasm: A New Health System for the 21st Century*. Washington, DC: The National Academies Press; 2001.

3. Oracle. Temperature Check, Healthcare Provider Community Perceptions on the Road to Electronic Health Records. Oracle "Healthcare Provider Examination" Survey, February 13, 2006.

4. Institute of Medicine Committee on the Consequences of Uninsurance. *Insuring America's Health: Principles and Recommendations*. Washington, DC: The National Academies Press; 2004.

5. Oregon Health Plan. Available at: http://www.oregon.gov/DHS/healthplan/index.shtml Accessed August 18, 2006.

6.  Single Payer Rhode Island (SPRI). Available at: http://www.everybodyinnobodyout.org/ri/. Accessed August 4, 2006.

7.  Vermont Health Care for All. Available at: http://www.vthca.org/index.php. Accessed August 4, 2006.

8.  Curtin K, Beckman H, Pankow G, Milillo Y, Greene RA. ROI in P4P: A diabetes case study. *Health Manag*. In press.

9.  MedPac. www.medpac.gov/

10. American Medical Association. National legislative activities – Medicare. Available at: www.ama-assn.org/ama/pub/category/6583.html. Accessed August 4, 2006.

11. Congressional Budget Office. An Analysis of the Literature on Disease Management Programs. October 13, 2004. Available at: www.cbo.gov/showdoc.cfm?index=5909&sequence=0. Accessed July 13, 2006.

# Index

# Index

## A

Academic practice, 226
Access, 227-228
Accountability, 7, 9, 10
Accounting, 323-336
Accreditation, 234
Active listening, 54, 118-119
Adherence, 95, 100
Advanced access scheduling, 243-255
Adverse medical events, 188, 190, 191, 195
Antitrust, 144, 145, 146, 150
Appeals, 163, 268-270, 272-274
Authorization, 259-262, 266-268, 272

## B

Bar-designated specialty, 131
Billing, 353-356, 372
    Balance billing, 267
Brand identity, 95
Budgeting, 329
Business plan, 311
Business systems, 305

## C

Capital investment, 303
Cash flow, 326, 332
Centers for Medicare and Medicaid Services (CMS), 173
    Medicaid, 180-183
    Medicare, 173-179
    State Children's Health Insurance Plan (SCHIP), 183
Civil penalties, civil suits, civil claims, 130
Clinical practice guidelines (CPG), 36

Communication, 53, 94-107, 116-119, 122, 229-230
    and adverse medical events, 192-193, 195
    Asynchronous communication, 101, 103
    Email, 101-104
    Interpersonal communication, 67-70 99-100
    and Referrals, 261-263
    and Risk Management, 116-117, 118-119,122-123, 264-265
Compensation, 306, 317
    Compensation versus value paradox,  380
    Cash-based compensation (CBC), 386
Computerized Physician Order Entry (CPOE), 83, 87
Concierge medicine (CM), 387
Consultation, 261, 264-265
Consumer-directed health care, 163-165
    Consumer-directed health plans (CDHP), 387
Control charts, 19
Corporate issues, 144 -149
Coverage, 303-304
    Covered benefit, 260,266
Credentialing, 232-233
Criminal penalties (see HIPAA)
Cultural competency, 49
Cultural sensitivity, 51
Culture of safety, 20

# D

Demand management, 261
Denial, 269-270
Disease management, 204-222
    Defined, 204-205
    Programs, 212-214
Documentation
    Guidelines, 353-355, 358, 360-365
    and risk management, 124-125, 193, 196-198
    and telephone communication, 122-123

# E

Electronic health record (EHR) (see *Health information technology*)
Electronic medical record (EMR) (see *Health information technology*)
Email (see *Communication*)
Encrypted, 102-103
E-newsletter, 95-96
Evaluation and management services, 354-355, 370
Evidence-based care, 34, 40, 41

# F

Financing, 86, 323-336
Five C's of communication, 66
Fraud and abuse, 131, 133, 145

# G

Goodwill conundrum, 379
Group practice, 301-319

# H

Health care team, 55, 65-67
Health information technology (HIT),10, 56-57, 78-87
  Electronic health record (EHR), 78-89, 103
  Electronic medical record (EMR), 41, 78-89, 105, 210-211
  Interoperability, 79, 81, 87-88
Health Insurance Portability and Accountability Act (HIPAA), 102, 131,160
  Criminal penalties under HIPAA, 131, 141-142
  Fraud and abuse, 131, 133
  HIPAA Privacy Rule, 132,
  Mental health care record, 135-136, 137, 138
  Patient rights under HIPAA, 132, 137-141
  Protected health information, 135
Health literacy, 54
Health outcomes, 2-3, 53
Health reimbursement accounts (HRAs), 163
Health savings accounts (HSAs), 163
History, 356-358
Hospital-based practice, 234-237
Hospitalist, 236

# I

Idealized Design of Clinical Office Practices (IDCOP), 245
Indemnity insurance, 156, 157
Independent contractor (IC), 383
Independent review organization (IRO), 270
Informed consent, 123
Institute for Healthcare Improvement (IHI), 9

# L

Lean health care, 237-238
Legal duty (see *Medical malpractice*)
Liability, 115, 143, 144, 194, 196
Liability insurance, 130, 151
Locum tenens practitioner (LTP), 386

# M

Managed care, 156
    Managed care organization (MCO), 269
    Managed care plans, 157
    Health maintenance organization (HMO), 156, 157, 159, 267-268
    Point of service (POS), 159, 258
    Preferred provider organization (PPO), 157,159, 258
Market share, 309
Medical coding, 160-161
Medical error, 16-18
Medical ethics, 150
Medical malpractice, 114-116, 130, 142, 143, 144, 187-201
    Legal duty, 132, 189-190
    Tort reform, 142-144
Medical necessity, 266-267, 269-270
Medical record documentation, 124-125
Medical staff organization (MSO), 232-234
Medline Plus®, 97
Mental health care record (see *Health Insurance Portability and Accountability Act*)
Military medicine, 237

# N

National Committee for Quality Assurance (NCQA), 269, 271
National Health Information Network (NHIN), 79
Negligence, 115-116, 190, 194, 198-199
Negligent referral, 265
Negotiating, 318-319
Nonqualified deferred compensation plans (NQDCP), 384

# O

Open access scheduling, 243-255 (see also *advanced access scheduling*)

# P

Patient expectations, 50
Patient portal, 102-103
Patient safety, 15-25
Patient satisfaction, 57-58
Patient-centered care, Patient-centered practice , patient-centeredness, patient-centered, 33, 34, 35, 48
Pay for performance (P4P), 8, 80, 86, 89, 179, 208, 210, 230
Payment policies, 157, 163
Patient-physician relationship, 48, 55
Patient-provider relationship, 56, 99, 103
Performance measurement, 4-6
Physician advocacy 150-151
Physician buy-in, XXX
Physician-patient relationship, 114-115, 116, 120-121 (see also *patient-physician relationship and patient-provider relationship*)
Payor satisfaction, 39-42
Practice management, 160
    Physician practice management companies (PPMCs), 384
Prior authorization, 260-262, 266-268

# Q

Qualified deferred compensation plan (QDCP), 381
Quality of care, 1-10

# R

Rabbi trust, 21
Reconsideration, 269
Referral, 257-276
Regional health information organization (RHIO), 79
Regulatory issues, 144 -149
Reimbursement, 160
Return on investments (ROI), 85-86, 333
Risk, risk management, 308, 310
Root cause analysis, 17, 19

# S

Secular trust, 21
Sentinel events, 18
Severity adjustment, 6
Shared decision making, 50
Solo practice, 301-319
Staff satisfaction, 38-39
State Children's Health Insurance Plan (SCHIP), (see *Centers for Medicare and Medicaid Services*)
Systems-based practice, 65

# T

Telephone tag, 100-101
Tiered networks, tiered benefits, 165-166, 210
Transparency, 163
Trust, 51, 192
Truth-telling, 195-196

# U

Utilization management, 259, 266

# V

Value-based health insurance (VBHI), 281-286, 387
Value chain, 281-283
    Primary activities, 281-283
    Supporting activities, 281-283
Value equation, 284

Printed in the United States
74746LV00006B/1-66

9 780924 674990